ANALYTICAL PROCEDURES
for THERAPEUTIC DRUG MONITORING and EMERGENCY TOXICOLOGY
SECOND EDITION

RANDALL C. BASELT, Ph.D.

Director, Chemical Toxicology Institute
Foster City, California

PSG Publishing Company, Inc.

Littleton, Massachusetts

Published by
YEAR BOOK MEDICAL PUBLISHERS • INC.

Library of Congress Cataloging-in-Publication Data

Baselt, Randall C.
  Analytical procedures for therapeutic drug
monitoring and emergency toxicology.

  Includes bibliographies and indexes.
  1. Drugs – Analysis. 2. Poisons – Analysis.
3. Body fluids – Analysis. I. Title. [DNLM:
1. Body Fluids – analysis. 2. Drugs – analysis.
3. Poisons – analysis. QV 25 B324a]
RS189.B34 1987   615.9′07   86-30237
ISBN 0-88416-722-4

Published by:
PSG PUBLISHING COMPANY, INC.
545 Great Road
Littleton, Massachusetts 01460

Printed in the United States of America

International Standard Book Number: 0-88416-722-4

Library of Congress Catalog Card Number: 86-30237

Last digit is the print number: 9 8 7 6 5 4 3 2 1

CONTENTS

INTRODUCTION

The methods employed in the analysis of biological specimens for drugs and chemicals differ sufficiently from other clinical chemical methods that a few words of guidance are in order. While the experienced analyst is well aware of these considerations, those with less familiarity with this field would do well to acquaint themselves with the advice offered in several selected references.[1-3]

Substance Concentrations. The concentrations of substances in stock solutions as well as those in body fluids are expressed in terms of free acid or base, if the substance is a weak electrolyte, or of the free anion or cation, if an ionic species. Thus, to prepare a 1 mg/mL solution of methadone, for instance, one must prepare a solution that contains 1.12 mg/mL of methadone hydrochloride. An easy method to determine this ratio is to divide the molecular weight of the salt by the molecular weight of the species of interest. One must remember to take into account the relative proportion of each moiety (ie, two amphetamine molecules for every sulfuric acid molecule in amphetamine sulfate) as well as any water of hydration.

Pure Standards. The pure drug standards obtained from pharmaceutical companies are rarely assayed and may vary widely in purity from batch to batch. It is preferable in most instances to obtain these materials from commercial suppliers who can verify their purity, although some substances, especially drug metabolites, are not available from other than the drug houses.

Calibration Standards. For most assays, it is desirable to prepare calibration standards in a fluid that resembles as closely as possible the specimen to be analyzed. This serves the dual purpose of duplicating test interferences by endogenous materials and of mimicking the effect of these materials on the analytical recovery of the analyte. Analytes that are present in significant amounts in normal biological fluids, such as the essential trace elements, must understandably be prepared in aqueous solution for use as standards.

Calculations. For an assay that is reproducible from day to day and that is suited to quality control techniques, it is sufficient to perform a calibration of the assay every 3 to 6 months. This is done by analyzing a negative specimen and three to five standards that cover the linear concentration range of the method, and by preparing a standard curve. From this standard curve may be determined a response factor, which is a number representing the expected instrumental response to a specimen containing a given concentration of the analyte. For instance, the response factor for secobarbital using a spectrophotometric procedure would be expressed as the absorbance obtained when a plasma specimen containing 1 mg/L of the analyte is processed; using a gas chromatographic method, the factor would be expressed as the secobarbital peak height resulting from analysis of the same specimen divided by the internal standard peak height. The response factor should be determined from the slope of a standard curve rather than from the mean value of a single standard. Once the factor is obtained, it may be used to calculate the concentrations of the daily patient specimens, providing the result of the quality control specimen is acceptable. If the cumulative quality control results begin showing a bias, or if proficiency testing indicates the method is inaccurate, then the method should be re-calibrated and a new response factor calculated.

Quality Control. A substantial number of assays for drugs or chemicals are not subject to the usual quality control procedures due to the instability of the analyte in biological fluids or even in aqueous solution. This requires that a separate calibration curve be prepared each time the assay is performed. These situations have been duly noted in the text.

References:

1. J.J. Thoma. Quality Assurance in Toxicology. In Guidelines for Analytical Toxicology Programs, Vol. 1 (J.J. Thoma, P.B. Bondo and I. Sunshine, eds.), CRC Press, Cleveland, 1977, pp. 133–168.
2. P.H. Field, B.J. Basteyns, M.A. Evenson and R.H. Laessig. Clinical Toxicology. In Quality Assurance Practices for Health Laboratories (S.L. Inhorn, ed.), American Public Health Association, Washington, D.C., 1978, pp. 1033–1096.
3. R.V. Blanke. Quality control in the toxicology laboratory. Clin. Tox. 13: 141–151, 1978.

ACETAMINOPHEN

Serum Concentrations (mg/L)		
Therapeutic	Toxic	T½
2–13	30–300	2 hr

Acetaminophen analysis is often requested for confirmation of suspected overdosage. An increased serum half-life is considered to be the best indicator of serious toxicity and may be estimated by analyzing at least three specimens, each drawn 2 hours apart. Three procedures are presented: a rapid colorimetric assay and both gas and liquid chromatographic assays. For concentrations of less than 50 mg/L the chromatographic techniques are recommended, since the colorimetric assay is known to yield misleadingly high values in this range. Two other chromatographic procedures for the simultaneous determination of phenacetin and its metabolite, acetaminophen, in plasma are included in the section on phenacetin (p. 225).

Serum Acetaminophen by Colorimetry

Principle:
A trichloroacetic acid filtrate of serum is prepared. Sodium nitrite is added to the clear supernatant, forming a nitro-compound with acetaminophen. Ammonium sulfamate and sodium hydroxide are added to produce a yellow chromophore and the absorbance is measured at 430 nm using a visible spectrophotometer.

Reagents:
Stock solution – 1 mg/mL acetaminophen in methanol
Serum standards – 50, 100, 200 and 300 mg/L
10% Trichloroacetic acid – 10 g/100 mL H_2O
10% Sodium nitrite – 10 g/100 mL H_2O
15% Ammonium sulfamate – 15 g/100 mL H_2O
50% Sodium hydroxide – 50 g NaOH/100 mL H_2O
6 mol/L Hydrochloric acid – 26 mL conc. HC1/100 mL H_2O

Instrumental Conditions:
Visible double-beam spectrophotometer set to 430 nm

Procedure:
1. Transfer 1.0 mL of serum to a test tube.
2. Add 2.0 mL of 10% trichloroacetic acid, vortex and let stand at least 5 minutes. Centrifuge at 2000 rpm for 10 minutes.

3

3. Transfer 2.0 mL of the clear supernatant to a clean tube. Perform the following operations in the hood.
4. Add 0.5 mol/L HC1 to the serum supernatant.
5. Carefully, dropwise, add 0.5 mL 10% sodium nitrite to the tube. The mixture will foam. Agitate by hand to mix. Let stand 2 minutes.
6. Carefully, dropwise, add 0.5 mL 15% ammonium sulfamate to each tube. The mixture will foam.
7. Add 0.5 mL 50% NaOH to each tube.
8. Centrifuge at 2000 rpm for 3–5 minutes to clear. Spin even if the solution "looks" clear.
9. Read at 430 nm against a drug-free serum processed in the same manner.

Calculation:

Calculation is based on a response factor derived from a standard curve. A quality control serum containing 100 mg/L acetaminophen is analyzed daily.

Evaluation:

Sensitivity: 10 mg/L
Linearity: 50–600 mg/L
C.V.: not established
Relative recovery: not established

Interferences:

Phenacetin causes negligible interference; salicylamide will produce an absorbance of 20% of an equal amount of acetaminophen, but it is highly unlikely that it will be present in serum in amounts that will result in significant interference.

Reference:

C.B. Walberg. Determination of acetaminophen in serum. J. Analyt. Tox 1: 79–80, 1977.

Serum Acetaminophen by Gas Chromatography

Principle:

Only 200 µL of serum are required for this assay, which utilizes 2-acetamidophenol as internal standard. Both substances are derivatized with acetic anhydride and are chromatographed isothermally on 3% SP2250–DA, with detection by flame-ionization.

Reagents:

Stock solution – 5 mg/mL acetaminophen in methanol
Serum standards – 50, 100, 250 and 500 mg/L
Internal standard – 100 mg/L 2-acetamidophenol (Aldrich) in water
Ammonium sulfate
Dichloromethane
Acetic anhydride
Pyridine

Instrumental Conditions:

Gas chromatograph with flame-ionization detector
0.9 m × 2 mm i.d. glass column containing 3% SP2250–DA on 100/120 mesh Supelcoport
   (Supelco) or equivalent OV–17 on Chromosorb W
Injector, 300°C.; column, 180°C.; detector, 275°C.
Nitrogen flow rate, 40 mL/min

Procedure:

1. Add 0.2 mL internal standard to 0.2 mL serum in a 15 mL screw-cap tube. Add 0.3 g
    solid ammonium sulfate and vortex for 5 seconds.
2. Add 5 mL dichloromethane, cap and shake for 3 minutes. Centrifuge for 2 minutes.
3. Aspirate upper aqueous layer and decant organic layer into a 5 mL conical tube.
4. Add 25 µL acetic anhydride and 5 µL pyridine to the conical tube and evaporate to
    dryness in a 40°C. water bath under a stream of nitrogen.
5. Dissolve the residue in 30 µL of dichloromethane and inject 1 µL into the gas
    chromatograph.

	Retention time (min)
internal standard	1.2
acetaminophen	3.2

Calculation:

Calculation is based on a response factor derived from a standard curve. A quality control
serum containing 100 mg/L acetaminophen is analyzed daily.

Evaluation:

Sensitivity: 5 mg/L
Linearity: 50–500 mg/L
C.V.: 4.8% within-run, 7.4% day-to-day
Relative recovery: not established

Interferences:

Meprobamate has a retention time of 3.4 minutes. Nineteen other drugs, including
salicylate and caffeine, were found not to interfere. Phenacetin is detected but is well
separated at a retention time of about 2.0 minutes.

Reference:

J.J. Thoma, M. McCoy, T. Ewald and N. Myers. Acetaminophen – an improved gas chromatographic assay.
J. Analyt. Tox. 2: 226–228, 1978.

Serum Acetaminophen by Liquid Chromatography

Principle:

As little as 50 µL of serum may be analyzed in this procedure, which is based on a liquid
chromatographic assay for theophylline. An internal standard dissolved in acetonitrile is

added directly to serum, causing protein precipitation. An aliquot of the supernatant is injected onto a reversed-phase column and detection is performed at 254 nm.

Reagents:

Stock solution – 1 mg/mL acetaminophen in water

Serum standards – 50, 100, 200 and 400 mg/L

Internal standard – 400 mg/L β-hydroxyethyltheophylline (Pierce) in acetonitrile

Sodium acetate buffer – 0.01 mol/L $Na_2C_2H_3O_2$ (820 mg of sodium acetate in 900 mL water; adjust to pH 4.0 with glacial acetic acid, bring volume to 1000 mL and filter through Millipore 0.4 micron filter)

Acetonitrile – Mallinckrodt Nanograde or Burdick-Jackson

Mobile phase – 93% sodium acetate buffer/7% acetonitrile

Instrumental Conditions:

Liquid chromatograph with 254 nm wavelength detector μBondapak C_{18} reversed-phase column (Waters Associates)

Column temperature, ambient

Solvent flow rate, 3 mL/min

Procedure:

1. Add 100 μL internal standard to 100 μL serum and vortex for 10 seconds.
2. Centrifuge for 10 minutes at 3000 rpm and inject 10 μL of the supernatant into the liquid chromatograph.

	Retention time (min)
acetaminophen	3.0
internal standard	5.3

Calculation:

Calculation is based on a response factor derived from from a standard curve. A quality control serum containing 50 mg/L acetaminophen is analyzed daily.

Evaluation:

Sensitivity: 25 mg/L

Linearity: 25–400 mg/L

C.V.: not established

Relative recovery: not established

Interferences:

None encountered. Theophylline elutes just after acetaminophen.

Reference:

M. Black and K. Sprague. Rapid micromethod for acetaminophen determination in serum. Clin. Chem. 24: 1288–1289, 1978.

ACETYLMETHADOL

	Maintenance Plasma Level	T½
acetylmethadol	0–0.10 mg/L	6 hr
noracetylmethadol	0.06–0.37 mg/L	31–42 hr
dinoracetylmethadol	0.08–0.37 mg/L	100 hr

Acetylmethadol is a long-acting narcotic analgesic that is used for the maintenance therapy of opiate addiction. The plasma concentrations of this drug and its two active metabolites, nor- and dinor-acetylmethadol, may need to be determined for the assessment of treatment failure or drug toxicity. A gas chromatographic procedure is presented that has sufficient sensitivity to measure plasma concentrations developed during maintenance therapy.

Plasma Acetylmethadol by Gas Chromatography

Principle:

Acetylmethadol and its active metabolites are extracted from plasma with chlorobutane. Following a back extraction into hydrochloric acid, the metabolites are converted to their corresponding amides by alkali-catalyzed rearrangement. The three drugs are simultaneously analyzed by flame-ionization gas chromatography.

Reagents:

Stock solutions – 4 mg/L solutions of acetylmethadol, noracetylmethadol and dinoracetyl-
    methadol in water
Plasma standards – 0.05, 0.10, 0.20 and 0.40 mg/L for each of the above drugs
Internal standard – 20 mg/L SKF–525A in water
1–Chlorobutane
1–Octanol
Hexane
Chloroform
Phosphate buffer – 1 mol/L K_2HPO_4 adjusted to pH 7.4
Hydrochloric acid – 0.2 mol/L HCl
Sodium hydroxide – 50 g NaOH q.s. to 100 mL with water

Instrumental Conditions:

Gas chromatograph with flame-ionization detector
2 m × 2 mm i.d. glass column containing 3% SE–30 (OV–1) on 80/100 mesh Gas Chrom Q
Injector, 275°C.; column, 235°C.; detector, 295°C.

Procedure:

1. To 2 mL of plasma in a 15 mL screw-cap tube are added 50 μL internal standard, 1 mL of pH 7.4 phosphate buffer and 1 drop of 1-octanol. Vortex briefly.

7

2. Add 9 mL 1-chlorobutane, shake for 1 minute and centrifuge. Transfer the upper solvent layer to a clean tube.
3. Add 5 mL of 0.2 mol/L HCl and shake for 1 min. Centrifuge and discard upper solvent layer.
4. Add 5 mL hexane, shake briefly, centrifuge and discard hexane.
5. Add 4 drops of 50% NaOH to the aqueous phase and incubate at 70°C. for 30 min. Allow to cool.
6. Extract into 4 mL chloroform by shaking. Centrifuge, discard aqueous phase and transfer solvent to a clean tube. Evaporate to dryness on a 50°C. water bath under a stream of nitrogen.
7. Rinse the sides of the tube with 50 μL of chloroform and allow to evaporate. Dissolve the residue in 20 μL of chloroform and inject 4 μL into the gas chromatograph.

	Retention time (min)
acetylmethadol	1.8
internal standard	2.5
dinoracetylmethadol (amide)	3.6
noracetylmethadol (amide)	4.2

Calculation:

Calculation is based on a response factor derived from a standard curve. A quality control plasma containing 0.10 mg/L acetylmethadol and 0.20 mg/L of the two metabolites is analyzed daily.

Evaluation:

Sensitivity: 0.01 mg/L (acetylmethadol and dinoracetylmethadol) 0.02 mg/L (noracetyl-methadol)
Linearity: 0.05–0.40 mg/L
C.V.: 5%
Relative recovery: 86–105%

Interferences:

Normal plasma components do not interfere. Other drugs were not tested for interferences.

Reference:

R.F. Kaiko, N. Chatterjie and C.E. Inturrisi. Simultaneous determination of acetylmethadol and its active biotransformation products in human biofluids. J. Chrom. 109: 247–258, 1975.

ACID AND NEUTRAL DRUG SCREEN

| | Plasma Concentrations (mg/L) | | |
	Therapeutic	Toxic (nonfatal)	T½
amobarbital	1–2	8–66	24 hr
butabarbital	1–2	20–40	?
butalbital	?	?	?
ethchlorvynol	2–8	20–135	24 hr
glutethimide	2–6	5–120	12 hr
meprobamate	6–12	60–240	11 hr
methaqualone	1–7	6–17	33–38 hr
methyprylon	8–10	50–100	4–5 hr
pentobarbital	1–3	13–28	20–30 hr
phenobarbital	10–30	65–134	4 days
phenytoin	10–20	45–112	12–36 hr
primidone	1–14	40–95	6–12 hr
secobarbital	1–2	3–67	23–29 hr

For the purposes of emergency toxicology, the acid and neutral drugs consist largely of a group of chemically-related sedatives and hypnotics that develop relatively high blood concentrations even after administration of therapeutic doses. Urine is generally not a good specimen in which to detect these drugs, since most of them are extensively metabolized and only a minor percentage of the dose is excreted unchanged. Methaqualone, a very weak base, is included in these procedures since it behaves like a neutral substance and will be easily detected if present in the specimen. The three assays presented include thin-layer chromatography, a qualitative test that can be used alone or as a confirmatory tool for one of the other techniques, and gas chromatography and high-pressure liquid chromatography, both of which are suitable for quantitative and qualitative purposes.

Serum Acid and Neutral Drug Screen by Thin-Layer Chromatography

Principle:

A serum or plasma specimen is extracted for thin-layer chromatography at pH 5 with chloroform. Alternatively, the extract from the acid and neutral drug GC screen may be applied directly to TLC to confirm the GC results. The heptabarbital in each sample will act as an internal standard for the TLC procedure. The drugs are visualized with a silver acetate and diphenylcarbazone spray combination.

Reagents:

TLC standards – three separate methanol solutions containing 1 mg/L of the following drugs:

9

    A. phenobarbital, heptabarbital, amobarbital, secobarbital, glutethimide
    B. barbital, butabarbital, pentobarbital, meprobamate
    C. phenytoin, primidone, methyprylon, ethchlorvynol

Internal standard – 100 mg heptabarbital/500 mL H_2O (Ciba-Geigy Corporation)

Phosphate buffer – 50% saturated KH_2PO_4

TLC plates – glass or plastic plates coated with a 250 micron thick silica gel G layer. Store in
    a 75°C. oven.

Developing solvent – ethyl acetate methanol ammonium hydroxide, 85:10:5 (prepare fresh
    daily)

Diphenylcarbazone spray – dissolve 10 mg diphenylcarbazone in 50 mL acetone and 50 mL
    H_2O (prepare weekly)

1% Silver acetate spray – 1 g silver acetate/100 mL H_2O (stable indefinitely)

Procedure:

1. To 2 mL serum in a 15 mL screw-cap tube, add 0.5 mL phosphate buffer, 50 µL internal
    standard and 5 mL chloroform. Shake for 30 seconds to extract.
2. Centrifuge to separate layers and discard aqueous layer. Transfer the chloroform to a
    5 mL conical centrifuge tube and evaporate to low volume (25–50 µL) under a stream of
    dry air while warming in a 40°C. water bath.
3. Spot one-half of the concentrated extract to the origin of a TLC plate. Also spot several
    microliters of one or more standard mixtures.
4. Place the plate into the ethyl acetate methanol ammonia tank and allow the solvent to
    rise to a height of 10 cm.
5. Remove the plate, allow it to air dry, and spray with the silver acetate solution.
6. Spray with the diphenylcarbazone solution and note the color and location of any spots.
    Compare to spotted standards.

Drug	Rf	Color
theophylline	.09	pink
phenobarbital	.20	violet
barbital	.25	violet
phenytoin	.30	blue
internal standard	.33	violet
butalbital	.34	blue
butabarbital	.36	violet
primidone	.37	blue-gray
amobarbital	.39	violet
pentobarbital	.41	violet
secobarbital	.42	blue
meprobamate	.60	gray
4-OH-glutethimide	.62	violet
methyprylon	.66	blue-black
glutethimide	.70	violet
methaqualone	.72	violet
ethchlorvynol	.76	rose

Evaluation:

Sensitivity: 2 mg/L for most drugs
Linearity: not applicable

C.V.: not applicable
Relative recovery: not applicable

Interferences:

Many other drugs and drug metabolites will produce chromatographic spots that may hinder interpretation. Results should be considered presumptive until confirmed by other techniques.

References:

1. K.K. Kaistha and J.H. Jaffe. TLC techniques for identification of narcotics, barbiturates, and CNS stimulants in a drug abuse urine screening program. J. Pharm. Sci. 61: 679–689, 1972.
2. S.J. Mule. Identification of narcotics, barbiturates, amphetamines, tranquilizers and psychotomimetics in human urine. J. Chrom. 39: 302–311, 1969.

Serum Acid and Neutral Drug Screen by Gas Chromatography

Principle:

An internal standard, heptabarbital, is added to patient serum and the solution is extracted at pH 5 with a small volume of chloroform. An aliquot of the chloroform is injected onto the OV-1 column of the gas chromatograph, utilizing flame-ionization detection. Confirmation of results is obtained with the OV-17 column.

Reagents:

Stock solutions –
    10 mg/mL methyprylon (100 mg/10 mL methanol)
    10 mg/mL butabarbital (110.8 mg Na salt/10 mL methanol)
    10 mg/mL amobarbital (110.2 mg Na salt/10 mL methanol)
    10 mg/mL pentobarbital (110.2 mg Na salt/10 mL methanol)
    10 mg/mL secobarbital (109.7 mg Na salt/10 mL methanol)
    10 mg/mL meprobamate (100 mg/10 mL methanol)
    10 mg/mL glutethimide (100 mg/10 mL methanol)
    10 mg/mL phenobarbital (109.9 mg Na salt/10 mL methanol)
    10 mg/mL methaqualone (114.7 mg HC1 salt/10 mL methanol)
    10 mg/mL phenytoin (109.2 mg Na salt/10 mL methanol)
Serum standards – 2, 5, 10 and 20 mg/L for each of the above drugs
Quality control serum – 10 mg/L of all of the above except phenobarbital and phenytoin (20 mg/L) and methyprylon, meprobamate, glutethimide and methaqualone (5 mg/L)
Internal standard – 100 mg heptabarbital (Ciba-Geigy Corporation) in 500 mL H_2O
Phosphate buffer – 50% saturated KH_2PO_4
Chloroform

Instrumental Conditions:

Gas chromatograph with dual flame-ionization detectors
2 m × 2 mm i.d. glass columns containing 2% OV-1 or OV-17 on 100/120 mesh Chromosorb G-HP

Column temperature: initial, 170°C. (4 min)

> 16°C./min increase
> final, 250°C. (4 min)

Injector, 250°C.; detector, 300°C.

Nitrogen flow rate, 33 mL/min

Procedure:

1. Pipet 2 mL of serum into a 5 mL centrifugal separator tube (Kontes Glass Co., K-414400) fitted with a blind hole rubber stopper (K-774200-22). Add 100 µL of the internal standard and 0.5 mL phosphate buffer and vortex briefly.
2. Add 100 µL of chloroform to the tube with no mixing. Stopper the tube, secure with a rubber band, and place on a slow (3 rpm) tilted rotator for 20 minutes.
3. Centrifuge tubes for several minutes and withdraw 4 µL of the lower chloroform layer by piercing the rubber septum with a 10 µL syringe. Inject onto the OV-1 column.

Drug	OV-1 Retention time (min)
methyprylon	1.6
butabarbital	2.5
amobarbital	3.2
pentobarbital	3.5
secobarbital	4.3
meprobamate	4.8
glutethimide	5.0
4-OH-glutethimide	5.5
phenobarbital	6.6
internal standard	7.6
methaqualone	8.2
phenytoin	9.7

Calculation:

Calculation is based on a response factor derived from a standard curve for each drug. A quality control serum prepared as described is analyzed daily.

Evaluation:

Sensitivity: 2 mg/L
Linearity: 2–20 mg/L
C.V.: not established
Relative recovery: not established

Interferences:

Many other drugs and drug metabolites will be detected by this procedure if they are present in sufficiently high concentrations. The results obtained with this technique should be considered semi-quantitative and should be qualitatively confirmed using another method (i.e., Serum Acid and Neutral Drug Screen by Thin-Layer Chromatography).

Reference:

J.A. Wright and R.C. Baselt. Unpublished results, 1974.

Serum Acid and Neutral Drug Screen by Liquid Chromatography

Principle:

Serum proteins are precipitated by addition of acetonitrile containing the internal standard. The supernate is injected onto a reversed-phase column and the eluted drugs are detected by absorption at 195 nm. A sensitivity of 1 mg/L is attained with specimen volumes as low as 25 μL.

Reagents:

Stock solutions – 10 mg/mL methanol solutions of the following drugs: primidone, methyprylon, phenobarbital, butabarbital, butalbital, ethchlorvynol, pentobarbital, amobarbital, phenytoin, glutethimide, secobarbital and methaqualone

Serum standards – 5, 10, 20 and 50 mg/L for each of the above drugs

Quality control serum – 10 mg/L of all of the above except primidone, phenobarbital and phenytoin (5 mg/L)

Internal standard – 5 mg 5-(p-methylphenyl)-5-phenylhydantoin (Aldrich) in 100 mL acetonitrile

pH 4.4 Phosphate buffer – 300 μL of 1 mol/L KH_2PO_4 and 50 μL of 0.9 mol/L phosphoric acid in 1800 mL H_2O

Mobile phase – 785 mL phosphate buffer plus 215 mL acetonitrile

Acetonitrile – spectrophotometric grade

Instrumental Conditions:

Liquid chromatograph with 195 nm wavelength detector

25 cm × 4.6 mm i.d. μBondapak C_{18} reversed-phase column (Waters Associates)

Column temperature, 50°C.

Solvent flow rate, 3 mL/min

Procedure:

1. Add 200 μL of internal standard solution to 200 μL of serum and vortex (smaller specimens may be used if desired).
2. Centrifuge and inject 20 μL of supernate into the chromatograph.

Drug	Retention time (min)
primidone	2.9
methyprylon	4.0
phenobarbital	4.4
butabarbital	5.4
butalbital	6.5
ethchlorvynol	8.5
pentobarbital	9.7
amobarbital	10.5
phenytoin	11.2
glutethimide	12.0
secobarbital	13.7
methaqualone	19.5
internal standard	22.0

Calculation:

Calculation is based on a response factor derived from a standard curve for each drug. A quality control serum prepared as described is analyzed daily.

Evaluation:

Sensitivity: 0.25–1.0 mg/L
Linearity: 5–100 mg/L
C.V.: 4–9% within day, 4–10% day-to-day
Relative recovery: 93–112%

Interferences:

Many other drugs will be detected by this procedure, including xanthine derivatives and most anticonvulsants. A number of antihistamines, benzodiazepines and tricyclic antidepressants were found not to interfere.

Reference:

P.M. Kabra, H.Y. Koo and L.J. Marton. Simultaneous liquid-chromatographic determination of 12 common sedatives and hypnotics in serum. Clin. Chem. 24: 657–662, 1978.

ALPRAZOLAM/TRIAZOLAM

	Serum Concentrations (µg/L)		
	Therapeutic	Toxic	T½
alprazolam	10–50	>75	10–15 hr
triazolam	2–16	?	2–4 hr

Alprazolam and triazolam are newer, more potent members of the benzodiazepine class of drugs that are employed as orally-administered hypnotics. Doses and therefore serum concentrations are very low for both drugs and very sensitive methods must be used to assay these compounds. The following liquid chromatographic technique is applicable for either drug in the absence of the other.

Serum Alprazolam/Triazolam by Liquid Chromatography

Principle:

The drugs are extracted from alkalinized serum with toluene and the extract is evaporated to dryness, re-dissolved and analyzed by liquid chromatography with ultraviolet detection at 221 nm.

Reagents:

Stock solution – 1 mg/mL alprazolam in methanol 1 mg/mL triazolam in methanol
Serum standards – 2, 5, 10, 20, and 50 µg/L for each drug
Internal standards – 25 µ/L alprazolam or triazolam in acetonitrile
4 mol/L Sodium hydroxide
Mobile phase – acetonitrile/isopropanol/water, 94:5:1

Instrumental Conditions:

Liquid chromatograph with 221 nm absorbance detector
25 cm × 5 mm i.d. µBondapak C_{18} column (Waters Associates)
Solvent flow rate, 0.75 mL/min
Column temperature, ambient

Procedure:

1. Transfer 1 mL of the appropriate internal standard to a 15 mL screw-cap tube and evaporate the acetonitrile to dryness at 50°C. under a stream of nitrogen.
2. Add 1 mL of serum to the tube and vortex for 20 seconds. Add 2 mL of 4 mol/L NaOH and vortex briefly.
3. Add 5 mL of toluene and place on a rotator for 10 minutes. Centrifuge to separate phases and transfer the toluene to a conical centrifuge tube.

15

4. Evaporate the toluene to dryness at 50°C. under a stream of nitrogen. Dissolve the residue in 300 μL of acetontrile and inject 250 μL into the chromatograph.

	Retention time (min)
alprazolam	11.7
triazolam	9.1

Calculation:

Calculation is based on a response factor derived from a standard curve. A quality control specimen containing the appropriate drug at a mid-level concentration is analyzed daily.

Evaluation:

Sensitivity: 1 μg/L
Linearity: 6–100 μg/L
C.V.: 2–12% (day-to-day)
Relative recovery: 97–112%

Interferences:

No interference was found due to endogenous serum constituents. Other drugs were not studied for potential interference.

Reference:

W.J. Adams. Specific and sensitive high performance liquid chromatographic determination of alprazolam or triazolam. Anal. Lett. 12: 657–671, 1979.

AMIKACIN

Serum Concentrations (mg/L)		
Therapeutic	Toxic	T½
15–25	>32 (peak)	1.9–2.8 hr
	>10 (trough)	

Amikacin is a frequently used aminoglycoside antibiotic. Reagents are commercially available for determination of the drug in serum by radioimmunoassay, EMIT and fluorescence immunoassay, but occasionally it may be necessary to use a technique with more specificity. The following liquid chromatographic method is well suited for the routine assay of amikacin.

Serum Amikacin by Liquid Chromatography

Principle:

An internal standard, kanamycin, dissolved in acetonitrile is added to serum, causing protein precipitation. The supernatant is treated with a derivatizing reagent to form a trinitrophenyl derivative of amikacin and the internal standard. The drugs are isolated using a Bond-Elut extraction column and analyzed by liquid chromatography with detection at 340 nm.

Reagents:

Stock solution – 1 mg/mL amikacin in water
Serum standards – 5, 10, 25 and 50 mg/L
Internal standard – 25 mg kanamycin per L of acetonitrile
Tris buffer – 2 mol/L Trizma base (Sigma), pH 10.3 (dissolve 24.2 g in 100 mL water)
Derivatizing reagent – 2,4,6-trinitrobenzene-1-sulfonic acid, 250 g/L (dissolve 2.5 g in 10 mL acetonitrile)
Wash buffer – 10 mmol/L K_2HPO_4 (1.82 g in 1 L water, adjust to pH 8.6 with H_3PO_4)
Acetonitrile – Burdick-Jackson
Methanol – Burdick-Jackson
Mobile phase – 520 mL acetonitrile plus 480 mL 20 mmol/L pH 3.0 phosphate buffer (dissolve 2.68 g KH_2PO_4 in 1 L water and adjust to pH 3.0 with H_3PO_4)

Instrumental Conditions:

Liquid chromatograph with 340 nm wavelength detector
Ultrasphere Octyl 5 micron column, 25 cm × 4.6 mm i.d. (Altex Scientific)
Column temperature, 50°C.

Solvent flow rate, 2.0 mL/min

Vac-Elut vacuum chamber with Bond-Elut C_{18} extraction columns (Analytichem International)

Procedure:

1. Transfer 50 µL serum to a disposable plastic microtube and add 25 µL Tris buffer and 100 µL internal standard. Vortex and centrifuge at 15,000 × g for 1 min.
2. Decant the supernatant into a clean microtube and add 30 µL derivatizing reagent. Cap and vortex and heat at 70°C. for 30 min.
3. Pretreat the Bond-Elut column with 2 column volumes of methanol and 2 of water. Disconnect the vacuum and fill column with 700 µL of wash buffer followed by 250 µL of derivatized sample.
4. Turn on the vacuum and add 3 volumes of wash buffer to the column. Disconnect the vacuum and place a 10 × 75 mm glass tube under the column.
5. Elute the drugs from the column with 300 µL acetonitrile and inject 50 µL of the eluate into the chromatograph.

Calculation:

Calculation is based on a response factor derived from a standard curve. A quality control specimen containing 20 mg/L amikacin is analyzed daily.

Evaluation:

Sensitivity: 0.5 mg/L
Linearity: 2.5–50 mg/L
C.V.: 2.8–3.1% day-to-day
Relative recovery: 93–98%

Interferences:

None of the more than 30 drugs studied, including gentamicin and tobramycin, was found to interfere. The method correlated well with a commercial radioimmunoassay (American Diagnostic).

Reference:

P.M. Kabra, P.K. Bhatnager and M.A. Nelson. Liquid chromatographic determination of amikacin in serum with spectrophotometric detection. J. Chrom. 307: 224–229, 1984.

AMPHETAMINES

Drug	Concentrations After Single Dose (mg/L)		Concentrations in Abuse Situations (mg/L)	
	Plasma	Urine	Plasma	Urine
amphetamine	0.02–0.12	1–5	0.2–3.0	25–250
chlorphentermine	0.10–0.40	5–25	?	?
diethylpropion	0.001–0.010	1	?	?
ephedrine	0.05–0.10	2–30	?	?
fenfluramine	0.03–0.30	1–30	0.6–1.0	50–100
methamphetamine	0.01–0.05	0.5–4	0.2–0.6	25–300
p-methoxyamphetamine	<0.2	<5	0.3–2.0	5–200
methylenedioxyamphetamine	<0.4	<10	5–25	50–150
phendimetrazine	0.03–0.25	1–20	?	?
phenmetrazine	0.06–0.25	5–30	0.5–4.0	50–300
phentermine	0.03–0.09	5–25	0.9	50
phenylpropanolamine	0.05–0.10	5–50	2	?
tranylcypromine	0.01–0.10	0.2–4	4	25

Amphetamine, or β-phenylisopropylamine, is a potent central nervous system stimulant that is subject to frequent abuse. It is the prototype of a class of phenylethylamine derivatives known as the amphetamines, which includes other stimulants (i.e., methamphetamine), anorexigenic drugs (i.e., fenfluramine and phenmetrazine), antidepressant agents (i.e., methylphenidate and tranylcypromine), decongestants (i.e., ephedrine and phenylpropanolamine) and the methoxylated hallucinogens (i.e., p-methoxyamphetamine). Many of these basic amines may be simultaneously analyzed using gas chromatographic screening techniques; both flame-ionization and electron-capture detection schemes are presented and are suitable for drug abuse screening and the monitoring of plasma concentrations after single doses, respectively. For strictly qualitative purposes, most of the compounds are detectable in urine using the Serum Basic Drug Screen by Thin-Layer Chromatography. Quantitative analyses for methylphenidate and tranylcypromine at therapeutic concentrations are presented separately (see Index). A gas chromatography-mass spectrometry method is included for improved specificity, which is especially important in forensic situations.

Reagents are commercially available for determination of the amphetamines by EMIT and radioimmunoassay. These assays are designed primarily for amphetamine in urine specimens; the radioimmunoassay is relatively specific for amphetamine but the EMIT procedure exhibits significant cross-reactivity with a number of amphetamine derivatives.

N-n-propylamphetamine is a useful internal standard for amphetamine analysis by gas chromatography and may be easily synthesized according to the following procedure.

Synthesis of N-Propylamphetamine

Principle:

This useful internal standard may be easily prepared from amphetamine. The N-propionyl derivative of amphetamine is first formed and is then reduced to N-propylamphetamine with lithium aluminum hydride. Crystals of the hydrochloride salt are finally collected by filtration.

Reagents:

Amphetamine – free base form
Propionic anhydride
Lithium aluminum hydride ($LiAlH_4$)
Ether
1 mol/L Sodium hydroxide
0.5 mol/L Hydrochloric acid
2 mol/L Hydrochloric acid

Procedure:

1. Dissolve 5 g amphetamine base (liquid) in 200 mL ether and add 10 g propionic anhydride. Let stand for 1 hr at room temperature.
2. Wash ether with 50 mL of each of the following in sequence: 1 mol/L NaOH, 0.5 mol/L HCl, H_2O. Dry ether by shaking with anhydrous Na_2SO_4 or Na_2CO_3.
3. Transfer ether to a refluxing apparatus, add 4 g $LiAlH_4$ slowly and reflux for 2 hours.
4. Cool and add 25 mL H_2O. Extract precipitate with 100 mL ether, discard aqueous phase and filter ether to remove precipitate.
5. Extract ether with 25 mL 2 mol/L HCl.
6. Wash HCl layer once with 50 mL ether. Discard ether. Store aqueous layer at 4°C. overnight and collect crystals by filtration. Dry in desiccator (m.p. 158°). Yields about 4 g of the hydrochloride salt of N-propylamphetamine.

Reference:

J. Wright. Personal communication, 1976.

Plasma and Urine Amphetamines by Flame-Ionization Gas Chromatography

Principle:

The amphetamines are extracted into chloroform from alkalinized plasma or urine following the addition of an internal standard, N-propylamphetamine. The internal standard and the majority of the drugs are converted into amides by addition of acetic anhydride; the extract is concentrated by evaporation and an aliquot is injected onto an OV-17 column, with subsequent flame-ionization detection.

Reagents:

Stock solutions –
    1 mg/mL amphetamine (13.64 mg sulfate salt/10 mL methanol)

1 mg/mL methamphetamine (12.44 mg HC1 salt/10 mL methanol)

1 mg/mL methanol solutions of other drugs as required

Plasma or urine standards – 0.5, 2.0 and 5.0 mg/L for each drug

Internal standard – 25 mg N-propylamphetamine HC1/100 mL H_2O (synthesize according to preceding procedure)

10 mol/L Sodium hydroxide – 200 g NaOH/500 mL H_2O

Chloroform

Acetic anhydride

Instrumental Conditions:

Gas chromatograph with flame-ionization detector

2 m × 2 mm i.d. glass columns containing 2% OV-17 or OV-1 on 100/200 mesh Chromosorb G-HP

Column temperature: 175°C. (OV-17) or 155°C. (OV-1)

Injector, 250°C.; detector, 300°C.

Nitrogen flow rate, 33 mL/min

Procedure:

1. Pipet into a 35 mL screw-cap tube 3 mL of the plasma or urine specimen.
2. Add 100 µL internal standard, 3 drops 10 mol/L NaOH and 20 mL chloroform.
3. Stopper and shake for 30 seconds. Unstopper, allow layers to separate, aspirate and discard aqueous layer and filter chloroform layer through a folded filter paper into a 50 mL beaker.
4. Add 100 µL acetic anhydride to the beaker and place on a 50–70°C. hot plate, allowing chloroform to evaporate to a volume of 1–2 mL. Transfer chloroform to a 5 mL conical centrifuge tube and continue evaporation using an airstream until a volume of approximately 100 µL is attained.
5. Inject 2 µL of the chloroform onto a 6′ OV-17 column at 175°C., using the OV-1 column for confirmation of positive results. Quantitation may be performed on either column. Some of the less volatile compounds may require higher column temperatures for best results.

	Retention time (min)		
Drug	OV-17	OV-1 (155°C.)	OV-1 (185°C.)
phendimetrazine		3.1	
amphetamine-OAc	2.3	3.5	
diethylpropion		3.7	
phentermine-OAc		3.7	
propylhexedrine-OAc		5.0	
methamphetamine-OAc	3.2	5.1	
mephentermine-OAc		5.5	
internal standard-OAc	4.3	9.7	
tranylcypromine-OAc	5.4		2.5
chlorphentermine-OAc			2.9
phenylpropanolamine-OAc			3.2
ephedrine-OAc			3.4
phenmetrazine-OAc			4.6
methylenedioxyamphetamine-OAc			5.1
4-methyl-2,5-dimethoxyamphetamine-OAc			6.7

Calculation:

Calculation is based on a response factor derived from a standard curve for each drug. A quality control specimen containing 0.5 mg/L (plasma) or 5.0 mg/L (urine) of the drug of interest is analyzed daily.

Evaluation:

Sensitivity: 0.1 mg/L for most drugs under optimal conditions
Linearity: 0.5–5 mg/L; prepare suitable standards for higher concentrations
C.V.: 5% within run
Relative recovery: not established

Interferences:

Many other neutral and basic substances will be extracted and detected by this procedure. Methyprylon and meperidine are known to have the same OV-17 retention times as the acetyl derivatives of methamphetamine and tranylcypromine, respectively. Positive results should be confirmed on an OV-1 column or, preferably, by another separation technique such as thin-layer chromatography.

References:

1. P. Lebish, B.S. Finkle and J.W. Brackett, Jr. Determination of amphetamine, methamphetamine, and related amines in blood and urine by gas chromatography with hydrogen-flame ionization detector. Clin. Chem. 16: 195–200, 1970.
2. R. Baselt and C. Stewart. Unpublished results, 1976.

Plasma Amphetamines by Electron-Capture Gas Chromatography

Principle:

This is a sensitive technique specifically designed for the determination of therapeutic plasma levels of certain anorexigenic amphetamine analogues. It is similar in principle to the previous technique, but involves the formation of halogenated derivatives of the drugs with subsequent electron-capture detection. It is applicable to any of the amphetamines that will form amide derivatives with heptafluorobutyric anhydride.

Reagents:

Stock solutions – 1 mg/mL methanol solutions of amphetamine, chlorphentermine, fenfluramine and methamphetamine
Plasma standards – 25, 50, 75 and 100 µg/L for each of the above drugs
Internal standard – 0.5 mg N-propylamphetamine in 100 mL H_2O
2 mol/L Sodium hydroxide
Pentane
Sodium sulfate (anhydrous)
Heptafluorobutyric anhydride

Instrumental Conditions:

Gas chromatograph with electron-capture detector

2 m × 2 mm i.d. glass column containing 5% OV-1 on 100/120 mesh Gas Chrom Q, conditioned by four injections of 5 µL of a 1:4 dilution of heptafluorobutyric anhydride in pentane followed by 2 hours of heating at 200°C.

Injector, 250°C.; column, 110°C.; detector, 250°C.

Nitrogen flow rate, 30 mL/min

Procedure:

1. Add 100 µL internal standard to 5.0 mL of plasma in a 35 mL screw-cap tube. Add 5 mL water and 1 mL 2 mol/L NaOH. Vortex.
2. Extract with 15 mL pentane by shaking for 30 seconds. Centrifuge to separate layers and pass the pentane layer through anhydrous Na_2SO_4.
3. Evaporate the pentane to dryness in a conical centrifuge tube under a stream of nitrogen.
4. Add 100 µL heptafluorobutyric anhydride and let stand for 30 minutes. Evaporate to dryness.
5. Cool the tube in an ice bath and add 0.5 mL 2 mol/L NaOH. Extract with 10 mL pentane and centrifuge.
6. Filter the pentane layer through anhydrous Na_2SO_4 and evaporate to dryness in a clear centrifuge tube.
7. Dissolve residue in 200 µL pentane and inject 2–4 µL into the gas chromatograph.

Heptafluorobutyryl derivative	Retention time (min)
amphetamine	3
methamphetamine	5
fenfluramine	6
internal standard	7
chlorphentermine	9

Calculation:

Calculation is based on a response factor derived from a standard curve for each drug. A quality control plasma containing 50 µg/L of the drug of interest is analyzed daily.

Evaluation:

Sensitivity: 20 µg/L
Linearity: 20–100 µg/L
C.V.: not established
Relative recovery: 97–105%

Interferences:

No interfering peaks were observed in an extract of control plasma. It was necessary to heat the column to 270°C. after four injections in order to volatilize the accumulated impurities.

Reference:

R.B. Bruce and W.R. Maynard, Jr. Determination of amphetamine and related amines in blood by gas chromatography. Anal. Chem. 41: 977–979, 1969.

Blood Amphetamines by Gas Chromatography-Mass Spectrometry

Principle:

The drugs are extracted into an organic solvent from alkalinized blood and trifluoroacetic acid derivatives are formed. The residue is chromatographed on a capillary column and detection is accomplished by selected ion monitoring using a dedicated mass spectrometer.

Reagents:

Stock solution – 1 mg/mL methanol solutions of amphetamine, ephedrine, methamphetamine, β-phenethylamine, phenylpropanolamine and phentermine
Blood standards – 25, 50, 100 and 200 µg/L for each of the above drugs
Internal standard – 0.5 mg N-propylamphetamine in 100 mL H_2O
Ammonium hydroxide – conc. NH_4OH
Extraction solvent – butyl chloride/chloroform, 4:1
Trifluoroacetic anhydride
Hexane
N,O-bis(trimethylsilyl)trifluoroacetamide – BSTFA (Pierce Chemical Co.)
Ethyl acetate

Instrumental Conditions:

Gas chromatograph with mass selective detector (Hewlett-Packard 5970B MSD or equivalent)
12 m × 0.20 mm i.d. methylsilicone capillary column (Hewlett-Packard)
Injector, 300°C.; transfer line, 250°C.
Column temperature program: initial, 90°C. (2 min)
$\qquad\qquad\qquad\qquad\qquad$ 10°C./min increase
$\qquad\qquad\qquad\qquad\qquad$ final, 150°C. (2 min)
Helium flow rate, 1 mL/min
Splitless on time, 0.7 min
Solvent delay time, 3.0 min
Election multiplier voltage, 2000
Ions monitored, 140.05, 154.05, 182.10 m/z

Procedure:

1. Transfer 1 mL blood to a 15 mL screw-cap glass tube. Add 100 µL internal standard and 50 µL conc. NH_4OH and vortex.
2. Add 3 mL extraction solvent and vortex for 30 seconds. Centrifuge and transfer organic layer to a 5 mL Reacti-vial (Pierce Chemical Co.).
3. Add 100 µL trifluoroacetic anhydride and heat at 70°C. for 15 min in a heating block. Allow to cool to room temperature and evaporate to low volume under a stream of dry air.
4. Add 20 µL heptane, vortex, and inject 1 µL into the gas chromatograph.

Trifluoroacetyl derivative	Retention time (min)	Base peak (m/z)
β-phenethylamine	4.9	104
amphetamine	5.0	140
phentermine	5.5	154
phenylpropanolamine	5.7	140
methamphetamine	6.1	154
ephedrine	6.1	154
pseudoephedrine	6.5	154
internal standard	7.5	182

Separation of methamphetamine and ephedrine:
1. Extract specimen as described in steps 1 and 2 above. Evaporate organic layer to dryness under a stream of air.
2. Add 100 µL BSTFA and 100 µL ethyl acetate and heat at 80°C. for 10 min in a heating block. Evaporate residue to near dryness, reconstitute in 20 µL hexane and inject 1 µL into the gas chromatograph. Monitor for m/z 58.

Drug	Retention time (min)	Base peak
methamphetamine (no derivative)	5.5	58
ephedrine-TMS derivative	7.1	58

Calculation:

Calculation is based on a response factor derived from a standard curve for each drug. A quality control blood containing 50 µg/L of the drug of interest is analyzed daily.

Evaluation:

Sensitivity: 20 µg/L
Linearity: 25–200 µg/L
C.V.: not established
Relative recovery: 95–104%

Interferences:

Very high concentrations of β-phenethylamine (a protein decomposition product) may obscure the presence of a low amphetamine concentration. Methamphetamine and ephedrine cannot be distinguished through their trifluoroacetyl derivatives; it is necessary to utilize BSTFA as derivatizing reagent (methamphetamine does not form a derivative) to separate these drugs.

Reference:

M.A. Peat. Unpublished results, 1984.

ANTICONVULSANTS

Drug or Metabolite	Therapeutic Serum Conc. (mg/L)	T½
carbamazepine	4–8	8–12 hr
ethosuximide	40–100	29 hr
mephenytoin	5–15	?
normephenytoin	15–40	?
mephobarbital	8–15	1–3 hr
phenobarbital	10–30	4 days
methsuximide	<1	1.5 hr
normethsuximide	10–40	28–36 hr
phenobarbital	10–30	4 days
phenytoin	10–20	12–36 hr
primidone	1–15	6–12 hr
phenylethylmalonamide	7–10	29–36 hr
phenobarbital	15–30	4 days

Specimens for anticonvulsant drug analysis are normally drawn just prior to the next drug dose in order to insure that the "trough" serum concentration is within the therapeutically effective range. Due to the large number of therapeutic agents available, the various active metabolites that are produced and the popularity of multiple-drug therapy, it is desirable to use the broadest possible approach to the analysis of anticonvulsant drugs. Two highly suitable procedures are presented, one utilizing gas chromatography and the other, liquid chromatography. Clonazepam and valproic acid, which present special problems to the analyst, are dealt with individually (see Index). Radioimmunoassay kits are available for the determination of phenobarbital and phenytoin, while the EMIT system is available for carbamazepine, ethosuximide, phenobarbital, phenytoin and primidone.

Serum Anticonvulsants by Gas Chromatography

Principle:
The anticonvulsant drugs and suitable internal standards are extracted from serum with an organic solvent. The concentrated extract is analyzed without derivatization by flame-ionization gas chromatography. Temperature-programming of the column allows the separate quantitation of at least twelve of the common anticonvulsants and metabolites.

Reagents:
Stock solutions – 1 mg/mL solutions of the appropriate drugs and their active metabolites in methanol

Serum standards – Standards are prepared in serum to contain the following concentrations of the drugs: 5, 10 and 20 mg/L (carbamazepine, mephenytoin, primidone, phenyl-

ethylmalonamide); 10, 12 and 40 mg/L (normephenytoin, normethsuximide, phenobarbital, phenytoin); 40, 80 and 160 mg/L (ethosuximide).

Internal standard mixture – 100 mg/L α-methyl-α-propylsuccinimide (for ethosuximide) and
50 mg/L 4-methylprimidone (for all other drugs) in pH 1.4 0.1 mol/L HC1/KC1 buffer
(internal standards from Aldrich Chemical Co.)

1.5 mol/L Ammonium sulfate

3 mol/L Hydrochloric acid

Dichloromethane

Isoamyl acetate

Instrumental Conditions:

Gas chromatograph with flame-ionization detector

0.9 m × 2 mm i.d. glass column containing 2% SP 2110 and 1% SP 2510-DA on 100/120
mesh Supelcoport (Supelco, Inc.)

Column temperature: initial, 130°C.
15°C./min increase
final, 260°C. (3 min)

Injector, 300°C.; detector, 270°C.

Nitrogen flow rate, 40 mL/min

Procedure:

1. Combine 0.5 mL serum and 0.1 mL internal standard in a 15 mL screw-cap tube. Add
   0.5 mL 1.5 mol/L ammonium sulfate and vortex.
2. Add 3 drops of 3 mol/L HC1 and vortex. Add 5 mL of dichloromethane and shake for
   1 min. Centrifuge to separate layers.
3. Discard the upper aqueous phase and decant the organic layer into a 5 mL conical tube.
   Add 30 μL isoamyl acetate to reduce the loss of ethosuximide.
4. Evaporate the solvent under nitrogen at 40–50°C. until only the isoamyl acetate
   remains. Add 30 μL dichloromethane, vortex and inject 1 μL into the gas
   chromatograph.

	Retention time (min)
ethosuximide	1.3
internal standard	1.8
normethsuximide	4.6
mephenytoin	5.0
phenylethylmalonamide	5.9
normephenytoin	6.8
phenobarbital	6.9
carbamazepine	7.7
primidone	8.5
internal standard	8.9
phenytoin	9.4

Calculation:

Calculation is based on a response factor derived from a standard curve for each drug. A
quality control serum containing the appropriate drugs at concentrations intermediate in
the therapeutic ranges is analyzed daily.

Evaluation:

Sensitivity: 2 mg/L for most drugs
Linearity: to about twice the upper limit of the therapeutic range for each drug
C.V.: 1.2% within-run, 5% day-to-day
Relative recovery: 100–102%

Interferences:

Extraction at a low pH in the presence of ammonium sulfate eliminates much of the usual interference from serum fatty acids and plasticizers. Cholesterol is eluted after the last drug, phenytoin. Normephenytoin (Nirvanol), a mephenytoin metabolite, elutes just prior to phenobarbital and may appear as a shoulder on the phenobarbital peak. Nordiazepam, if present in high concentrations, may interfere with phenytoin.

Reference:

J.J Thoma, T. Ewald and M. McCoy. Simultaneous analysis of underivatized phenobarbital, carbamazepine, primidone and phenytoin by isothermal gas-liquid chromatography. J. Analyt. Tox. 2: 219–225, 1978.

Serum Anticonvulsants by Liquid Chromatography

Principle:

This convenient procedure allows the use of very small serum specimens for the simultaneous analysis of the common anticonvulsants. Proteins are precipitated by addition of the internal standard solution and the supernatant is chromatographed directly on a reversed-phase column. Detection is by ultraviolet absorption at 195 nm.

Reagents:

Stock solutions – 1 mg/mL solutions of the appropriate drugs and their active metabolites in methanol
Serum standards – see previous procedure
Internal standard – 5 mg 5-(p-methylphenyl)-5-phenylhydantoin (Aldrich Chemical Co.) in 100 mL acetonitrile
Acetonitrile – UV grade (Burdick and Jackson Laboratories)
pH 4.4 Phosphate buffer – 0.3 mL of 1 mol/L KH_2PO_4 and 50 μL of 0.9 mol/L H_3PO_4 in 1800 mL of water
Mobile phase – 210 mL of acetonitrile plus 790 mL of the phosphate buffer

Instrumental Conditions:

Liquid chromatograph with 195 nm wavelength detector
25 cm × 4.6 mm i.d. μBondapak C_{18} reversed-phase column (Waters Associates)
Column temperature, 50°C.
Solvent flow rate, 3.0 mL/min

Procedure:

1. Add 200 μL internal standard solution to 200 μL serum in a disposable plastic microtube (as little as 25 μL of each may be used if necessary). Vortex and centrifuge for 1 min at 8000 × g.

2. Inject 20 µL of the supernatant into the chromatograph.

	Retention time (min)
phenylethylmalonamide	1.9
ethosuximide	2.1
primidone	2.4
normephenytoin	3.8
ethotoin	4.1
phenobarbital	4.1
normethsuximide	4.7
carbamazepine-10,11-epoxide	5.3
mephenytoin	6.4
methsuximide	8.1
mephobarbital	9.2
phenytoin	10.0
carbamazepine	11.7
internal standard	21.0

Calculation:

Calculation is based on a response factor derived from a standard curve for each drug. A quality control serum containing the appropriate drugs at concentrations intermediate in the therapeutic ranges is analyzed daily.

Evaluation:

Sensitivity: 1 mg/L for most drugs
Linearity: 2–100 mg/L
C.V.: 2–5% within-run, 2–8% day-to-day
Relative recovery: 88–102%

Interferences:

No interferences are seen with normal, hemolyzed, lipemic or icteric drug-free serum specimens. Over 30 drugs were studied for possible interference; ethotoin co-elutes with phenobarbital and pentobarbital elutes just after mephobarbital. None of the other drugs studied was found to interfere.

Reference:

P.M. Kabra, D.M. McDonald and L.J. Marton. A simultaneous high-performance liquid chromatographic analysis of the most common anticonvulsants and their metabolites in the serum. J. Analyt. Tox. 2; 127–133, 1978.

ANTIHISTAMINES

	Therapeutic Plasma Conc. (mg/L)	T½
brompheniramine	0.005–0.015	?
chlorpheniramine	0.004–0.017	12–15 hr
diphenhydramine	0.009–0.112	5–8 hr
methapyrilene	0.010–0.050	?
orphenadrine	0.050–0.200	?
tripelennamine	0.020–0.060	?

The antihistamines are all weakly basic tertiary amines that produce very low plasma concentrations with normal usage. They are often present in nonprescription cold and allergy remedies and are occasionally subject to abuse. For detection of toxic levels of the antihistamines in plasma or urine, the Basic Drug Screens utilizing gas chromatography and thin-layer chromatography are appropriate. In order to measure therapeutic plasma concentrations, however, a very sensitive method is required; the following procedure provides the necessary sensitivity through the use of a nitrogen-phosphorus detector.

Plasma Antihistamines by Nitrogen-Specific Gas Chromatography

Principle:
The drugs are isolated by extraction from alkalinized plasma into an organic solvent. The concentrated extract is injected directly into the gas chromatograph, which is equipped with a nitrogen-sensitive detector. Orphenadrine is used as internal standard but may be replaced with another antihistamine if it is to be measured itself.

Reagents:
Standard solutions – 1 mg/mL solutions of the appropriate drugs in methanol
Plasma standards – 10, 20, 40 and 80 µg/L for each drug
Internal standard – 10 mg/L orphenadrine in water
0.1 mol/L Sodium hydroxide
Heptane
Chloroform
Methanol

Instrumental Conditions:
Gas chromatograph with nitrogen-phosporus detector
2 m × 2 mm i.d. glass column containing 3% OV-17 on Chromosorb W-HP

Injector, 260°C.; column, 220°C.; detector, 280°C.
Helium flow rate, 50 mL/min

Procedure:

1. To 2 mL of plasma are added 15 μL of internal standard solution and 2 mL 0.1 mol/L NaOH. Add 12 mL heptane and shake to extract.
2. Centrifuge and transfer 8 mL of the organic layer to a clean tube. Evaporate to dryness under nitrogen at 40°C.
3. Dissolve the residue in 500 μL of chloroform and transfer to a Reacti-vial (Pierce Chemical). Evaporate to dryness under nitrogen at 40°C.
4. Dissolve the residue in 10 μL methanol and inject 4 μL into the gas chromatography

	Retention time (min)
diphenhydramine	1.6
internal standard	2.0
tripelennamine	3.8
chlorpheniramine	3.9
methapyrilene	4.0
brompheniramine	4.6

Calculation:

Calculation is based on response factors derived from standard curves for each drug. A quality control plasma containing the appropriate drugs at mid-range concentrations is analyzed daily.

Evaluation:

Sensitivity: 1 μg/L
Linearity: 10–100 μg/L
C.V.: 3–5% within-run
Relative recovery: not established

Interferences:

Normal plasma specimens should be checked for possible interfering substances. Many other basic drugs will be detected by this procedure; these substances have not been studied as potential interferences.

References:

1. W. Bilzer and U. Gundert-Remy. Determination of nanogram quantities of diphenhydramine and orphenadrine in human plasma using gas-liquid chromatography. Eur. J. Clin. Pharm. 6: 268–270, 1973.
2. K.S. Albert, E. Sakmar, J.A. Morais et al. Determination of diphenhydramine in plasma by gas chromatography. Res. Comm. Chem. Path. Pharm. 7: 95–103, 1974.

ARSENIC

Arsenic Concentrations in Human Specimens (mg/L or mg/kg)			
	Normal	Chronic Poisoning	Acute Poisoning
Blood	0.002–0.062	0.01–0.5	0.6–9.3
Hair	<1	1–47	200 (after 6 days)
Urine	0.01–0.03	0.05–5	1–20

Arsenic is a trace element that is present in all human tissues. Arsenic concentrations may be elevated in specimens from persons who are occupationally or environmentally exposed to this toxic metalloid. Occasionally, acute accidental or intentional poisoning occurs in children and adults. Chronic poisoning is best diagnosed by the analysis of hair, whereas blood and urine are usually the preferred specimens for the early confirmation of acute poisoning.

A colorimetric technique is described that is simple enough to be performed in nearly any laboratory. A more sensitive and specific procedure based on atomic absorption spectrometry is also included. Since most methods of arsenic determination require prior destruction of organic matter, procedures for both wet and dry ashing of biologic specimens will be first presented. Wet ashing does not require special equipment (other than a fume hood), but is suitable only for inorganic arsenic; dry ashing requires a muffle furnace and is the preferred procedure for total arsenic (inorganic plus organic) determination.

Wet Ashing of Biologic Specimens

Principle:
Biologic fluids or tissues are reduced to inorganic matter by heating with nitric, sulfuric and perchloric acids. Inorganic arsenic that is present is oxidized to As_2O_3. The resulting colorless liquid is suitable for analysis by a number of different procedures.

Reagents:
Acid mixture – 3 parts conc. HNO_3, 1 part conc. H_2SO_4 and 1 part conc. $HClO_4$ by volume
Nitric acid – conc. HNO_3
Perchloric acid – conc. $HClO_4$

Procedure:
1. Transfer 5 mL or 5 g of the biologic specimen to a 125mL Erlenmeyer flask. Add 5 mL of the acid mixture. Perform all of the following operations in a well-vented safety hood.
2. Warm gently on a hot plate until the frothing subsides.
3. Heat at 130–150°C. until solution boils and darkens. Add 1–2 mL nitric acid and continue heating.

4. Repeat nitric acid addition until solution remains clear. It may be necessary to occasionally add several drops of perchloric acid if solution does not clarify.
5. Continue heating until white fumes of sulfur trioxide are evolved and the solution is free of nitric acid. The resulting volume should be approximately 5 mL.
6. Transfer the cooled solution quantitatively to a 10 mL volumetric flask, rinsing the walls of the digestion flask with water. Adjust the final volume to 10 mL with water.

Reference:

NIOSH Manual of Analytical Methods, 2nd ed., Volume 1, National Institute of Occupational Safety and Health, Cincinnati, 1977, p. 140–141.

Dry Ashing of Biologic Specimens

Principle:

The organic matter of biologic specimens is destroyed by oxidation in a muffle furnace. Both inorganic and organic arsenic are converted to As_2O_3. The ash is dissolved in acid in preparation for analysis by any of the following procedures.

Reagents:

Magnesium oxide
Cellulose powder – Whatman CF-11 (Reeve Angel and Co.)
2 mol/L Hydrochloric acid

Procedure:

1. Transfer 5 mL or 5 g of the biologic specimen to a porcelain evaporating dish and dry in a 95°C. oven for 3–4 hours.
2. Add magnesium oxide to cover the specimen (1–2 g). Add cellulose powder to cover the magnesium oxide (about 5 mL).
3. Place specimen in cold muffle furnace. Set temperature to 550°C.; when furnace reaches operating temperature allow specimen to ash for 2–3 hours.
4. Remove from oven, cool and suspend residue in 5 mL 2 mol/L HC1. Transfer quantitatively to a 10 mL volumetric flask, using water to rinse the dish. Adjust the final volume to 10 mL with water.

References:

1. H.M. Stahr (ed.). Arsenic. In Analytical Toxicology Methods Manual, Iowa State University Press, Ames, Iowa, 1977, pp. 80–83.
2. G.M. George, L.J. Frahm and J.P. McDonnell. Dry ashing method for the determination of total arsenic in animal tissues: collaborative study. J. Asso. Off. Anal. Chem. 56: 793–797, 1973.

Arsenic by Colorimetry

Principle:

A previously ashed specimen is subjected to Zn-HC1 arsine generation following conversion of arsenic to the trivalent form. Hydrogen sulfide is removed with a glass wool plug soaked in lead acetate solution. The arsine is chelated with diethydithiocarbamate and the absorbance of the chelate measured in a spectrophotometer at 540 mm.

Reagents:

Stock solution – 1 mg/mL arsenic (Fisher reference standard SO-A-449) (or dissolve 1.32 g As_2O_3 in 10 mL of 40% NaOH and dilute to 1 L with water)

Arsenic standards – 0.5, 2, 5 and 10 mg/L in water

DDC solution – 0.5 g silver diethyldithiocarbamate in 100 mL pyridine (stable if stored in amber bottle)

Concentrated hydrochloric acid

Stannous chloride solution – 40 g $SnCl_2$ in 100 mL conc. HCl

15% Potassium iodide – 15 g KI/100 mL water

10% Lead acetate – 10 g $Pb(C_2H_3O_2)_2$/100 mL water

Zinc – 20 mesh, low arsenic

Arsine generator – Fisher Scientific Co. #1–405

Instrumental Conditions:

Double beam visible spectrophotometer set to 540 nm

Procedure:

1. Transfer 3.09 mL of the previously ashed specimen to the arsine generator flask and dilute to about 35 mL with water. A water blank and four aqueous standards, previously carried through the identical ashing procedure as the specimen, are to be analyzed in the same manner.
2. Add 5 mL conc. HCl, 2 mL 15% KI and 8 drops $SnCl_2$ solution. Swirl and allow to stand for 15 min.
3. Wet a pledget of glass wool in the lead acetate solution and place it loosely into the scrubber tube of the arsine generator. Lubricate all joints with stopcock grease. Add 3.0 mL DDC solution to the absorber tube.
4. Add 3 g zinc to the generator flask and immediately insert the scrubber-absorber assembly. Allow arsine evolution to continue for 2 hours.
5. Transfer the DDC solution to a 3 mL cuvette and measure the absorbance at 540 nm, using the negative control as a reference. (This solution may also be analyzed by graphite furnace atomic absorbtion spectrometry).

Calculation:

Prepare a standard curve of absorbance versus concentration of the aqueous standards.

Evaluation:

Sensitivity: 0.2 mg/L
Linearity: 0.2–10 mg/L
C.V.: 4–9% day-to-day
Relative recovery: 97–108%

Interferences:

Antimony will be detected as arsenic if it is present in sufficiently high concentrations, but this is unlikely. The antimony hydride, stibine, forms a chelate that has maximum absorbance at 510 nm. Chromium, copper and molybdenum may interfere with the evolution of arsine if present in high concentrations.

References:

1. NIOSH Manual of Analytical Methods, 2nd ed., Volume 1, National Institute for Occupational Safety and Health, Cincinnati, 1977, pp. 140–141.
2. H.M. Stahr (ed.). Arsenic. In Analytical Toxicology Methods Manual, Iowa State University Press, Ames, Iowa, 1977, pp. 80–83.
3. G.M. George, L.J. Frahm and J.P. McDonnell. Dry ashing method for the determination of total arsenic in animal tissues: collaborative study. J. Asso. Off. Anal. Chem. 56: 793–797, 1973.

Arsenic by Atomic Absorption Spectrometry

Principle:

A previously ashed specimen is treated to convert arsenic to the trivalent form. Arsenic is chelated with diethyldithiocarbamate, the chelate is extracted into chloroform, partitioned back into water and an aliquot analyzed by graphite furnace atomic absorption spectrometry at 193.7 nm.

Reagents:

Stock solution – 1 mg/mL arsenic (Fisher reference standard SO-A-449)
Arsenic standards – 0.2, 0.5, 1 and 2 mg/L in water
8 mol/L Hydrochloric acid
Saturated potassium iodide
Chloroform
DDC solution – 2% diethylammonium diethyldithiocarbamate in water (prepare fresh)
2 mol/L Nitric acid

Instrumental Conditions:

Atomic absorption spectrometer with graphic furnace
Arsenic electrodeless discharge lamp
Furnace program: dry 20 sec at 100°C.
              char 29 sec at 500°C.
              atomize 15 sec at 2100°C.
Measure absorption at 193.7 nm

Procedure:

1. Transfer 0.5 mL of a previously ashed specimen to a 15 mL centrifuge tube. A water blank and four aqueous standards, previously carried through the identical ashing procedure as the specimen, are to be analyzed in the same manner. Add 0.3 mL 8 mol/L HC1 and 0.1 mL saturated KI and vortex.
2. Add 2 mL chloroform and 0.1 mL DDC solution. Vortex for 15 sec and allow layers to separate.
3. Discard the upper layer and transfer 1.0 mL of the lower chloroform layer to a clean tube.
4. Introduce 10–30 μL of the aqueous phase into the graphite furnace.

Calculation:

Prepare a standard curve of absorption versus concentration of the aqueous standards. Determine the specimen concentration from this curve.

Evaluation:

Sensitivity: 0.1 mg/L
Linearity: 0.2–2.0 mg/L
C.V.: 10%
Relative recovery: not established

Interferences:

None known.

Reference:

P. Mushak, K. Dessauer and E.L. Walls. Flameless atomic absorption (FAA) and gas-liquid chromatographic studies in arsenic bioanalysis. Env. Health Persp. 19: 5–10, 1977.

BARBITURATES

The therapeutic and toxic plasma levels of the barbiturates are included under the Serum Acid and Neutral Drug Screen, as are specific qualitative and quantitative methods for their determination. The present colorimetric and ultraviolet spectrophotometric techniques are somewhat nonspecific and only semi-quantitative, but are convenient emergency procedures for the small clinical laboratory. Of the two, the ultraviolet procedure is the more specific and sensitive.

Commercial kits are also available for the determination of barbiturates in both serum and urine by radioimmunoassay and EMIT.

Serum Barbiturates by Colorimetry

Principle:
The barbiturates are extracted from serum with chloroform. A mercury-diphenylcarbazone chromogen is formed directly in the chloroform phase and the absorbance at 550 nm is determined in a colorimeter.

Reagents:
Stock solution – 10 mg/L secobarbital in methanol
Serum standards – 10, 20 and 40 mg/L
Chloroform
0.15 mol/L Phosphate buffer – 95.5 mL 0.15 mol/L Na_2HPO_4 and 5.5 mL 0.15 mol/L KH_2PO_4 (pH 8)
Mercuric nitrate solution – 100 mg $Hg(NO_3)_2$ and 20 µL conc. HNO_3 in 5 mL water, dilute to 250 mL with 0.15 mol/L phosphate buffer (stable at room temperature)
Diphenylcarbazone solution – 100 mg/100 mL chloroform (stable if stored in a dark bottle in the refrigerator)

Instrumental Conditions:
Visible spectrophotometer set to 550 nm

Procedure:
1. Transfer 0.5 mL serum and 5 mL chloroform to a test tube. Vortex for 15 seconds.
2. Filter through #31 Whatman paper into a clean tube.
3. Add 0.5 mL mercuric nitrate solution and vortex for 15 seconds. Filter through #31 Whatman paper into a clean tube.
4. Transfer 2.5 mL of the filtered chloroform to a cuvette and add 0.5 mL diphenylcarbazone. Mix and measure absorbance at 550 nm.

Calculation:

Calculation is based on a response factor derived from a standard curve of absorbance (corrected for a serum blank) versus concentration of the serum standards. A quality control serum containing 20 mg/L secobarbital is analyzed daily. Since each barbiturate has a different molar extinction coefficient, this procedure is only semi-quantitative. It can be fully quantitative if the identity of the drug is known and the proper standards are analyzed.

Evaluation:

Sensitivity: 5 mg/L for most barbiturates
Linearity: 10–100 mg/L
C.V.: not established
Relative recovery: not established

Interferences:

Phenytoin and mephenytoin react as barbiturates. Glutethimide and methyprylon react weakly and 27 other sedatives and tranquilizers were found not to interfere.

Reference:

D.M. Baer. A simple colorimetric method for detection of barbiturates, suitable for the small clinical laboratory. Amer. J. Clin. Path. 44: 114–117, 1965.

Serum Barbiturates by Ultraviolet Spectrophotometry

Principle:

The barbiturates are extracted from serum into chloroform and back-extracted into dilute sodium hydroxide. Aliquots of the alkaline fraction are adjusted to pH 10 and 13 and a differential spectrum is recorded from 280 to 226 nm in the ultraviolet region. The absorbance difference between 240 and 260 nm is proportional to the amount of barbiturate present.

Reagents:

Stock solution – 10 mg/mL secobarbital (109.7 mg Na salt/10 mL methanol)
Serum standards – 5, 10, 20 and 40 mg/L
0.5 mol/L Phosphate buffer – 50 mL 0.5 mol/L KH_2PO_4 plus 30 mL 0.1 mol/L NaOH, adjusted to pH 7.4 with 10% NaOH
Chloroform – spectral grade
0.45 mol/L Sodium hydroxide – 18 g NaOH/L of water
Ammonium chloride solution – 10.7 g NH_4Cl/100 mL water

Instrumental Conditions:

Double-beam scanning ultraviolet spectrophotometer

Procedure:

1. Transfer 3 mL serum to a 125 mL separatory funnel and add 2 mL 0.5 mol/L phosphate buffer and 25 mL chloroform. Shake for 1 min and allow layers to separate.

2. Drain 22 mL chloroform layer through filter into a 25 mL glass-stoppered graduated cylinder. Add 5 mL 0.45 mol/L sodium hydroxide, shake for 1 min and allow layers to separate.

3. Transfer 2 mL aliquots of the alkaline layer to two separate 3 mL quartz cuvettes. Add 0.5 mL of ammonium chloride solution to one to adjust the sodium to pH 10 (reference cuvette). Add 0.5 mL 0.45 mol/L sodium hydroxide to the other to maintain pH 13 (sample cuvette).

4. Place the cuvettes in the spectrophotometer and record the differential spectrum from 280 to 226 nm. Measure the absorbance difference between 240 and 260 nm.

Calculation:

Calculation is based on a response factor derived from a standard curve of absorbance difference versus concentration for a serum blank and the serum standards. A qualtiy control serum containing 20 mg/L secobarbital is analyzed daily. Since each barbiturate has a different molar extinction coefficient, this procedure is only semi-quantitative. It can be fully quantitative if the identity of the drug is known and the proper standards are analyzed.

Evaluation:

Sensitivity: 2–3 mg/L
Linearity: 5–100 mg/L
C.V.: 5.4% within-run
Relative recovery: 91–113%

Interferences:

The method is relatively specific for the barbiturates as a class. Twenty other drugs, including meprobamate and glutethimide, were found not to interfere.

References:

1. G.B. Schumann, K. Lauenstein, D. LeFever and J.B. Henry. Ultraviolet spectrophotometric analysis of barbiturates. Amer. J. Clin. Path. 66: 823–830, 1976.
2. P. Jatlow. Ultraviolet spectrophotometric analysis of barbiturates. Amer. J. Clin. Path. 59: 167–173, 1973.

BASIC DRUG SCREEN

	Toxic Concentrations (mg/L)	
	Plasma	Urine
amitriptyline	0.5–2.0	0.5–10
amphetamine	0.2–3.0	25–250
chlordiazepoxide	2–30	1–10
codeine	0.2–5.0	25–250
diazepam	2–20	1–10
diphenhydramine	0.2–5.0	2–20
doxepin	0.5–2.0	0.5–10
flurazepam	0.2–2.0	2–10
meperidine	0.5–5.0	25–250
methadone	0.1–2.0	1–50
methamphetamine	0.2–2.0	25–300
methaqualone	2–200	0.5–25
morphine	0.1–1.0	0.5–25
nordiazepam	2–20	1–10
norpropoxyphene	2–10	20–200
nortriptyline	0.5–2.0	10–100
pentazocine	0.2–2.0	3–30
phencyclidine	0.01–1.0	0.1–340
propoxyphene	0.5–2.0	2–30

The basic drugs are a group of weakly basic amino compounds consisting largely of the antihistamines, narcotic analgesics, phenothiazines, stimulants and tricyclic antidepressants, as well as several miscellaneous substances. The plasma and urine concentrations of the drugs commonly detected in clinical emergencies are listed above; many of the less common drugs are listed under the procedures for specific drugs or drug classes.

Most of the basic drugs achieve relatively high urine concentrations in contrast to their plasma concentrations, and so the following thin-layer chromatography screen for these drugs in urine is an excellent qualitative procedure to use for emergency purposes. The identification of a substance in urine by this procedure is not necessarily indicative of overdose, however, since even therapeutic doses of many compounds may be detected. For this reason, the gas or liquid chromatography screen, since they are quantitative and are performed on serum, may be more useful as an initial screening tool if a drug overdosage is suspected. Any of the procedures may be used in conjunction with another in order to confirm positive findings.

Urine Basic Drug Screen by Thin-Layer Chromatography

Principle:

Urine is extracted at pH 9.3 with an organic solvent to remove basic drugs and their metabolites. If heroin use is suspected, prior acid hydrolysis of the sample may be necessary to release conjugated morphine. The extract is evaporated to dryness and the residue spotted onto a thin-layer chromatography plate. After development, the plate is sprayed with various chromogenic reagents for visualization of the drugs.

Reagents:

Stock solutions –

    1 mg/mL amphetamine (13.64 mg SO_4 salt/10 mL methanol)

    1 mg/mL chlorpromazine (11.15 mg HCl salt/10 mL methanol)

    1 mg/mL codeine (14.19 mg PO_4 salt/10 mL methanol)

    1 mg/mL methadone (11.19 mg HCl salt/10 mL methanol)

    1 mg/mL methaqualone (11.47 mg HCl salt/10 mL methanol)

    1 mg/mL morphine (13.30 mg SO_4 salt/10 mL methanol)

    1 mg/mL nicotine (10 μL/10 mL methanol)

    1 mg/mL propoxyphene (11.09 mg HCl salt/10 mL methanol)

    1 mg/mL phencyclidine (11.50 mg HCl salt/10 mL methanol)

Urine standard – 1 mg/L of chlorpromazine, methadone, nicotine, propoxyphene; 2 mg/L of codeine, morphine, phencyclidine; 4 mg/L methaqualone; 5 mg/L amphetamine (prepared in drug-free urine containing 0.5% NaF; stable for 1 month if refrigerated or 1 year if frozen)

pH 9.3 Borate buffer – 950 mL saturated $Na_2B_4O_7$. 10 H_2O plus 50 mL 0.3 mol/L NaOH

Hydrochloric acid – conc. HCl

NH_4Cl/NH_4OH Buffer – 250 mL 50% saturated NH_4Cl plus 250 mL conc. NH_4OH

Methanol

Extraction solvent – chloroform/isopropanol, 4:1 by volume

TLC plates – glass or plastic plates coated with a 250 micron thick silica gel G layer. Store in a 75°C. oven.

Developing solvents – ethyl acetate/methanol/ammonium hydroxide, 82:13:5, and ethyl acetate/methanol, 98:2

Ninhydrin spray – 400 mg ninhydrin/100 mL of 0.1 mol/L K_2HPO_4. Adjust pH to 10 with 2 mol/L KOH (make fresh daily).

Phenylacetaldehyde spray – 0.5 mL phenylacetaldehyde/100 mL ethanol (stable for 3 months)

Iodoplatinate spray – 1 mL of 10% $PtCl_3$, 1 g KI and 0.5 mL 5 mol/L HCl per 100 mL H_2O

Procedure:

1. Transfer 10 mL of urine to a 125 mL separatory funnel. Add 5 mL of pH 9.3 borate buffer.
2. Add 25 mL of the extraction solvent, shake for 1 min, allow layers to separate and drain the solvent through filter paper into a 50 mL beaker.
3. Add 1 drop of conc. HCl to the beaker and evaporate the solvent to dryness on a 60°C. water bath inside a fume hood.

4. Dissolve the residue in 100 μL methanol and spot about 1/2 of this solution to the origin of a TLC plate.
5. Place the plate into the ethyl acetate/methanol/ammonia tank and allow the developing solvent to rise to a height of 7.5 cm.
6. Remove the plate, allow it to air dry and then place into the ethyl acetate/methanol tank. Allow the solvent to rise to a height of 15 cm.
7. Remove the plate, allow it to air dry and then dry completely in a 75°C. oven for several minutes. Examine the plate under long-wave UV light for quinine fluorescence.
8. Spray lightly with ninhydrin. Spray again with phenylacetaldehyde and let the plate stand at room temperature for 10–15 minutes. Observe amphetamine fluorescence under the long-wave UV light.
9. Spray plate with iodoplatinate solution and note the locations of all colored spots.

Acid hydrolysis technique for morphine:

1. To 10 mL of urine in a test tube, add 1 mL of conc. HC1. Place a marble over the top of the tube and heat in a boiling water bath for 1 hour.
2. Cool the specimen and transfer to a 125 mL separatory funnel. Extract with 25 mL of the extraction solvent.
3. Discard the solvent and add to the aqueous sample an equal volume of NH_4Cl/NH_4OH buffer (gives pH of 9.3). Now follow the procedure for unhydrolyzed samples beginning with step #2.

	Distance from Origin (cm)
methaqualone	12.5
phencyclidine	11.3
propoxyphene	10.0
cocaine	9.4
pentazocine	7.3
methadone	6.8
flurazepam	6.6
scopolamine	6.5
doxepin	6.3
methapyrilene	6.2
thioridazine	6.2
amitriptyline	5.7
chlorpromazine	5.4
methylphenidate	5.3
oxycodone	5.1
diphenhydramine	5.0
meperidine	4.5
imipramine	4.5
hydroxyzine	4.4
nalorphine	4.2
trifluoperazine	4.2
nicotine	4.2
desipramine	4.0
quinine	4.0
norpropoxyphene	3.9
dexbrompheniramine	3.9
prochlorperazine	3.8
amphetamine	3.5

oxymorphone	3.5
propranolol	3.3
methamphetamine	3.0
levorphanol	3.0
phenylpropanolamine	2.5
atropine	2.4
ephedrine	2.3
codeine	2.2
hydromorphone	1.8
morphine	1.3
phenylephrine	1.1

Calculation:

An aliquot of the urine standard is analyzed with each group of patient specimens. Other appropriate drug standards may be spotted as methanol solutions directly to the origin of the TLC plate when required for identification of unknown spots.

Evaluation:

Sensitivity: 1–2 mg/L for most drugs
Linearity: not applicable
C.V.: not applicable
Relative recovery: not applicable

Interferences:

Many drugs and drug metabolites other than the ones listed will produce chromatographic spots that may hinder interpretation. Results should be considered presumptive until confirmed by other techniques.

Reference:

R. Baselt and C. Stewart. Unpublished results, 1975.

Serum Basic Drug Screen by Gas Chromatography

Principle:

The basic drugs are extracted from alkalinized serum with chlorobutane, back-extracted into hydrochloric acid and finally partitioned into chloroform for injection into the gas chromatograph. Temperature programming and flame-ionization detection are utilized to provide a sensitivity limit of 0.2 mg/L for most basic drugs.

Reagents:

Stock solutions –
    1 mg/mL amitriptyline in methanol
    1 mg/mL chlordiazepoxide in methanol
    1 mg/mL diazepam in methanol
    1 mg/mL meperidine in methanol

1 mg/mL methadone in methanol
1 mg/mL norpropoxyphene in methanol
1 mg/mL nortriptyline in methanol
1 mg/mL phencyclidine in methanol
1 mg/mL propoxyphene in methanol

Serum standards – 0.5, 1.0 and 2.0 mg/L of the above drugs

Quality control serum – 0.5 mg/L meperidine, 1.0 mg/L amitriptyline, methadone, phencyclidine and propoxyphene, 2.0 mg/L norpropoxyphere and nortriptyline and 5.0 mg/L chlordiazepoxide and diazepam

Internal standard – 80 mg/L SKF-525A (Smith, Kline and French) in water

Ammonium hydroxide – conc. NH_4OH

1-Chlorobutane

1-mol/L Hydrochloric acid

Chloroform

Instrumental Conditions:

Gas chromatograph with flame-ionization detector

2 m × 2 mm i.d. glass columns containing 3% OV-17 or OV-1 on 80/100 mesh Chromosorb W-HP

Column temperature: initial, 170°C.
                        8°C./min increase
                        final, 270°C. (8 min.)

Injector, 200°C.; detector, 300°C.

Nitrogen flow rate, 30 mL/min

Procedure:

1. Transfer 2 mL serum to a 15 mL screw-cap tube. Add 50 µL internal standard and vortex.
2. Add 10 mL chlorobutane and 5 drops of conc. NH_4OH and place on a tilted rotator at slow speed for 5 min.
3. Centrifuge to separate layers and transfer 9 mL of the solvent layer to a clean tube. Add 5 mL of 1 mol/L HC1 and shake for 30 seconds.
4. Centrifuge and discard the upper solvent layer. Remove all traces of chlorobutane by evaporation with an airstream.
5. Transfer 4 mL of the acid layer to a 5 mL glass stoppered conical centrifuge tube and add 0.9 mL conc. NH_4OH. Vortex for 10 seconds and add 50 µL of chloroform. Stopper and shake for 15 seconds.
6. Centrifuge to separate layers. Remove and discard several mL of the upper aqueous phase to allow access to the lower chloroform layer.
7. Inject 4 µL of the chloroform layer onto the OV-17 column. Confirmation is performed on the OV-1 column.

	Retention times (min)	
	OV-17	OV-1
meperidine	5.4	3.4
phencyclidine	6.7	4.8
diphenhydramine	6.9	4.4

chlorpheniramine	8.6	5.8
methadone	10.0	7.2
propoxyphene	10.3	7.7
amitriptyline	10.8	7.7
imipramine	11.1	7.9
nortriptyline	11.3	7.8
doxepin	11.4	8.0
methaqualone	11.6	7.1
internal standard	12.0	8.4
norpropoxyphene amide	13.5	9.5, 9.7
codeine	14.1	9.4
diazepam	15.1	9.9
nordiazepam	17.0	10.4
chlordiazepoxide	17.3, 21.5	10.5, 11.6, 13.3

Calculation:

Calculation is based on a response factor for each drug derived from a standard curve. A quality control serum containing the most common drugs, as described under reagents, is analyzed daily.

Evaluation:

Sensitivity: 0.2 mg/L for most drugs
Linearity: 0.2–2.0 mg/L for most drugs
C.V.: 2–10% day-to-day
Relative recovery: 92–104% at 0.5 mg/L

Interferences:

Many basic drugs and their metabolites are detected by this procedure. Confirmation of results on the OV-1 column helps to improve specificity but the results should be considered presumptive until further confirmation is possible. The use of the Urine Basic Drug Screen by Thin-Layer Chromatography for the analysis of a urine specimen from the same patient is recommended in conjunction with this assay.

References:

1. E.H. Foerster, D. Hatchett and J.C. Garriott. A rapid, comprehensive screening procedure for basic drugs in blood or tissues by gas chromatography. J. Analyt. Tox. 2:50–55, 1978.
2. D.R. Clark. Personal communication, 1979.

Serum Basic Drug Screen by Liquid Chromatography

Principle:

Alkalinized serum is extracted with ether, the solvent is back-extracted with dilute acid, and the acid is made basic and re-extracted with ether. The solvent is evaporated to dryness, reconstituted in mobile phase and analyzed by liquid chromatography with dual-wavelength ultraviolet detection.

Reagents:

Stock solutions – 1 mg/mL methanol solutions of the appropriate drugs

Serum standards – 0.1, 0.2 and 0.5 mg/L (or other appropriate, concentrations)

Quality control serum – 0.2 mg/L meperidine, chlorpheniramine, diphenhydramine, amoxapine, desipramine, imipramine and diazepam

Internal standard – 30 mg/L methixene (Wander Pharmaceuticals, Bern, Switzerland) in water

pH 10.5 Buffer – 1 mol/L sodium bicarbonate

Ether

1 mol/L Hydrochloric acid

Ammonium hydroxide – conc. NH_4OH

Mobile phase – water/acetonitrile/methanol/pH 2.8 buffer (14 g anhydrous Na_2HPO_4, 17 mL H_3PO_4 and 10 mL diethylamine per L of water), 55:30:10:5 (adjust internal standard retention time to 14.2–14.7 min by adding 0.2 mL H_3PO_4 or 0.2 mL 50% NaOH per 4 L of mobile phase in order to decrease or increase retention time, respectively)

Instrumental Conditions:

Liquid chromatography with dual-wavelength ultraviolet detector set at 220/230 nm

30 cm × 4 mm i.d. µBondapak C^{18} column (Waters Associates)

Column temperature, 25°C.

Solvent flow rate, 2 mL/min

Procedure:

1. Add 2 mL serum, 50 µL internal standard and 1 mL pH 10.5 buffer to a 15 mL screw-up tube and vortex. Extract with 10 mL ether by shaking for 3 min and centrifuge.
2. Transfer the ether layer to a clean tube. Extract with 2 mL 1 mol/L HCl and centrifuge. Discard the ether layer by aspiration.
3. Add 0.5 mL conc. NH_4OH to the acid layer and vortex. Further add 1 mL pH 10.5 buffer and vortex. Extract with 5 mL ether and centrifuge.
4. Transfer the ether layer to a 12 mL conical centrifuge tube and evaporate to dryness under a stream of nitrogen. Reconstitute with 100 µL mobile phase and inject 50 µL into the chromatograph.

	Retention time (min)	Absorbance ratio (220/230 nm)
lidocaine	2.2	2.1
quinidine	2.3	1.0
disopyramide	2.6	2.2
8-hydroxyamoxapine	2.7	1.8
meperidine	2.7	2.1
cocaine	2.9	0.6
norchlordiazepoxide	3.0	0.8
8-hydroxyloxapine	3.2	1.8
chlorpheniramine	3.5	1.2
methapyrilene	3.6	0.6
pentazocine	3.6	1.5
chlordiazepoxide	3.6	0.8
propranolol	4.2	1.2
demoxepam	4.9	0.7

tripolidine	4.9	0.9
mesoridazine	4.9	1.1
diphenhydramine	5.2	2.2
flurazepam	5.2	0.9
carbamazepine	5.5	1.5
nordoxepin	5.8	1.7
doxepin	6.2	1.6
amoxapine	6.6	1.4
oxazepam	6.9	0.9
haloperidol	6.9	1.5
methaqualone	7.5	0.9
methadone metabolite	7.6	2.1
loxapine	7.6	1.5
hydroxyethylflurazepam	7.8	0.9
lorazepam	7.9	0.9
promazine	8.5	0.8
desipramine	9.1	2.4
flunitrazepam	9.1	1.3
protriptyline	9.2	1.3
desalkylflurazepam	9.5	0.9
norpropoxyphene	9.6	20
temazepam	9.8	0.9
cyclobenzaprine	9.9	1.1
imipramine	9.9	2.4
nordiazepam	10.2	0.9
maprotiline	10.2	3.2
nortriptyline	10.8	1.5
propoxyphene	10.9	20
amitriptyline	11.7	1.5
methadone	12.1	2.6
trimipramine	13.0	2.3
internal standard	14.4	
diazepam	16.3	0.9
chlorpromazine	16.7	1.2

Calculation:

Calculation is based on a response factor for each drug derived from a standard curve. A quality control serum containing the most common drugs, as described under reagents, is analyzed daily.

Evaluation:

Sensitivity: 0.2 mg/L for most drugs
Linearity: 0.2–2.0 mg/L for most drugs
C.V.: 2–10% day-to-day
Relative recovery: 92–104% at 0.5 mg/L

Interferences:

Many basic drugs and their metabolites are detected by this procedure. The use of an absorbance ratio helps to improve specificity but the results should be considered presumptive until further confirmation is possible. The use of the Urine Basic Drug Screen by Thin-Layer Chromatography for the analysis of a urine specimen from the same patient is recommended in conjuction with this assay. Re-injection of the serum extract and liquid chromatographic analysis using slightly different conditions (detection at 250/260 nm; mobile phase: water/acetonitrile/methanol/pH 4.8 buffer, 40:40:10:10, the buffer consisting of 14 g sodium acetate trihydrate, 9 mL H_3PO_4 and 10 mL diethylamine per L of water) is recommended as an alternative means of confirmation of positive results.

Reference:

D.Demorest. Presented at the California Association of Toxicologists meeting, San Mateo, California, February 6, 1982

BENZODIAZEPINES

Drug or Metabolite	Therapeutic Plasma Conc. (mg/L)	T½ (hr)
bromazepam	0.08–0.17	12
chlordiazepoxide	0.5–1.0	7–14
norchlordiazepoxide	0.1–0.7	?
clorazepate	<0.02	?
nordiazepam	0.1–0.8	48
diazepam	0.1–1.5	21–37
nordiazepam	0.1–0.5	48
flunitrazepam	0.003–0.006	9–25
flurazepam	0–0.004	<2
desalkylflurazepam	0.01–0.11	47–100
lorazepam	0.05–0.24	12
medazepam	0.1–0.6	?
diazepam	0.03–0.07	21–37
nordiazepam	0.4–0.7	48
nitrazepam	0.03–0.09	25–28
oxazepam	0.2–1.4	4–18

The benzodiazepines are a group of structurally similar compounds used as sedative hypnotic and anticonvulsant drugs. They are all weak bases and produce relatively low plasma concentrations in therapeutic usage. The plasma concentrations produced by certain of these drugs, such as diazepam and chlordiazepoxide, in clinical emergencies can be detected using the Serum Basic Drug Screen by Gas Chromatography. The detection of these drugs as a class, however, requires a more specialized approach. The first two procedures presented, involving thin-layer chromatography and flame-ionization gas chromatography, are suitable for determination of the benzodiazepines in serum in clinical overdose cases and may be used in conjunction with one another for confirmation. The latter two methods, involving electron-capture gas chromatography and liquid chromatography, are more sensitive techniques and are suitable to the quantitation of therapeutic serum concentrations of the drugs.

Only a small fraction of a dose of most benzodiazepines is excreted unchanged in the urine, the majority being found as conjugated metabolites. An EMIT urine assay has been designed to detect usage of the benzodiazepines that are excreted as oxazepam; this would include chlordiazepoxide, clorazepate, diazepam, medazepam, oxazepam and prazepam. An EMIT benzodiazepine assay for serum has recently been developed. Clonazepam, a benzodiazepine anticonvulsant, is dealt with in a separate section (see Index).

Serum Benzodiazepines by Thin-Layer Chromatography

Principles:

The benzodiazepines are extracted from serum with an organic solvent, which is then evaporated to dryness. The residue is spotted to a thin-layer plate and after development the drugs are visualized by spraying with Dragendorff's reagent. Alternatively, the extract from the Serum Benzodiazepines by Flame-Ionization Gas Chromatography method may be spotted directly to the plate.

Reagents:

Stock solutions –

    1 mg/mL chlordiazepoxide in methanol
    1 mg/mL desalkylflurazepam in methanol
    1 mg/mL diazepam in methanol
    1 mg/mL flurazepam in methanol
    1 mg/mL nordiazepam in methanol
    1 mg/mL oxazepam in methanol

Serum standards – 2 mg/L for each of the above drugs
Internal standard – 20 mg prazepam (Warner-Lambert) in 100 mL methanol
Ammonium hydroxide – conc. NH_4OH
1-Chlorobutane
Dragendorff's reagent –

    A: 0.2 g bismuth subnitrate and 25 mL acetic acid in 50 mL water
    B: 4 g KI in 70 mL water
    Mix A and B in a 1:1 ratio fresh as needed

Glass or plastic thin-layer plates coated with 250 micron thick layer of silica gel G
Developing solvent – acetone/benzene/chloroform, 25:40:50 by volume

Procedure:

1. Transfer 4 mL serum to a 15 mL screw-cap tube. Add 0.4 mL internal standard and vortex.
2. Add 2 drops conc. NH_4OH and 10 mL 1-chlorobutane and place on a tilted rotator at slow speed for 20 min. Centrifuge to separate layers.
3. Transfer upper organic layer to a 15 mL conical centrifuge tube and evaporate to dryness under a stream of air at 50°C.
4. Dissolve the residue in 50 μL methanol and spot about one-half to the origin of a thin-layer plate. Place into the developing solvent and develop to a height of 10 cm.
5. Remove plate from tank, allow it to air-dry and spray with Dragendorff's reagent.

	Rf
flurazepam	0.14
chlordiazepoxide	0.20
oxazepam	0.42
nitrazepam	0.56
desalkylflurazepam	0.57
nordiazepam	0.59
flunitrazepam	0.79
internal standard (prazepam)	0.81
diazepam	0.83
medazepam	0.87

Calculation:

Determine the presence of benzodiazepines in the patient specimen by comparison of spot color and location with the drugs in the serum standard, extracted in an identical manner. Other benzodiazepines may be spotted directly to the origin as methanol solutions if required. The internal standard in each specimen acts as a check on extraction efficiency.

Evaluation:

Sensitivity: 1 mg/L for most drugs
Linearity: not applicable
C.V.: not applicable
Relative recovery: not applicable

Interferences:

Many other basic drugs will be extracted and detected by this method. It is most useful as a confirmation technique following initial detection of a benzodiazepine by the Basic Drug Screen by Gas Chromatography or the Benzodiazepines by Flame-Ionization Gas Chromatography procedures.

Reference:

R.C. Baselt, C.B. Stewart and S.J. Franch. Toxicological determination of benzodiazepines in biological fluids and tissues by flame-ionization gas chromatography. J. Analyt. Tox. 1: 10–13, 1977.

Serum Benzodiazepines by Flame-Ionization Gas Chromatography

Principle:

The benzodiazepines are extracted from aqueous alkaline solution with 1-chlorobutane, put through a clean-up procedure, and analyzed by gas chromatography with flame-ionization detection. The drugs and their major metabolites are well separated except for the chlordiazepoxide metabolites, norchlordiazepoxide and demoxepam, which are not detected by this method.

Reagents:

Stock solutions –
    1 mg/L chlordiazepoxide (11.22 mg HCl salt/10 mL methanol)
    1 mg/mL desalkylflurazepam (10 mg/10 mL methanol)
    1 mg/mL diazepam (10 mg/10 mL methanol)
    1 mg/mL flurazepam (11.88 mg HCl salt/10 mL methanol)
    1 mg/mL nordiazepam (10 mg/10 mL methanol)
    1 mg/mL oxazepam (10 mg/10 mL methanol)
Serum standards – 0.2, 0.5, 1.0 and 2.0 mg/L for each of the above drugs
Quality control sera – 2.0 mg/L of diazepam, nordiazepam, flurazepam, desalkyl-
    flurazepam and oxazepam; 2.0 mg/L of chlordiazepoxide
Internal standard – 20 mg prazepam (Warner-Lambert) in 100 mL methanol

1 mol/L Hydrochloric acid – 40 mL conc. HCl/500 mL H_2O
Ammonium hydroxide – conc. NH_4OH
1-Chlorobutane
Chloroform

Instrumental Conditions:

Gas chromatography with dual flame-ionization detectors
2 m × 2 mm i.d. glass columns containing 2% OV-17 on 100/120 mesh Chromosorb G-HP
Injector, 250°C.; column, 260°C.; detector, 300°C.
Nitrogen flow rate, 33 mL/min

Procedure:

1. Pipet 4.0 mL serum into a 15 mL screw-cap glass tube. Add 0.4 mL internal standard and vortex.
2. Add 2 drops conc. NH_4OH and 10 mL 1-chlorobutane and place on a tilted rotator at slow speed for 20 min. Centrifuge for 5 min at 2000 rpm.
3. Transfer the upper organic layer to a clean 15 mL graduated glass-stoppered centrifuge tube. Add 5 mL 1 mol/L HCl, stopper and shake for 1 min to extract. Centrifuge for 1 min at 2000 rpm after removing stopper.
4. Discard by aspiration and evaporation all traces of the upper organic layer. Add 0.5 mL conc. NH_4OH and 100 µL $CHCl_3$, stopper and shake for 15 seconds to extract. Centrifuge for 5 min at 2000 rpm after removing stopper.
5. Remove several mL of the upper aqueous phase by aspiration to allow access to the lower $CHCl_3$ layer. Inject 2–4 µL of the $CHCl_3$ layer onto the OV-17 column at 260°C. Confirmation is performed on OV-1 at 240°C. or by thin-layer chromatography.

	Retention time (min)	
	OV-17 at 260°	OV-1 at 240°
oxazepam	3.8	2.5
diazepam	5.3	3.2
desalkylflurazepam	6.0	3.2
nordiazepam	7.1	3.7
chlordiazepoxide	7.5	3.7
internal standard	8.8	5.5
flurazepam	10.8	7.8

Calculation:

Calculation is based on a response factor derived from a standard curve for each drug. The quality control specimens prepared as described are analyzed daily.

Evaluation:

Sensitivity: 0.2 mg/L
Linearity: 0.2–22.0 mg/L
C.V.: 5–22% day-to-day
Relative recovery: 92–105%

Interferences:

Normal patient serum specimens do not contain interfering substances. Many other basic drugs may be detected by this procedure and results should be considered presumptive until confirmed by another technique.

References:

1. R.C. Baselt, C.B. Stewart and S.J. Franch. Toxicological determination of benzodiazepines in biological fluids and tissues by flame-ionization gas chromatography. J. Analyt. Tox. 1: 10–13, 1977.
2. J.C. Garriott and N. Latman. Drug detection in cases of "driving under the influence." J. For. Sci. 21: 398–415, 1976.

Serum Benzodiazepines by Electron-Capture Gas Chromatography

Principle:

The benzodiazepines are extracted from alkalinized serum with an organic solvent, and an aliquot of the extract is injected directly into the gas chromatograph. The electron-capture detector allows determination of therapeutic concentrations of most of the drugs using small sample volumes.

Reagents:

Stock solutions –
> 1 mg/mL chlordiazepoxide in methanol
> 1 mg/mL desalkylflurazepam in methanol
> 1 mg/mL diazepam in methanol
> 1 mg/mL flurazepam in methanol
> 1 mg/mL nordiazepam in methanol

Serum standards – 0.1, 0.2, 0.5 and 1.0 mg/L for the above drugs
Quality control serum – 0.2 mg/L of chlordiazepoxide, diazepam, desalkylflurazepam, flurazepam and nordiazepam
Internal standard – 2 mg/100 mL flunitrazepam (Hoffman-La Roche, Inc.) in methanol
Borate buffer – saturated solution of sodium borate
Extraction solvent – toluene/heptane/isoamyl alcohol, 76:20:4 by volume

Instrumental Conditions:

Gas chromatograph with electron-capture detector
1.2 m × 3.2 mm i.d. glass column containing 3% OV-17 on 100/120 mesh Gas Chrom Q
Injector, 300°C; column, 240°C; detector, 300°C.
Nitrogen flow rate, 50 mL/min

Procedure:

1. Transfer 1 mL serum to a centrifuge tube, add 10 μL internal standard and vortex briefly.
2. Add 1 mL borate buffer and 1 mL extraction solvent and vortex for 15 seconds.

3. Centrifuge to separate layers and inject 2 µL of the upper solvent layer into the gas chromatograph.

	Retention time (min)
diazepam	2.2
desalkylflurazepam	2.5
nordiazepam	3.3
internal standard	3.8
flurazepam	4.6
chlordiazepoxide	10.0 (major peak)

Calculation:

Calculation is based on a response factor derived from a standard curve for each drug. A quality control serum prepared as described is analyzed daily.

Evaluation:

Sensivity: 0.1 mg/L for most drugs
Linearity: 0.1–1.0 mg/L
C.V.: not established
Relative recovery: not established

Interferences:

Normal patient plasma was found to be free of interfering substances. Other drugs may interfere and results should be considered presumptive until confirmed by another technique.

Reference:

M.A. Peat and L. Kopjak. The screening and quantitation of diazepam, flurazepam, chlordiazepoxide and their metabolites in blood and plasma by electron-capture gas chromatography and high pressure liquid chromatography. J. For. Sci. 24: 46–54, 1979.

Serum Benzodiazepines by Liquid Chromatography

Principle:

The benzodiazepines are taken through a series of extraction steps to concentrate and purify the drugs. The final extract is analyzed by liquid chromatography on a reversed-phase column with detection at 240 nm, using prazepam as internal standard.

Reagents:

Stock solutions –
    1 mg/mL chlordiazepoxide in methanol
    1 mg/mL desalkylflurazepam in methanol
    1 mg/mL diazepam in methanol
    1 mg/mL nordiazepam in methanol
    1 mg/mL oxazepam in methanol

Serum standards – 0.2, 0.5, 1.0 and 2.0 mg/L for each of the above drugs
Internal standard – 2 mg prazepam (Warner-Lambert) in 100 mL ethanol
1 mol/L Phosphate buffer – 136.1 g anhydrous KH_2PO_4/L, adjusted to pH 7.0 with 1 mol/L
    K_2HPO_4
Ether
6 mol/L Hydrochloric acid
6 mol/L Sodium hydroxide
Ethanol
Mobile solvent – acetonitrile/0.01 mol/L pH 4.6 sodium acetate buffer, 35:65 by volume

Instrumental Conditions:

Liquid chromatograph with 240 nm absorbance detector
25 cm × 4.5 mm i.d. Partisil-10 ODS column (Reeve Angel)
Solvent flow rate, 2.0 mL/min
Column temperature, ambient

Procedure:

1. Transfer 2 mL serum to a 35 mL screw-cap tube. Add 2 mL 1 mol/L phosphate buffer
    and 2 mL internal standard. Vortex briefly.
2. Add 20 mL ether and shake for 30 seconds. Centrifuge and transfer the ether phase to a
    clean tube.
3. Add 2.5 mL 6 mol/L HC1, shake for 30 seconds and centrifuge. Discard the ether layer.
4. Add 2.5 mL 6 mol/L NaOH and 2 mL 1 mol/L phosphate buffer. Extract with 20 mL
    ether and centrifuge.
5. Transfer the ether phase to a clean conical centrifuge tube and evaporate to dryness in
    a 40°C. water bath under a stream of nitrogen.
6. Dissolve the residue in 30 µL ethanol and inject 10–15 µL into the liquid
    chromatograph.

	Retention time (min)
oxazepam	4.0
desalkyflurazepam	4.5
chlordiazepoxide	5.2
nordiazepam	5.5
diazepam	7.5
internal standard	12.0
flurazepam	not eluted

Calculation:

Calculation is based on a response factor derived from a standard curve for each drug. A
quality control specimen containing 1 mg/L of oxazepam, nordiazepam and diazepam is
analyzed daily.

Evaluation:

Sensitivity: 0.05 mg/L
Linearity: 0.05–2.0 mg/L
C.V.: 3.7–6.3% within-run, 2.8–9.6% day-to-day
Relative recovery: 91–116%

Interferences:

Twelve other common basic drugs were checked for interfence with the benzodiazepines. Carbamazepine interferes with oxazepam analysis and amitriptyline, if present in sufficient concentration, many interfere with diazepam analysis.

References:

1. P.M. Kabra, G.L. Stevens and L.J. Marton. High-pressure liquid chromatographic analysis of diazepam, oxazepam and N-desmethyldiazepam in human blood. J. Chrom. 150: 355–360, 1978.
2. M.A. Peat and L. Kopjak. The screening and quantitation of diazepam, flurazepam, chlordiazepoxide, and their metabolites in blood and plasma by electron-capture gas chromatography and high pressure liquid chromatography. J. For. Sci. 24: 46–54, 1979.

BORATE

Serum Concentrations (mg/L)		
Normal	Toxic	Fatal
0–7.1	20–150	200–1600

Boric acid is frequently used as an antiseptic for external use and is found in eyewashes, mouthwashes, skin powders, ointments and irrigating solutions in concentrations of 0.5–5%. Borates are found in low concentrations in normal plasma. Boric acid applied externally as an antiseptic may be absorbed through broken skin surfaces, resulting in toxicity. A convenient colorimetric method is described for the determination of toxic levels of borate in serum, utilizing carminic acid for color development.

Serum Borate by Colorimetry

Principle:
Serum is deproteinized and allowed to react with a chromogen that is relatively specific for borate ion. The absorbance of the solution is measured at 600 nm in a spectrophotometer.

Reagents:
Stock solution – 2 mg/mL borate ion (210 mg boric acid/100 mL water)
Serum standards – 20, 50, 100 and 200 mg/L borate ion
Ammonium sulfate solution – 4 g $(NH_4)_2SO_4$/100 mL water
Sulfuric acid – conc. H_2SO_4
Carminic acid reagent – 10 mg carminic acid/100 mL conc. H_2SO_4 (stable indefinitely)

Instrumental Conditions:
Visible spectrophotometer set to 600 nm

Procedure:
1. Transfer 1 mL serum and 5 mL ammonium sulfate solution to a 15 mL centrifuge tube. Vortex and place into a boiling water bath for 15 min.
2. Centrifuge and decant the supernatant into a 10 mL volumetric flask. Suspend the precipitate in 2 mL water, vortex, centrifuge and add the second supernatant to the first.
3. Adjust the contents of the volumetric flask to 10 mL with water. Transfer 1 mL to a 15 mL centrifuge tube.
4. Add 5 mL sufuric acid and vortex. Add 5 mL carminic acid solution and vortex.

5. Transfer solution to a cuvette, stopper and allow to stand for 10 min. Determine absorbance at 600 nm, using as reference solution a negative control serum processed in the same manner.

Calculation:

Calculation is based on a response factor derived from a standard curve. A quality control serum containing 50 mg/L borate ion is analyzed daily.

Evaluation:

Sensitivity: 10 mg/L
Linearity: 20–200 mg/L
C.V.: 6%
Relative recovery: 92–104%

Interferences:

High concentrations of antimony, iron, copper and oxidizing acids may interfere.

Reference:

F. Rieders. Borate. In Manual of Analytical Toxicology (I. Sunshine, ed.), CRC Press, Cleveland, 1971, pp. 53–55.

BROMIDE

Serum Concentrations (mg/L)		
Therapeutic	Toxic	T½
75–100	>500	12–15 days

Inorganic bromide salts are occasionally used for their sedative and anticonvulsant effects in man. Organic bromide compounds (such as carbromal) used as sedatives and alkyl bromides used as industrial fumigants can also produce substantial amounts of inorganic bromide.

A simple but somewhat insensitive colorimetric procedure is presented for the determination of toxic levels of bromide in serum.

Serum Bromide by Colorimetry

Principle:

A protein-free filtrate of blood is prepared. A colored complex is then formed which is measured in the visible spectrophotometer.

Reagents:

Stock solution – 100 mg/mL bromide ion (1.489 g KBr/10 mL water)
Serum standards – 100, 200, 500 and 1000 mg/L
10% Trichloroacetic acid
0.5% Gold chloride – 500 mg $HAUCl_4$/100 mL water

Instrumental Conditions:

Visible spectrophotometer set to 440 nm

Procedure:

1. Transfer 2 mL serum to a 15 mL centrifuge tube. Add 8 mL 10% trichloroacetic acid and vortex. Wait 15 min and centrifuge.
2. Filter 4 mL of the supernatant through Whatman #1 filter paper into a clean tube and add 0.5 mL of the gold chloride solution.
3. Determine absorbance of this solution immediately at 440 nm. Use as a reference a negative control serum processed in the same manner.

Calculation:

Calculation is based on a response factor derived from a standard curve. A quality control specimen containing 500 mg/L bromide ion is analyzed daily.

Evaluation:

Sensitivity: 150 mg/L
Linearity: 150–600 mg/L
C.V.: 5.9% within-run
Relative recovery: 90–105%

Interferences:

Substances that lend obvious visible color to the specimen, such as hemoglobin or dyes used in liver function tests, will interfere with the procedure leading to a false positive. Physiological serum bromide concentrations average 3–4 mg/L in adults and are undetectable by this method.

Reference:

O. Wuth. Rational bromide treatment. J. Amer. Med. Asso. 88: 2013–2017, 1927.

CADMIUM

Blood Concentrations (mg/L)		Urine Concentrations (mg/L)	
Normal	Toxic	Normal	Toxic
0.001–0.005	0.1–3.0	0.0001–0.0002	0.1–1.0

The general population is exposed to cadmium via food, water, air and cigarette smoke; daily intake of 2–200 µg of the metal occurs in normal individuals and much of this amount is accumulated in lungs, liver and kidney. Elevated blood or urine concentrations can be indicative of either acute or chronic poisoning. Blood generally contains about twice as much cadmium as plasma or serum.

Two atomic absorption procedures are described for the determination of cadmium in body fluids, involving both flame and flameless detection. The former procedure is more suitable for the detection of toxic levels of the metal, while the latter is sufficiently sensitive to measure blood and urine concentrations of cadmium in healthy persons. Special precautions must be taken in performing these analyses due to the very low concentrations of cadmium in normal biological specimens and the presence of the metal in common laboratory reagents and glassware.

Blood and Urine Cadmium by Flame Atomic Absorption Spectrometry

Principle:
Cadmium is chelated in blood and urine specimens with sodium diethyldithiocarbamate. The chelate is extracted into an organic solvent and the solvent is aspirated into an oxidizing flame. Detection is at 228.8 nm. The sensitivity is adequate for measurement of toxic levels of cadmium.

Reagents:
Stock solution – 1 mg/mL cadmium ion (Fisher reference standard)
Aqueous standards – 0, 0.005, 0.01, 0.05, 0.1 and 0.5 mg/L dilutions of stock solution in 1% nitric acid (prepared weekly)
5% Trichloroacetic acid
2.5 mol/L Sodium hydroxide
DDC solution – 1% sodium diethyldithiocarbamate in water
Methyl isobutyl ketone

Instrumental Conditions:

Atomic absorption spectrophotometer with air-acetylene oxidizing flame
Cadmium hollow cathode lamp
Measure absorption at 228.8 nm

Sample Preparation:

All glassware is to be soaked overnight in 25% nitric acid and rinsed throughly in deionized water prior to use.

Blood:

1. Transfer 4 mL blood to a centrifuge tube and add 8 mL 5% trichloroacetic acid. Vortex and let stand 1 hour.
2. Centrifuge and transfer 10 mL supernatant into a 15 mL screw-cap tube. Adjust pH to 6.0–7.5 with 2.5 mol/L NaOH

Urine:

1. Transfer 10 mL urine to a 15 mL screw-cap tube. Adjust pH to 6.0–7.5 with 2.5 mol/L NaOH.

Procedure:

1. To prepared specimen add 1 mL DDC solution and vortex. Add 2.5 mL methyl isobutyl ketone and shake for 2 min.
2. Centrifuge, transfer the solvent layer to a sample tube and aspirate the solvent into the flame. Determine absorption at 228.8 nm.

Calculation:

Prepare a standard curve of absorption versus concentration of the aqueous standards. Determine the specimen concentration from this curve.

Evaluation:

Sensitivity: 0.002 mg/L
Linearity: 0.005–0.5 mg/L
C.V.: not established
Relative recovery: 98–110%

Interferences:

This procedure has high specificity for cadmium. Reagents and glassware must be checked carefully for cadmium contamination by analyzing water blanks. Some investigators have reported better results using plastic tubes that were soaked overnight in 5% Triton X-100 prior to use. Urine specimens that are to be stored prior to analysis should contain 1% conc. HCl to prevent precipitation of cadmium.

Reference:

E. Berman. Determination of cadmium, thallium and mercury in biological materials by atomic absorption. At. Abs. Newsl. 6: 57–60, 1967.

Blood and Urine Cadmium by Graphite-Furnace Atomic Absorption Spectrometry

Principle:

Blood and urine specimens are wet-ashed to destroy organic matter. The dry residue is dissolved in dilute nitric acid and analyzed by electrothermal atomic absorption spectrometry at 228.8 nm. Excellent sensitivity is achieved with this procedure.

Reagents:

Stock solution – 1 mg/mL cadmium ion (Fisher reference standard)
Aqueous standards – 0, 0.0002, 0.0005, 0.001 and 0.003 mg/L dilutions of stock solution
    in 1% nitric acid (prepare weekly)
Nitric acid – conc. HNO_3 (ultrapure grade)
30% Hydrogen peroxide
1% Nitric acid

Instrumental Conditions:

Atomic absorption spectrometer with graphite furnace
Cadmium hollow cathode lamp
Furnace program: dry 30 sec at 150°C.
               char 60 sec at 300°C.
               atomize 8 sec at 1950°C.
Argon purge gas in interrupt mode
Measure absorption at 228.8 nm

Procedure:

Pyrex digestion tubes are decontaminated by conducting six blank digestions with 0.5 mL 70% perchloric acid prior to use.
1. Blood – transfer 0.5 mL to a digestion tube and add 1 mL conc. HNO_3. Urine – transfer 1 mL to a digestion tube and add 0.2 mL conc. HNO_3.
2. Place tube in a heating block and digest for 3 hr at a temperature just below boiling.
3. When the specimem volume is reduced to one-third of the original, add 0.4 mL 30% H_2O_2.
4. Cool tube and dissolve residue in 5 mL (blood) or 2 mL (urine) 1% nitric acid. Inject 20 µL of this solution into the graphite furnace for analysis.

Calculation:

Prepare a standard curve of absorption versus concentration of the aqueous standards. Dilute specimens that exceed the range of the standard curve. Determine the specimen concentration from this curve.

Evaluation:

Sensitivity: 0.0001 mg/L
Linearity: 0.0002–0.003 mg/L
C.V.: 7–14% within-run
Relative recovery: 85–110%

Interferences:

This procedure has high specificity for cadmium. Reagents and glassware must be checked carefully for cadmium contamination by analyzing water blanks. Some investigators have reported better results using plastic tubes that were soaked overnight in 5% Triton X-100 prior to use. Urine specimens that are to be stored prior to analysis should contain 1% conc. HC1 to prevent precipitation of cadmium.

Reference:

E.F. Perry, S.R. Koirtyohann and H.M. Perry, Jr. Determination of cadmium in blood and urine by graphite furnace atomic absorption spectrophotometry. Clin. Chem. 21: 626–629, 1975.

CANNABINOIDS

| | Urine Concentrations (µg/L) | |
	Within 24 hr After Single Use	T½
COOH-THC	50–250	25–50 hr

Marijuana plant material (Cannabis sativa) contains variable amounts of a psychoactive principle, delta-9-tetrahydrocannabinol (THC), that causes sedation, euphoria, and temporal distortion when orally ingested or smoked. A major metabolite of THC, 11-nor-9-carboxy-delta-9-THC (COOH-THC), may be present in urine as a glucuronide conjugate or in the unconjugated form. It is pharmacologically inactive and therefore its detection in urine serves as an indicator of usage but not of the state of impairment. Passive exposure to marijuana smoke is not considered to produce urine cannabinoid levels exceeding 80 µg/L by immunoassay or 20 µg/L (of COOH-THC) by a specific chromatographic method.

Commercial reagent kits are available for the detection of cannabinoids in urine by radioimmunoassay and EMIT. These kits are often employed with a cut-off value of 100 µg/L total cross-reacting cannabinoids. The antibodies in the kits react with a variety of cannabinoids and their metabolites and so the semi-quantitative values obtained often exceed those produced by a more specific method by three- or four-fold.

Since immunoassay is considered a presumptive test, a confirmatory technique must be performed before a positive result is released. Two chromatographic methods are described that are specific for COOH-THC in urine; the simplest and most economical is based on thin-layer chromatography while a more definitive but complex procedure utilizes gas chromatography-mass spectrometry.

Urine COOH-THC by Thin-Layer Chromatography

Principle:
Urine is subjected to alkaline hydrolysis to cleave the glucuronide conjugate of COOH-THC. The hydrolysate is acidified and extracted using a commercial bonded-phase extraction column. COOH-THC is eluted with an organic solvent and identified by thin-layer chromatography.

Reagents:
Stock solution – 1 mg/mL 11-nor-9-carboxy-delta-9-THC (Applied Science or Research Triangle Institute) in methanol
Urine standards – 20, 50 and 100 µg/L
10 mol/L Sodium hydroxide

Hydrochloric acid – conc. HC1
Methanol
0.1 mol/L Hydrochloric acid
50 mmol/L Phosphoric acid containing 10% acetonitrile
Dichloromethane
Hexane
Acetone
Chromogenic spray – 50 mg Fast Blue RR (Calbiochem-Behring, San Diego, CA) in 10 mL methanol/water, 1:1 (prepare fresh)
Thin-layer plates – 25 mm × 75 mm E Merck silica gel 60 plates (Applied Analytical, Wilmington, NC)
Developing solvent – ethyl acetate/methanol/water/conc. NH_4OH, 12:5:0.5:1
Bonded-phase columns – Bond-Elut THC columns, 500 mg (Analytichem International, Harbor City, CA)

Procedure:

1. Transfer 10 mL urine to a siliconized 15 mL screw-cap tube and add 0.9 mL 10 mol/L NaOH. Vortex and allow to stand for 15 min. Adjust to pH 1–3 by adding approximately 0.7 mL conc. HC1.
2. Prepare the bonded-phase column by rinsing sequentially with 1 column volume of methanol, water, methanol, and water. Add the urine from step 1 to the column and rinse with 10 mL of 0.1 mol/L HC1 and then with 25 mL of 50 mmol/L H_3PO_4 containing 10% acetonitrile.
3. Elute the column with 1 mL acetone, collecting the eluate in a siliconized 10 mm × 75 mm culture tube. Add 0.5 mL dichloromethane, vortex, centrifuge and discard upper layer.
4. Add 0.5 mL hexane, vortex, centrifuge and transfer the upper layer to a clean tube. Evaporate to dryness at 60°C. under a stream of nitrogen.
5. Dissolve the residue in 10 µL acetone and spot to the origin of a thin-layer plate. Develop the plate to a height of 5 cm (about 7 min) and allow the plate to air dry. Spray with the chromogenic spray to visualize the COOH-THC.

	Rf
COOH-THC	0.43–0.50 (red spot)

Calculation:

Determine the presence of COOH-THC in the unknown urine specimen by comparison of spot color and location with that of the urine standard, analyzed in an identical manner.

Evaluation:

Sensitivity: 20 µg/L
Linearity: not applicable
C.V.: not applicable
Relative recovery: not applicable

Interferences:

No interfering substances have been reported. The occasional highly-pigmented urine specimen may give ambiguous results.

Reference:

M.J. Kogan, E. Newman and N.J. Willson. Detection of marijuana metabolite 11-nor-delta-9-tetrahydro-cannabinol-9-carboxylic acid in human urine by bonded-phase adsorption and thin-layer chromatography. J. Chrom. 306: 441–443, 1984.

Urine COOH-THC by Gas Chromatography-Mass Spectrometry

Principle:

The procedure involves the hydrolysis of the glucuronide by alkali, extraction of the COOH-THC, derivatization of the carboxylic acid and phenolic groupings, and identification of the derivative by GC-MS in the SIM mode. Deuterated COOH-THC is used as internal standard.

Reagents:

Stock solution – 1 mg/mL 11-nor-9-carboxy-delta-9-THC (Applied Science or Research Triangle Institute) in methanol

Urine standards – 5, 10, 20, 50 and 100 μg/L

Internal standard – 0.5 μg/mL trideuterated COOH-THC in ethanol (Research Triangle Institute)

2 mol/L Sodium hydroxide

6 mol/L Hydrochloric acid

Hexane/isoamyl alcohol, 99.5:0.5

Hexane/ethyl acetate, 5:1

Hexafluoro-2-propanol (Aldrich)

Pentafluoropropionic anhydride (Aldrich)

Hexane

Ethyl acetate

Instrumental Conditions:

Gas chromatograph with mass selective detector (Hewlett-Packard 5970B MSD or equivalent)

12 m × 0.20 mm i.d. methylsilicone capillary column (Hewlett-Packard)

Injector, 300°C.; transfer line, 250°C.

Column temperature program: initial, 150°C. (1 min)
30°C./min increase
final, 300°C. (1 min)

Helium flow rate, 1 moL/min

Splitless on time, 0.7 min

Solvent delay time, 4.0 min
Election multiplier voltage, 2600
Ions monitored: 477.35, 489.39, 640.35 (COOH-THC)
480.35 (internal standard)

Procedure:

1. Transfer 5 mL urine to a siliconized 15 mL screw-cap glass tube and add 200 μL internal standard. Add 1 mL of 2 mol/L NaOH and vortex.
2. Add 8 mL hexane/isoamyl alcohol and place on a rotator for 30 min. Centrifuge and discard the organic solvent layer.
3. Add 0.5 mL 6 mol/L HCl to the aqueous layer, vortex and check that pH is less than 5. Add 3 mL hexane/ethyl acetate and place on rotator for 30 min. Centrifuge and transfer the organic solvent to a siliconized Reacti-Vial (Pierce Chemical).
4. Evaporate the solvent to dryness in a 50°C. heating block under a stream of dry air. Add 100 μL hexane, 50 μL hexafluoro-2-propanol, and 50 μL pentafluoropropionic anhydride.
5. Heat the mixture at 100°C. in a heating block for 10 min. Cool. Just prior to injection, evaporate to dryness under a stream of dry air. Dissolve the residue in 20 μL ethyl acetate and inject 1–2 μL into the gas chromatograph.

	Retention time (min)
COOH-THC derivative	4.51
internal standard derivative	4.50

Calculation:

Calculation is based on a response factor derived from a standard curve of peak area ratio (COOH-THC: internal standard) versus COOH-THC concentration. This procedure cannot be controlled by the usual methods due to the long-term instability of COOH-THC in physiological fluids.

Evaluation:

Sensitivity: 4 μg/L
Linearity: 5–100 μg/L
C.V.: not established
Relative recovery: not established

Interferences:

No interfering substances have been identified, but the presence of high concentrations of normal urinary constituents may cause difficulty in the interpretation of results with specimens of very low COOH-THC concentration.

To be considered positive, an unknown specimen must have a peak at a relative retention time of 1.002 to the deuterated internal standard with ion intensity ratios (489/477 and 640/477) within ±20% of that of the 100 μg/L standard analyzed with that batch. The ion intensity ratios of the 5 μg/L standard may differ by more than ±20%. Specimens with concentrations less than 10 μg/L should be compared to the 5 μg/L standard.

References:

1. R.L. Foltz. Analysis of cannabinoids in physiological specimens by gas chromatography/mass spectrometry. In Advances in Analytical Toxicology, Vol. 1 (R. Baselt, ed.), Biomedical Publications, Foster City, CA, 1984, pp. 125–157.
2. L. Karlsson, J. Johnson, K. Berg and C. Roos. Determination of delta-9-tetrahydrocannabinol-11-oic acid in urine as its pentafluoropropyl-pentafluoropropionyl derivative by GC/MS utilizing negative ion chemical ionization. J. Analyt. Tox. 7: 198–202, 1983.

CARBON MONOXIDE

Blood Carboxyhemoglobin Cencentration (% Saturation)		
Rural Nonsmokers	Urban Nonsmokers	Smokers
0.4–0.7%	1–2%	5–6%

Carbon monoxide is the most abundant air pollutant in the lower atmosphere, being produced wherever organic matter is burned. Cigarettes, automobile exhaust and residential fires represent the most frequent sources of exposure to this toxic gas. Carbon monoxide in blood is tightly bound to hemoglobin and thus whole blood is the required specimen for analysis. Concentrations are expressed in terms of the percentage saturation by carbon monoxide of the available hemoglobin in the specimen.

Both a spectrophotometric procedure, which requires a separate hemoglobin measurement, and a gas chromatographic technique are included for the determination of carbon monoxide in blood. The latter technique is the more sensitive and accurate of the two but requires more sophisticated equipment.

An instrument for the automated determination of carbon monoxide, the CO-Oximeter (Instrumentation Laboratory), is commercially available and is based on visible spectrophotometric measurement of carboxyhemoglobin.

Blood Carboxyhemoglobin by Visible Spectrophotometry

Principle:
This is a rapid and convenient technique for the estimation of whole blood carboxyhemoglobin concentrations in clinical emergencies. Blood is diluted with a hydrosulfite reagent to convert methemoglobin to normal hemoglobin and the absorbance of the carboxyhemoglobin pigment is measured spectrophotometrically at 540 nm.

Reagents:
Hydrosulfite reagent – 1 g sodium hydrosulfite and 1 g sodium carbonate per L water
Carbon monoxide lecture bottle

Instrumental Conditions:
Visible spectrophotometer set at 540 nm

Procedure:
1. Determine the hemoglobin concentration of the blood specimen using the cyanmethemoglobin procedure or an equivalent technique.

2. Transfer 100 μL blood to a 20 mL volumetric flask and dilute to volume with the hydrosulfite reagent. Mix by inversion.
3. Centrifuge 5 mL of the diluted specimen at 2500 rpm for 5 min. Determine the absorbance of the supernatant at 540 nm against a reagent blank.

Calculation:

Determine the carboxyhemoglobin saturation of the specimen using the following equation:

$$\%COHb = \frac{A\text{-}0.0322\,Hb}{0.0445\,Hb\text{-}0.0322\,Hb} \times 100,$$

where A represents the absorbance at 540 nm of the diluted blood specimen and Hb is the hemoglobin concentration of the original specimen in g/dL. Carboxyhemoglobin concentrations of less than 20% should be considered of uncertain significance due to the inaccuracy of the method at this level.

Evaluation:

Sensitivity: 10% saturation
Linearity: 10–60% saturation
C.V.: not established
Relative recovery: not applicable

Interferences:

This is a semi-quantitative technique that cannot be controlled by the usual means due to the difficulty of storing whole blood containing carboxyhemoglobin. It is relatively specific for carboxyhemoglobin but can give both false positive and false negative results at concentrations less than 20%.

Reference:

T. Hayashi and R. Nanikawa. Further study on spectrophotometric determination of CO-Hb in post-mortem blood. For Sci. 11: 127–134, 1978.

Blood Carboxyhemoglobin by Thermal-Conductivity Gas Chromatography

Principle:

A sample of whole blood is hemolyzed and divided into 2 portions, one of which is saturated with carbon monoxide gas. After removing excess gas, both portions are allowed to react with ferricyanide reagent. The carbon monoxide that is released from carboxyhemoglobin is then measured by gas chromatography using a molecular sieve column and a thermal-conductivity detector.

Reagents:

Sodium hydrosulfite – solid $Na_2S_2O_4$
0.25% Triton X-100 – 2.5 mL/L water

5% Potassium ferricyanide – 5 g/100 mL water
Carbon monoxide lecture bottle

Instrumental Conditions:

Gas chromatograph with thermal-conductivity detector
6′ × 1/8″ stainless steel column containing 45/60 mesh molecular sieve type 5A (reactivated
    by heating to 200°C. whenever sensitivity deteriorates)
Injector, 90°C.; column, 75°C.; detector, 95°C.
Helium flow rate, 26 mL/min

Procedure:

1. Add 5 mL blood to 15 mL 0.25% Triton X-100 in a beaker. Add a spatula-tip of
   $Na_2S_2O_4$ (10 mg) and mix. Draw 10 mL of the solution into each of two 35 mL plastic
   syringes labelled *sample* and *100%*.
2. Introduce 10 mL carbon monoxide gas from a lecture bottle into the *100%* syringe,
   stopper and shake for 10 minutes. Expel the gas and remove excess by shaking three
   times with 10 mL of air.
3. Draw 10 mL of helium into both syringes using a 23 gauge needle and the injection port
   of the gas chromatograph. Shake and expel.
4. Adjust volume of solution to 8.0 mL in each syringe. Draw up 5.0 mL of the
   ferricyanide reagent and introduce 10 mL of helium. Shake for 10 minutes.
5. Analyze each sample in duplicate by transferring 2.0 mL of the gas to a third syringe
   and injecting into the gas chromatograph (alternatively utilize a gas sampling loop
   attached to the gas chromatograph).

	Retention time (min)
oxygen	0.6
nitrogen	0.8
carbon monoxide	2.1

Calculation:

Calculate the percentage saturation of the unknown from the ratio of the peak height of the
unknown to the peak height of the saturated (100%) aliquot. For samples of less than 50%
saturation, it is more accurate to utilize standards of 25% or 50% saturation, made by
mixing 2.5 or 5.0 mL of the saturated standard with 7.5 or 5.0 mL, respectively, of 0.25%
Triton X-100.

Evaluation:

Sensitivity: 2% saturation
Linearity: 2–100% saturation
C.V.: 5.6% within-run
Relative recovery: not applicable

Interferences:

Nine other common gases were analyzed and found not to interfere.

References:

1. D.W. Hessel and F.R. Modglin. The determination of carbon monoxide in blood by gas-solid chromatography. J. For. Sci. 12: 123–131, 1967.
2. K.M. Dubowski and J.L. Luke. Measurement of carboxyhemoglobin and carbon monoxide in blood. Ann. Clin. Lab. Sci. 3; 53–65, 1973.

CHLORAL HYDRATE

Trichloroethanol Blood Concentration (mg/L)	
Therapeutic Level	Fatal Intoxication
2–12	20–640

Chloral hydrate is occasionally used as a sedative or hypnotic. Its usage is monitored by detection of its major active metabolite, trichloroethanol, in serum or blood. The two procedures presented, involving colorimetry and gas chromatography, are both suitable for quantitation of serum trichloroethanol concentrations ranging from the high therapeutic level to those observed following overdosage with chloral hydrate. The gas chromatographic procedure is also applicable to the determination of ethchlorvynol.

Serum Trichloroethanol by Colorimetry

Principle:
Serum is subjected to the Fujiwara reaction by heating in the presence of pyridine and potassium hydroxide. The yellow chromophore produced by trichloroethanol is measured at 440 nm in a spectrophotometer.

Reagents:
Stock solution – 10 mg/mL trichloroethanol in methanol
Serum standards – 15, 30, 60 and 120 mg/L
Pyridine
10 mol/L Potassium hydroxide

Instrumental Conditions:
Visible spectrophotometer set to 440 nm

Procedure:
1. Transfer 1 mL serum to a 15 mL centrifuge tube and add 5 mL pyridine. Vortex briefly.
2. Add 2 mL 10 mol/L KOH and vortex. Place in a boiling water bath for exactly 4 min and transfer immediately to an ice bath for 3–5 min.
3. Transfer 3 mL of the pyridine layer to a tube containing 0.5 mL water. Vortex and immediately read absorbance at 440 nm against a negative control serum processed in the same manner.

Calculation:
Calculation is based on a response factor derived from a standard curve. A quality control serum containing 30 mg/L trichloroethanol is analyzed daily.

Evaluation:

Sensitivity: 10 mg/L
Linearity: 15–120 mg/L
C.V.: not established
Relative recovery: not established

Interferences:

Other halogenated hydrocarbons present in the specimen may interfere with the analysis. Trichloroacetic acid, a pharmacologically inactive metabolite of chloral hydrate that accumulates in serum, shows absorbance maxima of 370 and 540 nm and thus does not interfere with the determination of trichloroethanol.

Reference:

P.J. Friedman and J.R. Cooper. Determination of chloral hydrate, trichloroacetic acid, and trichloroethanol. Anal. Chem. 30: 1674–1676, 1958.

Serum Trichloroethanol and Ethchlorvynol by Gas Chromatography

Principle:

A small volume of serum is mixed with a small amount of chloroform containing an internal standard. An aliquot of the chloroform is subjected to analysis by flame-ionization gas chromatography. Both trichloroethanol and ethchlorvynol are measured by this procedure.

Reagents:

Stock solutions –
    10 mg/mL trichloroethanol in methanol
    10 mg/mL ethchlorvynol in methanol
Serum standards – 5, 10, 20, 50 and 100 mg/L for both drugs
Quality control serum – 20 mg/L of both drugs
Internal standard – 40 mg/L 2-methylnaphthalene in chloroform

Instrumental Conditions:

Gas chromatograph with flame-ionization detector
1.5 m × 4 mm i.d. glass column containing 2% Carbowax 20 M and 5% KOH on 80/100
    Chromosorb W-HP
Injector, 150°C; column, 140°C; detector, 200°C.
Nitrogen flow rate, 60 mL/min

Procedure:

1. Transfer 200 μL serum to a 5 mL tapered conical centrifuge tube. Add 100 μL internal standard and vortex for 30 seconds.
2. Centrifuge to separate layers and inject 4 μL of the lower chloroform layer into the gas chromatograph.

	Retention time (min.)
trichloroethanol	2.0
ethchlorvynol	2.8
internal standard	4.0

Calculation:

Calculation is based on a response factor derived from a standard curve for each drug. A quality control serum prepared as described is analyzed daily.

Evaluation:

Sensitivity: 5 mg/L
Linearity: 5–100 mg/L
C.V.: not established
Relative recovery: not established

Interferences:

No interferences have been observed.

Reference:

R.J. Flanagan, T.D. Lee and D.M. Rutherford. Analysis of chlormethiazole, ethchlorvynol and trichloroethanol in biological fluids by gas-liquid chromatography as an aid to the diagnosis of acute poisoning. J. Chrom. 153: 473–479, 1978.

CHLORAMPHENICOL

Plasma Concentrations (mg/L)			
Therapeutic	Toxic	Fatalities	T½
5–25	<25	>100	2–3 hr

Chloramphenicol is an antibiotic agent that is administered orally or by intravenous injection. Although the plasma half-life is quite short in most subjects, it averages about 28 hours in neonates due to their inability to metabolize the drug and may also be prolonged in patients with hepatic and renal disease. Bone marrow depression is commonly associated with plasma chloramphenicol concentrations exceeding 25 mg/L, while aplastic anemia, which occurs rarely, does not appear to be dose-related. Each of the following procedures, colorimetric, gas chromatographic and liquid chromatographic, has been found to produce useful clinical results within a relatively short period of time. Chloramphenicol is customarily measured by microbiological assay, which involves a lengthy incubation period.

Plasma Chloramphenicol by Colorimetry

Principle:
The patient specimen is divided into two aliquots, one of which is treated to a reduction step to convert the nitro group of chloramphenicol to a primary amine. Both aliquots are then subjected to a diazotization reaction and the resulting color is measured spectrophotometrically at 555 nm. The difference in optical densities between the two portions of the specimen represents the absorbance due to chloramphenicol.

Reagents:
Stock solution – 1 mg/mL chloramphenicol in methanol
Plasma standards – 5, 10, 20 and 40 mg/L
0.5 mol/L Hydrochloric acid
Zinc dust
0.25 mol/L Hydrochloric acid
0.1% Sodium nitrite (prepare fresh)
0.5% Ammonium sulfamate
Coupling reagent – 0.1% N-(1-naphthyl)ethylenediamine dihydrochloride

Instrumental Conditions:
Visible spectrophotometer set to 555 nm

Procedure:

1. Transfer 1 mL plasma to each of two 12 mL graduated centrifuge tubes labeled A and B. Add 4 mL 0.5 mol/L HCl to each tube and about 50 mg zinc dust to tube A, and heat both tubes in a boiling water bath for 1 hour.
2. Cool and adjust volumes to 5 mL by adding water. Mix, centrifuge and transfer 1 mL portions of the supernatants to clean tubes.
3. To each tube add 4 mL 0.25 mol/L HCl and 0.5 mL 0.1% $NaNO_2$. Vortex and let stand exactly 5 min.
4. Add 0.5 mL 0.5% ammonium sulfamate, vortex and let stand 3 min. Add 0.5 mL coupling reagent, vortex and incubate at 38°C. for exactly 1 hour.
5. Transfer the solutions to cuvettes and read each in the spectrophotometer at 555 nm against a plasma blank treated in a parallel manner. Subtract the reading of tube B from that of tube A.

Calculation:

Calculation is based on a response factor derived from a standard curve. A quality control specimen containing 15 mg/L chloramphenicol is analyzed daily.

Evaluation:

Sensitivity: 4 mg/L
Linearity: 5–120 mg/L
C.V.: 4%
Relative recovery: not established

Interferences:

Although the diazotization reaction described in this method is susceptible to interference by primary amines, the running of a parallel determination on the patient specimen that omits the reduction step will greatly increase the selectivity of the procedure. Results using this technique correlate very well with those obtained using a gas chromatographic procedure that is specific for unchanged chloramphenicol.

Reference:

A.J. Glazko, L.M. Wolf and W.A. Dill. Biochemical studies on chloramphenicol (Chloromycetin). Arch. Biochem. 23: 411–418, 1949.

Plasma Chloramphenicol by Gas Chromatography

Principle:

Chloramphenicol is extracted from plasma with ethyl acetate containing an internal standard. The evaporated residue is dissolved in dilute acid, washed with hexane, and extracted with ethyl acetate. The final residue is treated to convert the drugs to their trimethylsilyl derivatives, which are analyzed by flame-ionization gas chromatography.

Reagents:

Stock solution – 1 mg/mL chloramphenicol in methanol
Plasma standards – 5, 10, 20 and 40 mg/L

pH 6.8 1 mol/L Phosphate buffer
Internal standard solution – 3 mg/L thiamphenicol (Sigma) in ethyl acetate
0.5 mol/L Hydrochloric acid
Hexane
Ethyl acetate
Derivatizing reagent – Trisil (Pierce Chemical Co.)

Instrumental Conditions:

Gas chromatograph with flame-ionization detector
1.2 m × 2 mm i.d. glass column containing 3% OV-1 on 100/200 mesh Gas Chrom Q
Injector, 250°C.; detector, 300°C.
Column temperature program: initial, 190°C.
                                      rate of increase, 16°C./min
                                      final, 270°C.
Nitrogen flow rate, 40 mL/min

Procedure:

1. Transfer 0.5 mL serum to a 15 mL screw-cap tube. Add 0.5 mL pH 6.8 phosphate buffer and 7 mL internal standard solution and shake mechanically for 10 min.
2. Centrifuge and transfer the upper organic layer to a clean tube. Evaporate to dryness under a stream of nitrogen at 40°C.
3. Dissolve the residue in 4 mL 0.5 mol/L HC1. Wash the aqueous layer twice with 7 mL hexane, centrifuging and discarding the hexane layer each time.
4. Extract the aqueous layer with 7 mL ethyl acetate. Centrifuge and transfer the upper organic layer to a 12 mL glass-stoppered conical centrifuge tube.
5. Evaporate to dryness under a stream of nitrogen at 40°C. Add 50 µL derivatizing reagent and vortex.
6. Stopper the tube and let stand for 8 min at room temperature. Inject 2 µL of the mixture into the chromatograph.

	Retention time (min)
chloramphenicol derivative	3
internal standard derivative	4

Calculation:

Calculation is based on a response factor derived from a standard curve. A quality control specimen containing 15 mg/L chloramphenicol is analyzed daily.

Evaluation:

Sensitivity: 0.5 mg/L
Linearity: 0.5–80 mg/L
C.V.: 5–9% run-to-run
Relative recovery: not established

Interferences:

Normal plasma components do not interfere in the assay. Other drugs were not studied for potential interference.

Reference:

C.J. Least, Jr., N.J. Wiegand, G.F. Johnson and H.M. Solomon. Quantitative gas-chromatographic flame-ionization method for chloramphenicol in human serum. Clin. Chem. 23: 220–222, 1977.

Plasma Chloramphenicol by Liquid Chromatography

Principle:

Chloramphenicol is extracted from a small volume of plasma with ethyl acetate containing an internal standard. The concentrated extract is analyzed by reverse-phase liquid chromatography, with detection at 280 nm.

Reagents:

Stock solution – 1 mg/mL chloramphenicol in methanol
Plasma standards – 5, 10, 20 and 40 mg/L
Internal standard solution – 20 mg/L thiamphenicol (Sigma) in ethyl acetate
Sodium chloride – solid NaCl
Methanol
Mobile phase – methanol/water, 40:60 by volume

Instrumental Conditions:

Liquid chromatograph with 280 nm ultraviolet detector
30 cm × 4 mm i.d. stainless-steel column containing μBondpak C_{18} (Waters Associates)
Column temperature, ambient
Solvent flow rate, 1.7 mL/min

Procedure:

1. Transfer 50 μL plasma to a 15 mL screw-cap tube. Add 5 mL internal standard solution and about 1 g NaCl and shake to extract.
2. Centrifuge and transfer the organic layer to a 12 mL conical centrifuge tube. Evaporate to dryness under a stream of nitrogen at 40°C.
3. Dissolve the residue in 40 μL methanol and inject 25 μL into the chromatograph.

	Retention time (min)
internal standard	4.0
chloramphenicol	7.5

Calculation:

Calculation is based on a response factor derived from a standard curve. A quality control specimen containing 15 mg/L chloramphenicol is analyzed daily.

Evaluation:

Sensitivity: 2 mg/L
Linearity: 2–80 mg/L
C.V.: 9% between-run
Relative recovery: not established

Interferences:

Normal plasma constituents do not interfere with the assay. Other drugs were not studied for potential interference.

Reference:

J. Crechiolo and R.E. Hill. Determination of serum chloramphenicol by high-performance liquid chromatography. J. Chrom. 162: 480–484, 1979.

CHLOROQUINE

Plasma Concentrations (mg/L)		
Therapeutic	Fatal	T½
0.010–0.100	3–6	2–5 days

Chloroquine is an oral antimalarial drug that is occasionally involved in accidental or intentional poisoning. A convenient ultraviolet spectrophotometric method is presented for the determination of toxic levels of the drug in plasma. Therapeutic concentrations may be measured with the more sensitive fluorometric procedure that follows.

Plasma Chloroquine by Ultraviolet Spectrophotometry

Principle:
Plasma is alkalinized and extracted with chloroform. Chloroquine is recovered from the chloroform by extraction with dilute acid and is measured in an ultraviolet spectrophotometer at 343 nm. The procedure is suitable for the measurement of toxic levels of chloroquine.

Reagents:
Stock solution – 1 mg/mL chloroquine in methanol
Plasma standards – 2, 5 and 10 mg/L
16 mol/L Potassium hydroxide
Chloroform
1 mol/L Hydrochloric acid

Instrumental Conditions:
Ultraviolet spectrophotometer set to 343 nm

Procedure:
1. Transfer 4 mL plasma to a 125 mL separatory funnel and add 3 drops of 16 mol/L potassium hydroxide.
2. Add 25 mL chloroform and shake to extract. Filter 21 mL of the lower chloroform layer into a 25 mL glass-stoppered graduated cylinder.
3. Extract the chloroform with 4 mL 1 mol/L hydrochloric acid and allow layers to separate. Transfer 3 mL of the aqueous layer to a cuvette and read in the spectrophotometer against a plasma blank.

Calculation:

Calculation is based on a response factor derived from a standard curve. A quality control plasma containing 5 mg/L chloroquine is analyzed daily.

Evaluation:

Sensitivity: 1 mg/L
Linearity: 2–16 mg/L
C.V.: not established
Relative recovery: not established

Interferences:

Several of the oxidized metabolites of chloroquine may accumulate in plasma and would probably be detected by this procedure. Other basic drugs that absorb at 343 nm, including quinine, may interfere with the determination of chloroquine. The characteristic absorption spectrum of chloroquine in the range of 220–360 nm may be useful in enhancing the specificity of this assay.

References:

1. R.W. Prouty and K. Kuroda. Spectrophotometric determination and distribution of chloroquine in human tissues. J. Lab. Clin. Med. 52: 477–480, 1958.
2. A.E. Robinson, A.I. Coffer and F.E. Camps. The distribution of chloroquine in man after fatal poisoning. J. Pharm. Pharmacol. 22: 700–703, 1970.

Plasma Chloroquine by Fluorescence Spectrophotometry

Principle:

Chloroquine is extracted from deproteinized plasma with an organic solvent. The solvent is washed with an alkaline buffer to remove the chloroquine metabolites and then is extracted with dilute acid to remove chloroquine. The acid layer is adjusted to pH 9.8 and analyzed by spectrophotometry.

Reagents:

Stock solution – 1 mg/mL chloroquine in methanol
Plasma standards – 0.01, 0.02, 0.05 and 0.10 mg/L
Ethanol
Dichloromethane
pH 7.8 Phosphate buffer
0.1 mol/L Hydrochoric acid
0.1 mol/L Sodium hydroxide
pH 9.8 Buffer – 24.8 g Na_2CO_3 and 25.2 g $NaHCO_3$ in 500 mL water

Instrumental Conditions:

Fluorescence spectrophotometer set to excite at 335 nm
Read emission at 400 nm

Procedure:

1. Transfer 200 µL plasma to a 12 mL centrifuge tube and dilute to 2 mL with ethanol. Vortex and centrifuge.
2. Transfer 1 mL of the supernatant to a 30 mL screw-cap tube. Add 15 mL dichloromethane and 5 mL pH 7.8 phosphate buffer and shake.
3. Centrifuge and disgard the upper aqueous layer. Extract the organic phase with 5 mL 0.1 mol/L HC1.
4. Centrifuge and transfer 1 mL of the upper aqueous phase to a cuvette. Add 1 mL 0.1 mol/L NaOH and 1 mL pH 9.8 buffer.
5. Mix and analyze in the fluorometer under the described conditions. Subtract the fluorescence of a plasma blank.

Calculation:

Calculation is based on a response factor derived from a standard curve. A quality control specimen containing 0.05 mg/L chloroquine is analyzed daily.

Evaluation:

Sensitivity: 0.01 mg/L
Linearity: 0.01–0.10 mg/L
C.V.: not established
Relative recovery; not established

Interferences:

Normal plasma components do not interfere. Most of the interference from chloroquine metabolites is eliminated using the pH 7.8 aqueous buffer as a wash for the organic solvent. Other drugs have not been studied for potential interference.

References:

1. M. Rubin, N. Zvaifler, H. Bernstein and A. Mansour. Chloroquine toxicity. In Proceedings of the Second International Pharmacology Meeting, Vol. 4 (B.B. Brodie and J.R. Gillette, eds.), Pergamon Press, Oxford, England, 1965, pp. 467–487.
2. S.G. Schulman and J.F. Young. A modified fluorometric determination of chloroquine in biological samples. Anal. Chim. Acta 70: 229–232, 1974.

CHLORPROMAZINE

Therapeutic Plasma Concentrations (mg/L)

Gas Chromatographic Method	Spectrophotometric Methods
0.03–0.40	0.20–3.00

Chlorpromazine is an antipsychotic drug that is frequently administered in daily doses of 75–600 mg or more. As many as 10 metabolites of chlorpromazine, all believed to be less active than the parent drug, are known to accumulate in plasma. Most spectrophotometric methods yield results that represent the sum of the parent drug and its various metabolites (see Phenothiazines by Spectrophotofluorometry, p. 233). A more specific and more sophisticated technique involves electron-capture gas chromatography and allows the separate quantitation of chlorpromazine and its major metabolites.

Plasma Chlorpromazine by Electron-Capture Gas Chromatography

Principle:
Chlorpromazine and several of its metabolites are extracted from alkalinized plasma with an organic solvent. Following two additional extractions, the drugs are assayed by gas chromatography with electron-capture detection.

Reagents:
Stock solutions – 1 mg/mL solutions of chlorpromazine, norchlorpromazine, dinorchlorpromazine and chlorpromazine sulfoxide in methanol
Plasma standards – 0.025, 0.050, 0.100 and 0.250 mg/L for each drug
Quality control plasma – 0.100 mg/L chlorpromazine
Internal standard – 2 mg 2,4-dichlorpromazine (Smith, Kline & French) per L of water
1 mol/L Sodium hydroxide
Extraction solvent – heptane/isoamyl alcohol, 98.5:1.5 by volume
0.05 mol/L Hydrochloric acid
1 mol/L Ammonium hydroxide
Injection solvent – toluene/isoamyl alcohol/isovaleraldehyde, 85:15:0.1 by volume
All vessels used in the procedure must be previously soaked overnight in chromic acid cleaning solution, rinsed in water, soaked in 25% ammonium hydroxide for 1 hr and finally rinsed several times in distilled/deionized water.

Instrumental Conditions:
Gas chromatograph with electron-capture detector
2 m× 2 mm i.d. glass column containing 3% OV-17 on 80/100 mesh Chromosorb W-HP

Injector, 275°C.; column, 265°C.; detector, 300°C.
5% Methane in argon flow rate, 50 mL/min

Procedure:

1. Transfer 2 mL plasma to a 25 mL screw-cap polycarbonate tube. Add 10 µL internal standard and 1 mL 1 mol/L NaOH and vortex.
2. Add 10 mL extraction solvent and shake for 1 min. Centrifuge to separate layers.
3. Transfer 9 mL of the solvent layer to a 15 mL glass-stoppered conical centrifuge tube.
4. Discard upper solvent layer. Add 0.2 mL 1 mol/L NH₄OH to the aqueous phase and vortex.
5. Add 100 µL injection solvent and vortex for 30 seconds. Centrifuge.
6. Discard the lower aqueous layer by aspiration. Collect the organic layer in the tapered portion of the tube by centrifuging and re-aspirating if necessary.
7. Inject 10 µL of the organic layer into the gas chromatograph.

	Retention time (min)
chlorpromazine	4.0
norchlorpromazine	4.7
internal standard	6.7
dinorchlorpromazine*	8.0
chlorpromazine sulfoxide	11.9

* as an imine with isovaleraldehyde

Calculation:

Calculation is based on a response factor derived from a standard curve for each drug. A quality control plasma containing 0.100 mg/L chlorpromazine (and metabolites if desired) is analyzed daily.

Evaluation:

Sensitivity: 0.010 mg/L
Linearity: 0.20–0.250 mg/L
C.V.: 5.9% within-run
Relative recovery: not established

Interferences:

Only diazepam is known to interfere with the analysis of chlorpromazine. These two compounds may be separated by using an OV-225 column. Interference due to chlorpromazine itself has been observed as a result of adsorption of the drug to previously used extraction tubes. Thorough cleaning of vessels will prevent this problem.

References:

1. S.H. Curry. Determination of nanogram quantities of chlorpromazine and some of its metabolites in plasma using gas-liquid chromatography with an electron-capture detector. Anal. Chem. 40: 1251–1255, 1968.
2. S.H. Curry. Gas-chromatographic methods for the study of chlorpromazine and some of its metabolites in human plasma. Psychopharm. Comm. 2: 1–15, 1976.
3. D.R. Flint, C.R. Ferullo, P. Levandoski and B. Hwang. More sensitive gas-chromatographic measurement of chlorpromazine in plasma. Clin. Chem. 17: 830, 1971.

CIMETIDINE

Serum Concentrations (mg/L)		
Therapeutic	Toxic	T½
1–4 (peak)	>1.25 (trough)	1–4 hr
0.3–0.8 (trough)		

Cimetidine is a histamine H_2-receptor antagonist that is frequently employed in the treatment of duodenal ulcer. It is commonly administered orally, but can also be given by intramuscular or intravenous injection; daily doses range from 1200–2400 mg/day.

Cimetidine serum concentrations are often monitored just prior to administration of the next dose to prevent toxic accumulation of the drug in patients with real insufficiency (from one-third to one-half of a dose is excreted unchanged in the urine). The thermal instability of this drug makes liquid chromatographic analysis the obvious choice when monitoring serum levels.

Serum Cimetidine by Liquid Chromatography

Principle:

Cimetidine and ranitidine, added as an internal standard, are extracted from alkalinized serum with ethyl acetate. The solvent is back-extracted with dilute acid, an aliquot of which is directly analyzed by liquid chromatography on a cyanonitrile column with ultraviolet detection at 220 nm.

Reagents:

Stock solution – 1 mg/mL cimetidine in methanol

Serum standards – 0.5, 1, 2, 5 and 10 mg/L

Internal standard – 20 mg/L ranitidine (Glaxo Pharmaceuticals) in 0.2 mol/L sodium carbonate

Ethyl acetate

Dilute phosphoric acid (0.5 N) – 16 g conc. H_3PO_4 per L of water

Mobile phase – 33% acetontirile in water, containing 5 mmol/L triethylamine and adjusted to pH 3.0 with H_3PO_4

Instrumental Conditions:

Liquid chromatograph with 220 nm ultraviolet detection

10 cm × 8 mm i.d. Radial-Pak 10 micron CN column cartridge and RCM-100 cartridge compression module (Waters Associates)

Solvent flow rate, 2 mL/min

Column temperature, ambient

Procedure:

1. Transfer 100 µL serum to a 12 mL conical centrifuge tube and add 50 µL internal standard. Vortex and add 5 mL ethyl acetate. Vortex for 1 min and centrifuge to separate layers.
2. Transfer the upper organic layer to a clean tube and add 200 µL dilute phosphoric acid. Vortex for 1 min and centrifuge. Discard the upper organic layer and inject 100 µL of the aqueous phase into the chromatograph.

	Retention time (min)
cimetidine	7.5
internal standard	11.5

Calculation:

Calculation is based on a response factor derived from a standard curve. A quality control specimen containing 1.0 mg/L cimetidine is analyzed daily.

Evaluation:

Sensitivity: 0.02 mg/L
Linearity: 0.4–10 mg/L
C.V.: 2.6–2.9%
Relative recovery: not established

Interferences:

Normal serum components did not interfere with the assay. Other drugs were not studied for potential interference.

Reference:

H. Kubo, Y. Kobayashi and K. Tokunaga, Improved method for the determination of cimetidine in human serum by high-performance liquid chromatography. Anal. Lett. 18: 245–260, 1985.

CLONAZEPAM

	Therapeutic Plasma Concentrations (mg/L)	T½
clonazepam	0.025–0.075	19–42 hr
7-aminoclonazepam	0.020–0.140	?

Clonazepam is a benzodiazepine derivative that is used as an anticonvulsant drug in daily oral doses of 2–9 mg. The therapeutic plasma concentrations of the parent drug and its major active metabolite, 7-aminoclonazepam, a weak anticonvulsant, are so low that the usual analytical procedures for either the anticonvulsants or the benzodiazepine sedatives are unsuitable. The following procedure utilizes electron-capture detection for the analysis of underivatized clonazepam. An alternative method is presented for the liquid chromatographic determination of this drug that requires a normal-phase column.

Commercial reagent kits are available for the determination of clonazepam by radioimmunoassay and EMIT.

Plasma Clonazepam by Electron-Capture Gas Chromatography

Principle:

Clonazepam and an internal standard are extracted from alkalinized plasma into an organic solvent. Following concentration of the solvent, the drugs are analyzed by gas chromatography with electron-capture detection. The 7-aminoclonazepam metabolite requires a pH close to neutrality for extraction and is not detected by this procedure.

Reagents:

Stock solution – 1 mg/mL clonazepam in methanol
Plasma standards – 0.025, 0.050, 0.075 and 0.100 mg/L
Trisodium phosphate solution – saturated Na_3PO_4
Internal standard solution – 3 μg methylclonazepam (Hoffman-LaRoche, Inc.) per L of benzene/ethyl acetate, 1:1 by volume
Benzene/ethyl acetate, 1:1 by volume

Instrumental Conditions:

Gas chromatograph with electron-capture detector
2 m × 2 mm i.d. glass column containing 5% OV-17 on 100/200 mesh Gas Chrom Q
Injector, 300°C.; column, 290°C.; detector, 300°C.
5% Methane in argon flow rate, 30 mL/min.

Procedure:

1. Transfer 100 µL plasma to a 15 mL conical centrifuge tube and add 100 µL trisodium phosphate solution.
2. Add 1 mL internal standard solution and vortex for 30 seconds. Centrifuge.
3. Transfer the solvent layer to a 5 mL conical centrifuge tube and evaporate to dryness at 50–60°C. under a stream of nitrogen.
4. Dissolve the residue in 20 µL of benzene/ethyl acetate and inject 2 µL into the gas chromatograph.

	Retention time (min)
internal standard	11.0
clonazepam	15.6

Calculation:

Calculation is based on a response factor derived from a standard curve. A quality control specimen containing 0.050 mg/L clonazepam is analyzed daily.

Evaluation:

Sensitivity: 0.005 mg/L
Linearity: 0.005–0.100 mg/L
C.V.: 4.3% day-to-day
Relative recovery: not established

Interferences:

Of the other benzodiazepine derivatives, only chlordiazepoxide was found to interfere by co-eluting with clonazepam. The 7-aminoclonazepam metabolite can be distinguished under the chromatographic conditions used but is not extracted at an alkaline pH.

Reference:

E.B. Solow and C.P. Kenfield. A micromethod for the determination of clonazepam in serum by electron capture gas-liquid chromatography. J. Analyt. Tox. 1: 155–157, 1977.

Plasma Clonazepam by Liquid Chromatography

Principle:

Clonazepam and an internal standard are extracted from alkalinized plasma with an organic solvent. The extract is concentrated by evaporation and analyzed by liquid chromatography with detection at 254 nm.

Reagents:

Stock solution – 1 mg/mL clonazepam in methanol
Plasma standards – 0.025, 0.050, 0.075 and 0.100 mg/L
Internal standard – 0.5 mg 4,5-dihydrodiazepam (Hoffman-LaRoche, Inc.) per 100 mL of methanol

pH 10.5 Glycine buffer – 2.0 mol/L glycine in water
Extraction solvent – benzene/dichloromethane, 9:1 by volume
Mobile phase – cyclopentane/chloroform/acetonitrile/methanol, 29:55.5:15:0.5 by volume

Instrumental Conditions:

Liquid chromatograph with 254 nm absorbance detector
25 cm × 4.6 nm i.d. Partisil 5 column (Reeve Angel)
Solvent flow rate, 1.0 mL/min
Column temperature, ambient

Procedure:

1. Transfer 1 mL plasma to a 15 mL screw-cap tube. Add 10 µL internal standard and 0.5 mL glycine buffer and vortex.
2. Add 5 mL extraction solvent and shake for 1 min. Centrifuge to separate layers.
3. Transfer the organic layer to a 5 mL ReactiVial (Pierce Chemical) and evaporate to dryness at 55°C. under a stream of nitrogen.
4. Dissolve the residue in 70 µL of mobile phase and inject 20 µL into the chromatograph.

	Retention time (min)
internal standard	8
clonazepam	9

Calculation:

Calculation is based on a response factor derived from a standard curve. A quality control specimen containing 0.050 mg/L clonazepam is analyzed daily.

Evaluation:

Sensitivity: 0.010 mg/L
Linearity: 0.025–0.100 mg/L
C.V.: 5–6%
Relative recovery: not established

Interferences:

Other benzodiazepine derivatives including diazepam, nordiazepam, chlordiazepoxide, demoxepam and nitrazepam were found not to interfere. The 7-amino metabolite elutes at about 40 min and the 7-acetamido metabolite is not detected by this procedure.

Reference:

R.J. Perchalski and B.J. Wilder. Determination of benzodiazepine anticonvulsants in plasma by high-performance liquid chromatography. Anal. Chem. 50: 554–557, 1978.

COCAINE

	Therapeutic Concentrations (mg/L)		Fatal Concentrations (mg/L)	
	Plasma	Urine	Blood	Urine
cocaine	0.10–0.50	0–10	1–20	1–215
benzoylecgonine	<0.10	5–125	1–10	15–220

Cocaine is a local anesthetic drug that is frequently abused for its central nervous system stimulant and euphoric properties. The drug is rapidly hydrolyzed by esterases of the blood and liver to inactive metabolites, primarily benzoylecgonine and ecgonine. For the occasional need to determine unchanged cocaine in plasma following therapeutic usage, a gas chromatographic method is included that requires a sensitive nitrogen-specific detector. A more common requirement is the detection of urinary cocaine or benzoylecgonine as an indicator of drug abuse; both a flame-ionization gas chromatographic procedure and a gas chromatography-mass spectrometric method are presented for this purpose.

Both radioimmunoassay and EMIT reagents are commercially available for the determination of benzoylecgonine in urine. Unchanged cocaine cross-reacts strongly in the Roche radioimmunoassay but very poorly in the EMIT test.

Plasma Cocaine by Nitrogen-Specific Gas Chromatography

Principle:
Cocaine is extracted from alkalinized plasma with an organic solvent containing an internal standard. The drugs are back-extracted into aqueous acid and partitioned into a solvent prior to injection into the gas chromatograph. Nitrogen-sensitive detection provides excellent sensitivity.

Reagents:
Stock solution – 1 mg/mL cocaine in methanol
Plasma standards – 0.10, 0.20 and 0.50 mg/L (prepared just prior to extraction)
Internal standard – 1 mg ethylmorphine (Applied Science) per 100 mL water
pH 9.6 Carbonate buffer – mix together 20 g Na_2CO_3 and 17.5 g $NaHCO_3$; prior to use dissolve 700 mg of the solid mixture in 10 mL water
Heptane/isoamyl alcohol, 98:2 by volume
50 mmol/L Sulfuric acid
Sodium sulfate – anhydrous Na_2SO_4
Methanol

Instrumental Conditions:

Gas chromatograph with nitrogen-phosphorus detector
1.8 m × 2 mm i.d. glass column containing 3% OV-17 on 100/120 mesh Gas Chrom Q
Injector, 280°C.; column, 260°C.; detector, 300°C.
Flow rates: helium carrier, 20 mL/min; air, 400 mL/min; hydrogen, 1 mL/min

Procedure:

1. Transfer 2 mL plasma to a 15 mL glass-stoppered centrifuge tube (all glassware should be soaked overnight in 1 mol/L HCl and rinsed with heptane/isoamyl alcohol). Add 100 µL internal standard and 0.5 mL carbonate buffer solution and vortex.
2. Add 10 mL heptane/isoamyl alcohol and shake for 1 min to extract. Centrifuge and transfer the upper solvent layer to a clean 15 mL centrifuge tube.
3. Add 1 mL 50 mmol/L H_2SO_4 and shake for 1 min. Centrifuge and discard the solvent layer.
4. Wash the aqueous layer with 3 mL heptane/isoamyl alcohol, centrifuge and discard the solvent layer.
5. Add about 400 mg of the solid carbonate buffer to the aqueous layer and vortex. Extract with 2 mL heptane/isoamyl alcohol and centrifuge.
6. Transfer the solvent to a clean tube, add a small amount of solid Na_2SO_4 (300 mg) and vortex.
7. Transfer the solvent to a 5 mL conical centrifuge tube and evaporate to dryness under a stream of nitrogen at room temperature. Dissolve the residue in 10 µL methanol and inject 2 µL into the gas chromatograph.

	Retention time (min)
cocaine	3.5
internal standard	5.3

Calculation:

Calculation is based on a response factor derived from a standard curve.

Evaluation:

Sensitivity: 0.010 mg/L
Linearity: 0.05–0.50 mg/L
C.V.: 5.3% within-run
Relative recovery: not established

Interferences:

Specimens should be placed on ice immediately after drawing and should be analyzed within 1 hour to prevent extensive hydrolysis of cocaine. The usual quality control procedures are not applicable to this determination due to the instability of cocaine in plasma. Of more than 20 common basic drugs checked for interference, only methaqualone had the same retention time as cocaine. Atropine, desipramine, nortriptyline and pentazocine had retention times within 0.3 min of cocaine but were resolved from it.

References:

1. P.I. Jatlow and D.N. Bailey. Gas-chromatographic analysis for cocaine in human plasma, with use of a nitrogen detector. Clin. Chem. 21: 1918–1921, 1975.
2. B.H. Dvorchik, S.H. Miller and W.P. Graham. Gas chromatographic determination of cocaine in whole blood plasma using a nitrogen-sensitive flame ionization detector. J. Chrom. 135: 141–148, 1977.

Urine Cocaine and Benzoylecgonine by Flame-Ionization Gas Chromatography

Principle:

Cocaine and benzoylecgonine are extracted from urine using a chloroform/ethanol solvent mixture. One aliquot is analyzed directly by flame-ionization gas chromatography for cocaine, while another is subjected to methylation to convert benzoylecgonine to cocaine prior to chromatography. The difference between the two results represents the benzoylecgonine concentration.

Reagents:

Stock solutions –
    1 mg/mL cocaine in methanol
    1 mg/mL benzoylecgonine (Applied Science) in methanol
Urine standards – 1, 2, 5, and 10 mg/L for cocaine and 10, 20, 50 and 100 mg/L for benzoylecgonine
Quality control urine – 5 mg/L cocaine and 50 mg/L benzoylecgonine in urine containing 0.5% NaF and adjusted to pH 6 (stable for 1 month at 4°C.)
Internal standard – 50 mg/L butylanthraquinone (Aldrich) in chloroform
Extraction solvent – chloroform/ethanol, 80:20 by volume
Methylating reagent – add 1 volume conc. H_2SO_4 slowly to 2 volumes of methanol
Ether
Sodium bicarbonate – solid $NaHCO_3$

Instrumental Conditions:

Gas chromatograph with flame-ionization detector
1 m× 2 mm i.d. glass column containing 3% OV-17 on 80/100 mesh Supelcoport
Injector, 290°C.; column, 220°C.; detector, 290°C.
Nitrogen flow rate, 30 mL/min

Procedure:

1. Transfer 5 mL urine to a 50 mL glass-stoppered centrifuge tube and add 25 mL extraction solvent. Shake for 2 min and centrifuge to separate layers.
2. Discard the upper aqueous layer and transfer 10 mL aliquots of the solvent to two separate 15 mL conical centrifuge tubes. Evaporate both to dryness at 55°C. under a stream of air.
3. Cocaine determination: add 200 µL of the internal standard to one tube, rinsing the walls of the vessel to dissolve the residue. Inject 5 µL into the gas chromatograph.
4. Total cocaine/benzoylecgonine determination: add 0.6 mL methylating reagent to the second tube and vortex. Incubate at 85°C. for 10 min.

5. Cool and wash the solution twice with 10 mL portions of ether. Centrifuge each time and discard ether layers. Evaporate remaining traces of ether under a stream of air at 55°C.
6. Add 1 mL water and sufficient solid NaHCO₃ to neutralize the solution. Add 200 μL internal standard and vortex for 2 min.
7. Centrifuge to separate layers and inject 5 μL of the lower organic layer into the gas chromatograph.

	Retention time (min)
cocaine	3.7
internal standard	4.5

Calculation:

Calculation is based on a response factor derived from a standard curve. The benzoylecgonine concentration is obtained by subtracting the peak height ratio obtained in step 3 from that in step 7. A quality control specimen prepared as described is analyzed daily.

Evaluation:

Sensitivity: 0.2 mg/L
Linearity: 0.25–20 mg/L for cocaine, 0.5–100 mg/L for benzoylecgonine
C.V.: 5% within-run
Relative recovery: not established

Interferences:

Drug-free urine specimens yielded apparent cocaine concentrations averaging 0.14 mg/L. Propoxyphene and amitriptyline were found not to interfere in the procedure.

Reference:

J.E. Wallace, H.E. Hamilton, D.E. King et al. Gas-liquid chromatographic determination of cocaine and benzoylecgonine in urine. Anal. Chem. 48:34–38, 1976.

Urine Cocaine and Benzoylecgonine by Gas Chromatography-Mass Spectrometry

Principle:

The drugs and two internal standards, atropine and SKF-525A, are extracted from urine with an organic solvent mixture, which is washed with weak base and then evaporated to dryness. The residue is reacted with BSTFA to form the trimethylsilyl derivative of benzoylecgonine and atropine; the reaction mixture is analyzed for these two derivatives as well as for underivatized cocaine and SKF-525A by gas chromatography-mass spectrometry with selected ion monitoring.

Reagents:

Stock solutions – 1 mg/mL cocaine in methanol
                1 mg/mL benzoylecgonine (Applied Science) in methanol

Urine standards – 0.5, 1, 2, and 5 mg/L for cocaine and 2, 5, 10 and 25 mg/L for benzoylecgonine

Quality control urine – 2 mg/L cocaine and 10 mg/L benzoylecgonine in urine containing 0.5% NaF and adjusted to pH 5 (stable for 1 month at 4°C.)

Internal standard mixture – 1 mg/L atropine and SKF-525A (Smith, Kline & French) in water

Sodium bicarbonate

Extraction solvent – chloroform/ethanol, 80:20 by volume

0.01 mol/L Sodium hydroxide

Derivatizing reagent – BSTFA containing 1% TMCS (Pierce Chemical Co. #38831)

Ethyl acetate

Instrumental Conditions:

Gas chromatograph with mass selective detector (Hewlett-Packard 5970B MSD or equivalent)

12 m × 0.20 mm i.d. methylsilicone capillary column (Hewlett-Packard)

Injector, 275°C.; transfer line, 250°C.

Column temperature program: initial, 150°C. (1 min)
20°C./min increase
final, 300°C. (2 min)

Helium flow rate, 1 mL/min

Splitless on time, 1.0 min

Solvent delay time, 2.0 min

Electron multiplier voltage, 2200

Ions monitored, 82.10, 86.10, 124.15, 182.15, 240.20, 303.30, 361.30

Procedure:

1. Transfer 1 mL urine to a siliconized 15 mL screw-cap tube and add 100 μL internal standard solution. Saturate the solution with solid sodium bicarbonate.
2. Add 7 mL extraction solvent and place on a rotator for 30 min. Centrifuge to separate phases and discard the upper aqueous phase by aspiration.
3. Add 1 mL 0.01 mol/L NaOH and place on a rotator for 30 min. Centrifuge and discard the upper aqueous phase by aspiration.
4. Evaporate solvent layer to dryness under a stream of dry air at 50°C. Add 100 μL derivatizing reagent and 100 μL ethyl acetate, cap tube and heat at 80°C. for 30 min in a heating block.
5. Cool, centrifuge and inject 1 μL of the supernatant into the chromatograph.

	Retention time (min)	Principle ions (m/z)
cocaine	5.8	82, 182, 303
atropine-TMS	6.0	124
benzoylecganine-TMS	6.3	82, 240, 361
SKF-525A	6.7	86

Calculation:

Calculation is based on a response factor derived from a standard curve of ion chromatogram peak height ratio (182/86 ratio for cocaine/SKF-525A and 240/124 ratio for benzoylecgonine/atropine) versus drug concentration. A quality control specimen prepared as described is analyzed daily. Ion intensity ratios (82/182 and 303/182 for cocaine and 82/240 and 361/240 for benzoylecgonine) should compare well between standards and unknown to further confirm drug identification in the unknown specimens.

Evaluation:

Sensitivity: 0.02 mg/L
Linearity: 0.05–5 mg/L
C.V.: 8–10% day-to-day
Relative recovery: not established

Interferences:

Normal urine components do not interfere with the assay. Other commonly used or abused drugs have not been found to interfere.

References:

1. E.C. Griesemer, Y. Lin, R.D. Budd et al. The determination of cocaine and its major metabolite, benzoylecgonine, in postmortem fluids and tissues by computerized gas chromatography/mass spectrometry. J. For. Sci. 28:894–900, 1983.
2. M.A. Peat. Unpublished results, 1985.

COPPER

Total Serum Concentration (mg/L)			Urine Concentration (µg/day)
Children	Men	Women	General Population
0.1–1.5	0.7–1.4	0.7–1.6	15–64

Copper is an essential trace metal that is present in all human tissues. About 93% of normal serum copper is incorporated into ceruloplasmin (serum ferroxidase), an enzyme that plays an important role in the mobilization and transport of iron. Abnormally low serum copper concentrations are found in patients with Wilson's disease or with hypoproteinemia, while elavated concentrations are observed in copper poisoning due to ingestion of copper salts or during hemodialysis with units containing copper heating coils. A convenient flame atomic absorption procedure is presented that is suitable for the direct determination of total copper in serum and urine.

Serum and Urine Copper by Atomic Absorption Spectrometry

Principle:
Copper is measured directly in acidified urine and after dilution of serum by aspiration into the flame of an atomic absorption spectrometer. Signal suppression by inorganic urinary salts is overcome by preparing standards in a mixed salt solution.

Reagents:
Stock solution – 1 mg/mL copper (Fisher reference standard or dissolve 3.932 g $CuSO_4.5H_2O$ per L of water)

Standards for serum – 0.2, 0.5, 1.0 and 2.0 mg/L in water

Standards for urine – 10, 20, 50 and 100 µg/L in salt solution

Salt solution – 5.08 g NaCl, 2.86 g KCl, 0.31 g $CaCO_3$, 0.42 g $MgCl_2.6H_2O$, 0.67 mL conc. H_2SO_4, 8.7 mL conc. HCl and 3.09 g $NH_4H_2PO_4$ per L of water

0.1 mol/L Hydrochloric acid

Concentrated hydrochloric acid – low copper grade (<3 µg/L)

All plasticware used in this procedure should be soaked overnight in 5% nitric acid and rinsed several times in distilled/deionized water.

Instrumental Conditions:
Atomic absorption spectrometer with oxidizing air-acetylene flame and three slot burner head

Copper hollow cathode lamp

Measure absorption at 324.8 nm

Procedure:

Serum:

1. Collect blood in a disposable plastic syringe and transfer to a 5 mL plastic tube. Allow to clot, centrifuge and transfer 0.5 mL serum to a 15 mL plastic centrifuge tube. Also transfer 0.5 mL volumes of the serum standards to similar tubes.
2. Dilute serum and appropriate standards to 5 mL with 0.1 mol/L HCl and vortex. Use 0.1 mol/L HCl as a reagent blank.

Urine:

3. Collect a 24 hr urine specimen in an acid-washed 2.5 L polyethylene container. Acidify by adding 8.7 mL conc. HCl/L of urine. Urine standards are analyzed directly; the reagent blank for urine determinations consists of the salt solution.

Analysis:

4. Aspirate distilled/deionized water into the flame for 20 seconds, followed by the reagent blank for 20 seconds. Repeat this operation 5 times.
5. Perform a similar cycle but replace the reagent blank with the low standard solution. Repeat these cycles using standards of increasing concentration and finally the unknown. Average the 5 readings for each sample.

Calculation:

Calculation is based on a response factor derived from a standard curve. The value for the reagent blank should be subtracted from the standard and unknown readings prior to preparation of the curve. Quality control specimens consisting of pooled serum and urine are analyzed daily.

Evaluation:

Sensitivity: 0.02 mg/L for serum and 2 µg/L for urine
Linearity: 0.05–3.00 mg/L for serum and 10–300 µg/L for urine
C.V.: 3% within-run
Relative recovery: 91–104%

Interferences:

Care must be taken to minimize copper contamination from reagents and laboratory vessels. Suppression of the copper value in urine by inorganic salts is overcome by preparing urine standards in a synthetic salt mixture. No other interferences were found.

Reference:

J.B. Dawson, D.J. Ellis and H. Newton-John. Direct estimation of copper in serum and urine by atomic absorption spectroscopy. Clin. Chim. Acta 21: 33–42, 1968.

CYANIDE

	Cyanide Concentrations (mg/L)			
	Nonsmokers	Smokers	During Nitroprusside Therapy	Fatal Poisoning
plasma	0.004	0.006	0.010–0.060	?
blood	0.016	0.041	0.050–0.500	1–50

Cyanide is found in low concentrations in the tissues of healthy subjects as the result of normal metabolism, the ingestion of cyanogenetic foods and cigarette smoking. Higher concentrations are produced during intravenous administration of the hypotensive agent, nitroprusside, or following oral administration of laetrile, which contains a cyanogenetic glycoside. The majority of cyanide in whole blood is contained in the erythrocytes, and thus whole blood is preferred as a specimen for most emergency toxicology purposes. Two procedures are presented for the analysis of cyanide in whole blood; one is a colorimetric determination and the other utilizes a cyanide-specific electrode for the potentiometric measurement of the ion. The first method is designed primarily for the determination of toxic blood levels of cyanide, while the latter technique is sufficiently sensitive to measure plasma and blood concentrations of cyanide during nitroprusside administration. Both techniques require prior isolation of cyanide from blood by microdiffusion, a simple but somewhat time-consuming method.

Blood Cyanide by Colorimetry

Principle:

A blood specimen is pipetted into the outer circle of a Conway microdiffusion cell and cyanide is released by the addition of sulfuric acid. The released hydrocyanic acid is captured in sodium hydroxide solution in the central compartment of the dish during a several hour diffusion period. This solution is then reacted with a chromogenic reagent and the resulting color is measured in a spectrophotometer at 580 nm.

Reagents:

Stock solution – 1 mg/mL cyanide (25.0 mg KCN/10 mL water)
Blood standards – 0.5, 1, 2 and 5 mg/L (prepared fresh in whole blood)
0.1 mol/L Sodium hydroxide – 2 g NaOH/500 mL water
0.5 mol/L Sulfuric acid – 14 mL conc. H_2SO_4/500 mL water
1 mol/L Phosphate buffer – 68 g KH_2PO_4/500 mL water
0.25% Chloramine T – 250 mg/100 mL water (REFRIGERATE)
Pyridine-barbituric acid solution – 1.5 g barbituric acid, 7.5 mL pyridine and 1.5 mL conc. HCl in a 25 mL volumetric flask. Dilute to volume with water, warm mixture to dissolve and mix. Prepare fresh.

Instrumental Conditions:

Visible spectrophotometer set to 580 nm

Procedure:

1. Lubricate edges of Conway diffusion cells with stopcock grease. Add 3.0 mL 0.1 mol/L sodium hydroxide to the center well of all cells.
2. Add 4 mL of one of the following to the outer compartment of each cell: cyanide-free blood, blood standards and patient specimen.
3. Finally add 4 mL of 0.5 mol/L sulfuric acid to the outer compartment and rapidly close the cell. Tilt to mix and leave for 3–4 hours at room temperature (or for 1–2 hr in a 37°C. oven).
4. Pipet 1 mL of the reagent from the central compartment into a 15 mL centrifuge tube. Add 2 mL 1 mol/L phosphate buffer and 1 mL 0.25% chloramine T. Mix and let stand for 2–3 minutes.
5. Add 3 mL pyridine-barbituric acid solution. Mix and allow to stand for 10 minutes. Read in the visible spectrophotometer at 580 nm against the blood blank.

Calculation:

Calculation is based on a response factor derived from a standard curve. This procedure cannot be controlled by the usual methods due to the difficulty in storage of cyanide-containing blood specimens.

Evaluation:

Sensitivity: 0.2 mg/L
Linearity: 0.5–5 mg/L
C.V.: not established
Relative recovery: not established

Interferences:

Even freshly drawn whole blood contains a small quantity of cyanide. Both production and loss of cyanide can occur during storage of whole blood. Due to this phenomonen, it is suggested that patient specimens be kept at 4°C. until analysis and that analysis be performed as soon after drawing as is possible.

Reference:

M. Feldstein and N.C. Klendshoj. The determination of cyanide in biologic fluids by microdiffusion analysis. J. Lab. Clin. Med. 44: 166–170, 1954.

Blood Cyanide by Ion-Specific Potentiometry

Principle:

Cyanide is isolated from blood by microdiffusion according to the previous procedure. The concentration of the ion in the sodium hydroxide solution is determined by direct potentiometric measurement with a cyanide-specific electrode.

Reagents:
0.1 mol/L Sodium hydroxide
10% Lead acetate solution – 1 g $Pb(C_2H_3O_2)_2$ in 10 mL 0.1 mol/L NaOH

Instrumental Conditions:
pH Meter equipped with cyanide-specific electrode (Orion Research)

Procedure:
1. Process the blood blank, blood standards and patient blood specimen by Conway microdiffusion according to the previous procedure.
2. Stabilize the cyanide electrode by placing in 0.1 mol/L NaOH for 30 minutes or until a constant voltage reading is attained.
3. Determine the electrode response to the sodium hydroxide solution from the center well of the Conway cell of each of the processed specimens.
4. Add 1 drop 10% lead acetate solution to each sodium hydroxide sample after recording the initial reading. A significant change in electrode potential indicates the presence of sulfide as an interfering substance. In this case, record the electrode response to each of the solutions after adding lead acetate solution.

Calculation:
Calculation is based on a response factor derived from a standard curve. This procedure cannot be controlled by the usual methods due to the difficulty in storage of cyanide-containing blood specimens.

Evaluation:
Sensitivity: 0.01 mg/L
Linearity: 0.1–1.0 mg/L
C.V.: 5% within-run
Relative recovery: 100–109%

Interferences:
Although sulfide is known to interfere in this procedure, the addition of lead acetate to the final solution will insure its presence or absence. Since the blood used in the preparation of standards will probably contain a low level of cyanide, a blood blank must be analyzed and the result subtracted from those of the standards and patient specimen.

References:
1. B.H. McAnalley, W.T. Lowry, R. Oliver and J.C. Garriott. Determination of inorganic sulfide and cyanide in blood using specific ion electrodes. J. Analyt. Tox. 3: 111–114, 1979.
2. J.O. Egekeze and F.W. Oehme. Direct potentiometric method for the determination of cyanide in biological materials. J. Analyt. Tox. 3: 119–124, 1979.

CYCLOSPORINE

Blood Concentrations (μg/L)

Therapeutic	Toxic	T½
100–300 (trough)	>400 (trough)	10–40 hr

Cyclosporine is a naturally-occurring cyclic polypeptide that is frequently used as an immunosuppressive agent in organ transplant patients. The drug is administered either orally or by intravenous infusion. Daily oral doses of 15 mg/kg are often continued for one or two weeks after surgery and then gradually reduced by 5% per week to a daily maintenance dose of 5–10 mg/kg; intravenous doses are usually one-third that of the oral doses. Reagents for radioimmunoassay of cyclosporine are available from Sandoz, the manufacturer of the drug. A liquid chromatographic procedure is presented that is preferred by some analysts for its specificity in the presence of drug metabolites.

Blood Cyclosporine by Liquid Chromatography

Principle:
Cyclosporine and an internal standard, cyclosporin D, are extracted from acidified blood with ether, which is then washed with dilute alkali. The ether extract is evaporated to dryness, reconstituted in ammonium sulfate solution, washed with heptane, and analyzed by liquid chromatography. Ultraviolet detection is performed at 214 nm.

Reagents:
Stock solution – 1 mg/mL cyclosporine in methanol
Blood standards – 50, 100, 250, 500 and 1000 μg/L
Quality control blood – 200 μg/L cyclosporine
Internal standard – 10 mg/L cyclosporin D (Sandoz) in methanol
180 mmol/L Hydrochloric acid
Ether
95 mmol/L Sodium hydroxide
Ammonium sulfate solution – 76 mmol $(NH_4)_2SO_4$ per L of mobile phase
Heptane
Mobile phase – acetonitrile/water/methanol/0.757 mol/L ammonium sulfate, 470:350:180: 1.3 by volume

Instrumental Conditions:
Liquid chromatograph with 214 nm absorbance detector
7.5 cm × 4.6 mm i.d., 3 micron Supelcosil C-8 column (Supelco) with a 2 micron precolumn

filter and 3 feet of heated stainless steel delivery tubing (to allow temperature equilibration of the solvent prior to chromatography)

Solvent flow rate, 1.9 mL/min

Column temperature, 73°C.

Procedure:

1. Transfer 1 mL heparinized whole blood to a 15 mL screw-cap tube and add 75 µL internal standard. Add 1 mL 180 mmol/L HCl and vortex for 10 seconds.
2. Add 10 mL ether and place in a reciprocating shaker for 20 min. Centrifuge to separate layers and decant the upper ether layer into a clean tube.
3. Wash the ether with 1 mL 95 mmol/L NaOH by manually inverting 15 times. Centrifuge and transfer the ether layer to a conical 12 mL centrifuge tube. Evaporate to dryness under a stream of air at 45°C.
4. Dissolve the residue in 250 µL ammonium sulfate solution by vortexing for 30 sec. Wash the aqueous solution with 1 mL heptane by vortexing for 30 sec. Centrifuge, discard the upper heptane layer, and inject 50 µL of the aqueous layer into the chromatograph.

	Retention time (min)
cyclosporine	4.6
internal standard	6.1

Calculation:

Calculation is based on a response factor derived from a standard curve. A quality control specimen containing 200 µg/L cyclosporine is analyzed daily.

Evaluation:

Sensitivity: 10 µg/L

Linearity: 50–1000 µg/L

C.V.: 5.3–6.0% day-to-day

Relative recovery: not established

Interferences:

Many common therapeutic drugs, including amikacin, gentamicin, methotrexate, tobramycin, ketoconazole, azathioprene, and prednisone, were found not to interfere in the procedure.

Reference:

G.C. Kahn, L.M. Shaw and M.D. Kane. Routine monitoring of cyclosporine in whole blood and in kidney tissue using high performance liquid chromatography. J. Analyt. Tox. 10: 28–34, 1986.

DANTROLENE

Dantrolene is a hydantoin derivative used as a peripherally-acting skeletal muscle relaxant. Large overdoses are capable of producing unconsciousness and coma. The chemical instability and poor water solubility of the compound makes many of the usual analytical approaches unsuitable. A convenient technique for the determination of dantrolene in plasma is based on fluorescence spectrophotometry.

Plasma Dantrolene by Fluorescence Spectrophotometry

Principle:
Dantrolene is extracted from acidified plasma into a special solvent and read directly in the fluorimeter. Fluorescent emission is measured at 515 nm.

Reagents:
Stock solution – 0.1 mg/mL dantrolene (12.75 mg Na salt dissolved in 50 mL dimethylformamide, q.s. to 100 mL with H_2O)

Plasma standards – 0.5, 1, 2 and 4 mg/L (add 2.5, 5, 10 or 20 μL stock to 0.5 mL plasma as needed)

Saturated ammonium sulfate – 100 g $(NH_4)_2SO_4$/100 mL water

Extraction solvent – nitropropane/heptane, 1:1 by volume

Instrumental Conditions:
Fluorescence spectrophotometer set to excite at 400 nm

Record the emission spectrum over the range 470–560 nm and measure the emission peak at 515 nm

Procedure:
1. Pipet 0.5 mL plasma into a 15 mL screw-cap tube. Add 2 mL H_2O and 2 mL saturated $(NH_4)_2SO_4$.
2. Extract with 5 mL of the extraction solvent and centrifuge for 5 minutes at 2000 rpm.
3. Transfer 3.0 mL of the extraction solvent to a cuvette and read in the fluorimeter under the indicated conditions, subtracting the reading of a plasma blank from that of the patient specimen and plasma standards.

Calculation:

Calculation is based on a response factor derived from a standard curve. This assay cannot be controlled in the usual manner due to the instability of dantrolene in plasma.

Evaluation:

Sensitivity: 0.1 mg/L
Linearity: 0.2–8 mg/L
C.V.: not established
Relative recovery: not established

Interferences:

The dantrolene metabolite, 5-hydroxydantrolene, which is one-fifth as active as its parent and accumulates to a certain extent in plasma, is also measured by this technique. Other drugs have not been checked for possible interference.

References:

1. R.D. Hollifield and J.D. Conklin. A spectrophotofluorometric procedure for the determination of dantrolene in blood and urine. Arch. Int. Pharmaco. Ther. 174: 333–341, 1968.
2. R. Baselt and S. Voll. Unpublished results, 1978.

DICHLOROPHENOXYACETIC ACID

	Dichlorophenoxyacetic Acid Concentrations (mg/L)	
	Asymptomatic Exposed Individuals	Severe Intoxication
plasma	5–40	400–800
urine	50–100	200–400

The chlorinated phenoxyacid derivatives, 2,4-dichlorophenoxyacetic acid (2,4-D) and 2,4,5-trichlorophenoxyacetic acid (2,4,5-T), have been used abundantly as herbicides during the last 30 years. The use of 2,4,5-T has very recently been halted in the U.S. due to its suspected potential for producing miscarriages in exposed women. Commercially available 2.4-D, the most widely used herbicide in the U.S., is occasionally involved in accidental poisonings; a method for its determination in plasma or urine may therefore be useful in the diagnosis of suspected poisoning cases or to monitor urinary excretion of the agent. A convenient gas chromatographic method is presented that utilizes 2,4,5-T as internal standard.

Plasma and Urine Dichlorophenoxyacetic Acid by Gas Chromatography

Principle:

2,4-D and the internal standard, 2,4,5-T, are extracted from acidified plasma or urine with ether. A back extraction is performed into a methylating reagent and the methyl esters are chromatographed on OV-17, with detection by flame-ionization.

Reagents:

Stock solution – 10 mg/mL dichlorophenoxyacetic acid in methanol
Aqueous standards – 100, 200 and 400 mg/L
Internal standard – 400 mg trichlorophenoxyacetic acid in 100 mL methanol
1 mol/L Hydrochloric acid
Ether
Methylating reagent – 1:1 mixture of water and 0.2 mol/L trimethylanilinium hydroxide in methanol (prepared fresh)

Instrumental Conditions:

Gas chromatograph with flame-ionization detector
4' × 2 mm i.d. glass column containing 10% OV-17 on 100/120 mesh Gas Chrom Q
Injector, 310°C.; column, 200°C.; detector, 300°C.
Nitrogen flow rate, 60 mL/min

Procedure:

1. Transfer 1 mL plasma or urine to a 15 mL screw-cap tube and add 100 µL internal standard and 2 mL 1 mol/L HCl. Vortex.
2. Add 5 mL ether and shake to extract. Centrifuge.
3. Transfer the ether layer to a 15 mL glass-stoppered conical centrifuge tube. Add 100 µL of the methylating reagent and vortex for 30 seconds.
4. Centrifuge and inject 2 µL of the lower aqueous layer into the gas chromatograph.

	Retention time (min)
2,4-D	5
internal standard	7

Calculation:

Calculation is based on a response factor derived from a standard curve.

Evaluation:

Sensitivity: 1 mg/L
Linearity: 10–400 mg/L
C.V.: 5.3% within-run
Relative recovery: not established

Interferences:

The specimen should be analyzed with and without the internal standard to insure that 2,4,5-T is not one of the constituents of the ingested herbicide. Other chemical substances have not been studied for potential interference.

References:

1. J. Park, I. Darrien and L.F. Prescott. Pharmacokinetic studies in severe intoxication with 2,4-D and mecoprop. Proc. Eur. Soc. Tox. 18: 154–155, 1977.
2. L.F. Prescott, J. Park and I. Darrien. Treatment of severe 2,4-D and mecoprop intoxication with alkaline diuresis. Brit. J. Clin. Pharm. 7: 111–116, 1979.

DICUMAROL

Plasma Concentrations (mg/L)		
Therapeutic	Toxic	T½
8–30	40–100	21–96 hr

Dicumarol, or bishydroxycoumarin, is a vitamin K antagonist that is widely used as an oral anticoagulant. The rate of disappearance of the compound from the plasma has been found to be a function of both dosage and genetic difference; the plasma half-life in most subjects is 24 hours, but half-lives of up to 96 hours have been observed in some patients. For this reason it is important to control drug dosage by monitoring either prothrombin time or dicumarol plasma levels. The chemical characteristics of the compound allow a convenient ultraviolet spectrophotometric technique to be used for the latter purpose.

Plasma Dicumarol by Ultraviolet Spectrophotometry

Principle:
Dicumarol is extracted from acidified plasma into heptane. The solvent is back-extracted with dilute alkali and the concentration of dicumarol is determined by measurement at 315 nm in an ultraviolet spectrophotometer.

Reagents:
Stock solution – 1 mg/mL dicumarol in 0.1 mol/L NaOH (stable for 1 month at 4°C.)
Plasma standards – 5, 10, 20 and 40 mg/L
3 mol/L Hydrochloric acid
Heptane
2.5 mol/L Sodium hydroxide

Instrumental Conditions:
Ultraviolet spectrophotometer set to 315 nm

Procedure:
1. Transfer 3 mL plasma to a 35 mL screw-cap tube and add 0.5 mL 3 mol/L HCl.
2. Add 20 mL heptane and shake for 1 min. Centrifuge to separate layers.
3. Transfer 15 mL of the heptane phase to a 25 mL glass-stoppered graduated cylinder. Add 4 mL 2.5 mol/L NaOH and shake for 30 seconds.
4. Allow layers to separate and transfer 3 mL of the lower aqueous phase to a cuvette using a disposable pipet. Read at 315 nm in the spectrophotometer against a negative control plasma that has been processed in the same manner.

Calculation:

Calculation is based on a response factor derived from a standard curve. A quality control specimen containing 20 mg/L dicumarol is analyzed daily.

Evaluation:

Sensitivity: 1 mg/L
Linearity: 5–40 mg/L
C.V.: not established
Relative recovery: not established

Interferences:

There is a certain degree of interference in this procedure due to dicumarol metabolites in plasma, but this appears to be minimal. Of twelve acid and neutral drugs tested for possible interference, only thiopental and salicylate were found to present a serious problem. Due to the frequency of salicylate usage, the absence of this drug should be ascertained prior to reporting plasma level determinations of dicumarol by this procedure.

Reference:

J. Axelrod, J.R. Cooper and B.B. Brodie. Estimation of dicumarol, 3,3-methylenebis(4-hydroxycoumarin) in biological fluids. Proc. Soc. Biol. Med. 70: 693–695, 1949.

DISOPYRAMIDE

	Plasma Concentrations (mg/L)		T½
	Therapeutic	Toxic	
disopyramide	2–4	8–27	5–7 hr
nordisopyramide	0.5–1.5	2–6	?

Disopyramide is administered orally for the treatment of cardiac arrhythmias; its N-desmethyl metabolite is about one-half as active as the parent drug and probably need not be assayed for routine purposes. A convenient gas chromatographic procedure is described that allows determination of only the parent compound, while the succeeding liquid chromatographic method is suitable for the simultaneous measurement of both parent and metabolite.

Plasma Disopyramide by Gas Chromatography

Principle:
Disopyramide is extracted from alkalinized plasma with chloroform containing an internal standard. The extract is analyzed by gas chromatography with flame-ionization detection.

Reagents:
Stock solution – 1 mg/mL disopyramide in methanol
Plasma standards – 1, 2 and 4 mg/L
Internal standard solution – 2 mg p-chlorodisopyramide (Searle and Co.) in 100 mL chloroform
Tris buffer – 2 mol/L tris(hydroxymethyl)aminomethane in water

Instrumental Conditions:
Gas chromatograph with flame-ionization detector
1.5 m × 4 mm i.d. glass column containing 3% OV-1 on 80/100 mesh Supelcoport
Injector, 250°C.; column, 240°C.; detector, 300°C.
Nitrogen flow rate, 40 mL/min

Procedure:
1. Transfer 200 μL plasma to a 5 mL conical centrifuge tube. Add 20 μL tris buffer and 50 μL internal standard solution.
2. Vortex for 30 seconds and centrifuge to separate layers.

3. Inject 3 μL of the lower organic layer into the chromatograph.

	Retention time (min)
disopyramide	3
internal standard	5

Calculation:

Calculation is based on a response factor derived from a standard curve. A quality control specimen containing 2 mg/L disopyramide is analyzed daily.

Evaluation:

Sensitivity: 0.2 mg/L
Linearity: 0.5–8.0 mg/L
C.V.: 2–4% within-run
Relative recovery: not established

Interferences:

Eighteen other basic drugs were checked for interference in this assay and were not observed to hamper detection of disopyramide. The major metabolite, nordisopyramide, is unstable under the chromatographic conditions used and is not detected.

Reference:

A.M. Hayler and R.J. Flanagan. Simple gas-liquid chromatographic method for the measurement of disopyramide in blood-plasma or serum and in urine. J. Chrom. 153: 461–471, 1978.

Plasma Disopyramide and Nordisopyramide by Liquid Chromatography

Principle:

Disopyramide, its N-desalkyl metabolite and an internal standard are extracted from alkalinized plasma into chloroform. The concentrated extract is assayed by liquid chromatography with ultraviolet detection at 254 nm.

Reagents:

Stock solutions –
   1 mg/mL disopyramide in methanol
   1 mg/mL nordisopyramide in methanol
Plasma standards –
   1, 2 and 4 mg/L for disopyramide
   0.5, 1 and 2 mg/L for nordisopyramide
Internal standard – 40 mg/L p-chlorodisopyramide (Searle and Co.) in water
1 mol/L Sodium hydroxide
Chloroform
Mobile phase – 4 g sodium acetate, 40 g acetic acid and 150 mL methanol diluted to 1 L with water (adjust pH to 3.5 if necessary)

Instrumental Conditions:

Liquid chromatograph with 254 nm absorbance detector
25 cm × 5 mm i.d. µBondapak CN column (Waters Associates)
Solvent flow rate, 1.9 mL/min
Column temperature, ambient

Procedure:

1. Transfer 1 mL plasma to a 12 × 75 mm polypropylene tube. Add 50 µL 1 mol/L NaOH and 50 µL internal standard and vortex.
2. Add 1.2 mL chloroform and shake vigorously on a metabolic shaker for 10 min. Centrifuge to separate layers.
3. Discard the upper aqueous phase and evaporate the organic layer to dryness under a stream of nitrogen.
4. Dissolve the residue in 100 µL of mobile phase and inject 20 µL into the chromatograph.

	Retention time (min)
nordisopyramide	3.4
disopyramide	4.1
internal standard	6.3

Calculation:

Calculation is based on a response factor derived from a standard curve. A quality control specimen containing 2.0 mg/L disopyramide and 1 mg/L nordisopyramide is analyzed daily.

Evaluation:

Sensitivity: 0.05–0.08 mg/L
Linearity: 0.25–20.0 mg/L
C.V.: 2.6–4.6% for disopyramide, 6.6–12.0% for nordisopyramide
Relative recovery: 105–108%

Interferences:

Diazepam, furosemide, procainamide, NAPA and quinidine were found not to interfere with the analysis. Lidocaine co-elutes with nordisopyramide.

Reference:

J.J. Lima. Liquid chromatographic analysis of disopyramide and its mono-N-dealkylated metabolite. Clin. Chem. 25: 405–408, 1979.

DISULFIRAM

	Therapeutic Concentrations (mg/L)	
	Plasma	Urine
disulfiram	0	0
diethyldithiocarbamate	0.3–1.4	1–40
carbon disulfide	0.02–0.60	?

Disulfiram has been used for many years as an adjunct to aversion therapy for chronic alcoholism. The substance is administered in large daily oral doses but is rapidly reduced to diethyldithiocarbamate and carbon disulfide in the body. Treatment compliance or intoxication may be monitored by determining these metabolites in breath, blood or urine. Two procedures are presented that are applicable to the routine determination of diethyldithiocarbamate. The first involves flame-ionization gas chromatography for the measurement of plasma concentrations, while the second utilizes atomic absorption spectrometry for the assay of this metabolite in urine.

Plasma Diethyldithiocarbamate by Gas Chromatography

Principle:
Direct methylation of diethyldithiocarbamate (DDC) in plasma is performed prior to extraction with an organic solvent containing the internal standard. The concentrated extract is analyzed by flame-ionization gas chromatography.

Reagents:
Stock solution – 1 mg/mL diethyldithiocarbamate in methanol (prepared fresh from the sodium salt)
Plasma standards – 0.25, 0.50, 1.00 and 2.00 mg/L (prepared fresh and analyzed rapidly)
Methyl iodide
Extraction solvent – 0.2 mg/L bibenzyl (Aldrich Chemical Co.) in carbon tetrachloride

Instrumental Conditions:
Gas chromatograph with flame-ionization detector
1.8 m × 2 mm i.d. glass column containing 3% OV-1 on 80/100 mesh Chromosorb W-HP
Injector, 135°C.; column, 115°C.; detector, 140°C.
Nitrogen flow rate, 55 mL/min

Procedure:
1. Transfer 1 mL plasma to a 15 mL screw-cap tube, add 0.3 mL methyl iodide and vortex for 30 seconds.

2. Add 5 mL extraction fluid and mix by gentle inversion for 10 min. Centrifuge to separate layers.
3. Transfer approximately 4 mL of the organic phase to a 5 mL Reacti-Vial (Pierce Chemical). Concentrate the extract to about 40 μL under a stream of nitrogen.
4. Inject 2 μL of the concentrated extract into the gas chromatograph.

	Retention time (min)
DDC derivative	2.5
internal standard	5.2

Calculation:

Calculation is based on a standard curve. Due to the instability of diethyldithiocarbamate in aqueous solution this procedure cannot be controlled by the usual methods.

Evaluation:

Sensitivity: 0.2 mg/L
Linearity: the calibration curve for this assay is nonlinear
C.V.: 10.5%
Relative recovery: not established

Interferences:

Diethyldithiocarbamate added to human plasma has a half-life of about 70 minutes, and therefore patient specimens must be analyzed immediately after drawing. Other drugs have not been tested for interference with this procedure.

Reference:

J. Cobby, M. Mayersohn and S. Selliah. The rapid reduction of disulfiram in blood and plasma. J. Pharm. Exp. Ther. 202: 724–731, 1977.

Urine Diethyldithiocarbamate by Atomic Absorption Spectrometry

Principle:

Diethyldithiocarbamate in urine is complexed by addition of an excess of cupric ion. The copper chelate is extracted with an organic solvent and analyzed by atomic absorption spectrometry.

Reagents:

Stock solution – 1 mg/mL diethyldithiocarbamate in methanol (prepared fresh from the sodium salt)
Urine standards – 1, 2, 5 and 10 mg/L (prepared fresh and analyzed rapidly)
Copper solution – saturated $CuSO_4$
Phthalate buffer – saturated potassium hydrogen phthalate
Carbon tetrachloride

Instrumental Conditions:

Atomic absorption spectrophotometer with graphite furnace
Copper hollow cathode lamp
Furnace program: dry 15 sec at 100°C.

char 15 sec at 550°C.

atomize 7 sec at 2450°C.

Measure absorption at 324.5 nm

Procedure:

1. Transfer 2 mL urine to a 15 mL centrifuge tube. Add 50 µL copper solution and 1 mL phthalate buffer and vortex.
2. Add 2 mL CCl$_4$ and vortex for 1 min. Centrifuge to separate layers and discard aqueous layer.
3. Inject 50 µL of the organic layer into the graphite furnace and begin temperature program.

Calculation:

Calculation is based on a response factor derived from a standard curve. Due to the instability of diethldithiocarbamate in aqueous solution, this procedure cannot be controlled by the usual methods.

Evaluation:

Sensitivity: 0.5 mg/L
Linearity: 1–10 mg/L
C.V.: 7%
Relative recovery: not established

Interferences:

Diethyldithiocarbamate degrades readily in aqueous solution, especially under acidic conditions, and therefore patient specimens must be analyzed as soon as possible after sampling. Other metals (such as arsenic, iron, lead, mercury, nickel or thallium) that form stable chelates with diethyldithiocarbamate and that are present in substantial concentrations in urine will cause spuriously low results by this procedure.

Reference:

F.K. Martens and A. Heyndrickx. Analysis of sodium diethyldithiocarbamate (NaDEDC), a metabolite of tetraethylthiuramdisulfide (TETD) in human serum and urine. J. Analyt. Tox. 2: 269–274, 1978.

ETHCHLORVYNOL

Plasma Concentrations (mg/L)		
Therapeutic	Toxic	T½
2–8	20–135	1 hr

Ethchlorvynol is a frequently used sedative-hypnotic that is addressed in various procedures in this volume: Acid and Neutral Drug Screen by Thin-Layer Chromatography, Acid and Neutral Drug Screen by Liquid Chromatography, and Trichloroethanol and Ethchlorvynol by Gas Chromatography (the latter procedure being presented under the section on Chloral Hydrate). However, those analysts wishing to perform a quantitative analysis without resorting to chromatographic methods will find the presently described colorimetric technique convenient and reliable. Due to the cross-reactivity with ethchlorvynol metabolites in urine, the assay is best performed on plasma.

Plasma Ethchlorvynol By Colorimetry

Principle:
A protein-free supernatant is prepared from plasma or serum and is allowed to react with diphenylamine-sulfuric acid reagent. The ethchlorvynol chromogen is extracted into chloroform and its absorbance is measured in a spectrophotometer at 524 nm.

Reagents:
Stock solution – 1 mg/mL ethchlorvynol in methanol
Plasma standards – 5, 10, 20 and 30 mg/L
10% Trichloroacetic acid
Color reagent – 0.2 g diphenylamine in 50 mL conc. sulfuric acid, diluted to 100 mL with water (stable in refrigerator for 3 months)
Chloroform

Instrumental Conditions:
Visible spectrophotometer set to 524 nm

Procedure:
1. Add 3.5 mL cold 10% trichloroacetic acid to 0.5 mL plasma in a 15 mL centrifuge tube.
2. Decant the clear supernatant to a clean tube. Add 3 mL color reagent, vortex and let stand 5 min.
3. Add 3 mL chloroform and vortex for 30 seconds. Centrifuge to separate layers.
4. Discard the upper aqueous layer. Transfer the chloroform layer to a cuvette and read against a plasma blank in the spectrophotometer at 524 nm.

117

Calculation:

Calculation is based on a response factor derived from a standard curve. A quality control specimen containing 20 mg/L ethchlorvynol is analyzed daily.

Evaluation:

Sensitivity: 1 mg/L
Linearity: 1–35 mg/L
C.V.: 1.6% within-run
Relative recovery: not established

Interferences:

No other drugs have been found to interfere with this procedure. Ethchlorvynol metabolites will cause significant interference if the method is performed on urine specimens.

Reference:

P. Haux. Ethchlorvynol (Placidyl) estimation in urine and serum. Clin. Chim. Acta 43: 139–141, 1973.

ETHYLENE GLYCOL

Concentrations in Fatal Intoxication (mg/L)

Blood	Urine
300–4300	600–10,000

Ethylene glycol is a clear, odorless liquid that is a principle component of automotive antifreeze. Its sporific effects lead to its occasional abuse by persons unaware of its severe toxic effects. Either plasma or urine may be utilized in this convenient gas chromatographic technique in the clinical assessment of intoxication by ethylene glycol.

Determination of oxalic acid, a minor metabolite of ethylene glycol, is sometimes requested when ethylene glycol ingestion is suspected. A procedure for this substance is presented on p. 208.

Plasma And Urine Ethylene Glycol By Gas Chromatography

Principle:
Plasma or urine is diluted with an equal volume of water containing propylene glycol as an internal standard. An aliquot is analyzed directly by flame-ionization gas chromatography using a Porapak P column.

Reagents:
Stock solution – 10 mg/mL ethylene glycol in water
Aqueous standards – 50, 100, 200 and 400 mg/L
Internal standard solution – 200 mg/L propylene glycol in water

Instrumental Conditions:
Gas chromatograph with flame-ionization detector
2 m × 2 mm i.d. glass column containing 80/100 mesh Porapak P (Tenax-GC is also suitable as a packing material)
Injector, 220°C.; column, 180°C.; detector, 230°C.
Nitrogen flow rate, 40 mL/min.

Procedure:
1. To 1 mL plasma or urine in a 15 mL centrifuge tube add 1 mL internal standard solution and vortex. (Smaller volumes of specimen may be used if desired; reduce volume of internal standard solution accordingly.)

119

2. Inject 1 μL of the mixture into the gas chromatograph.

	Retention time (min)
ethylene glycol	3
internal standard	5

Calculation:

Calculation is based on a response factor derived from a standard curve. Ethylene glycol has been shown to be unstable in biological fluids and therefore the usual control procedures are not applicable.

Evaluation:

Sensitivity: 10 mg/L
Linearity: 50–400 mg/L
C.V.: not established
Relative recovery: not established

Interferences:

Other common volatile substances do not interfere with this procedure. Since propylene glycol is a minor component of biological systems and is present in certain commercial products, it is advisable to perform one analysis using only water as diluent to rule out the presence of this compound. Alternatively, diethylene glycol may be used as internal standard. Porapak Q has been recommended as a chromatographic support for ethylene glycol determination, but the high column temperature required may cause deterioration of the support after several weeks of operation. The use of Porapak P allows performance of the assay at lower temperatures.

References:

1. J.A. Kay, T.J. Siek and D.T. Teitelbaum. A rapid, non-extractive method for determination of ethylene glycol in biological fluids. Presented at the 31st annual meeting of the American Academy of Forensic Sciences, Atlanta, February 16, 1979.
2. C. Winek. Ethylene glycol poisoning. Presented at the 27th annual meeting of the American Academy of Forensic Sciences, Chicago, February 19, 1975.

FENOPROFEN

Therapeutic Plasma Concentrations (mg/L)	T½
20–65	2.5 hr

Fenoprofen is a non-narcotic analgesic that is administered in single oral doses of 300–600 mg; chronic therapy for rheumatoid arthritis may require doses of 2400–3400 mg daily. Therapeutic monitoring of fenoprofen plasma concentrations may be performed using a convenient gas chromatographic procedure. A liquid chromatographic method applicable to fenoprofen determination is described in the section on ibuprofen.

Plasma Fenoprofen by Gas Chromatography

Principle:
Fenoprofen and an internal standard are extracted from acidified plasma into hexane. After several partitioning steps the drug is converted to a trimethylsilyl ester and is assayed by flame-ionization gas chromatography.

Reagents:
Stock solution – 1 mg/mL fenoprofen in water
Plasma standards – 10, 20, 40 and 80 mg/L
Internal standard – 3 mg 2-(4-phenoxyphenyl)valeric acid (Eli Lilly and Co.) in 10 mL chloroform
10% Trichloroacetic acid
Hexane
0.1 mol/L Sodium hydroxide
Acetic acid
Derivatizing reagent – hexamethyldisilazane/carbon disulfide, 1:20 by volume

Instrumental Conditions:
Gas chromatograph with flame-ionization detector
0.9 m × 3 mm i.d. glass column containing 3.8% UCCW-982 on 80/100 mesh Diatoport-S
Injector, 220°C.; column, 175°C.; detector, 220°C.
Helium flow rate, 90 mL/min

Procedure:
1. Transfer 1 mL plasma to a 15 mL screw-cap tube. Add 50 µL internal standard and vortex.

2. Add 2 mL 10% trichloroacetic acid, vortex and allow to stand 10 min. Add 10 mL hexane and shake for 2 min.
3. Centrifuge to separate layers and transfer the upper organic layer to a clean tube. Add 4 mL 0.1 mol/L NaOH and shake for 2 min.
4. Centrifuge to separate layers and discard upper organic phase. Add 1.2 mL glacial acetic acid to the aqueous phase and re-extract with 8 mL hexane.
5. Transfer the hexane layer to a centrifuge tube and evaporate to dryness at 50°C. under a stream of nitrogen. Rinse the walls of the tube with 0.5 mL hexane and again evaporate to dryness.
6. Add 20 μL derivatizing reagent, sonicate for 30 seconds and inject 1 μL into the gas chromatograph.

	Retention time (min)
fenoprofen	4
internal standard	8.5

Calculation:

Calculation is based on a response factor derived from a standard curve. A quality control specimen containing 40 mg/L fenoprofen is analyzed daily.

Evaluation:

Sensitivity: 0.25 mg/L
Linearity: 10–80 mg/L
C.V.: 6–12%
Relative recovery: 95–102%

Interferences:

Normal plasma components do not interfere with the assay. Other drugs have not been checked for possible interference.

Reference:

J.F. Nash, R.J. Bopp and A. Rubin. GLC determination of dl-2-(3-phenoxyphenyl)propionic acid (fenoprofen) in human plasma. J. Pharm. Sci. 60: 1062–1064, 1971.

FLUORIDE

Normal Fluoride Concentrations (mg/L)	
Plasma	Urine
0.01–0.20	0.2–1.1

Fluoride is a trace element that is present in all human tissues. It is present in most water supplies, is added to many dentifrices and may be administered orally to children to prevent tooth decay and to adults for treatment of osteoporosis. Poisoning may occur as a result of accidental ingestion of pharmaceutical preparations, exposure to commercial fluoride-containing pesticides, or industrial accidents.

The following ion-specific electrode technique offers a convenient method for the direct determination of ionic fluoride in plasma and urine. A gas chromatographic procedure is included as a more specific and sensitive alternative.

Plasma and Urine Fluoride by Ion-Specific Potentiometry

Principle:
Plasma and urine specimens are diluted with a pH 5 buffer solution. Ionic fluoride is determined by direct ion-specific electrode potentiometry.

Reagents:
Stock solution – 100 mg/L fluoride (dissolve 221 mg NaF in one liter of water, store in a polyethylene container)
Aqueous standards – 0.01, 0.05, 0.10 and 0.20 mg/L (prepared fresh in buffer solution)
Buffer solution – dissolve 6.4 g NaCl in 1 L 0.05 mol/L pH 5.0 acetate buffer (store in a polyethylene container)

Instrumental Conditions:
Digital pH meter (Orion Research model 801) with fluoride-specific electrode (Orion Research model 94–09) and KCl reference electrode (Corning Glass Works)

Procedure:
1. Plasma: Dilute 1 mL plasma with 1 mL buffer solution.
   Urine: Dilute 1 mL urine with 9 mL buffer solution.
2. Place the electrode into the solution and allow 30 min equilibration prior to recording the ion potential.

Calculation:

Calculation is based on a response factor derived from a standard curve. Multiply urine values by 5 to correct for the additional dilution.

Evaluation:

Sensitivity: 0.01 mg/L
Linearity: 0.01–0.20 mg/L
C.V.: 5.6% within-run
Relative recovery: average 97%

Interferences:

Fluoride contamination by chemicals, water and glassware may be minimized by using high-purity reagents and polyethylene containers. Specimen containers should be checked for contamination by adding a volume of the buffer solution to the containers, allowing equilibration for several hours and analyzing the solutions for fluoride. Total fluoride concentrations in both plasma and urine are approximately twice those of ionic fluoride, which is measured by this technique; total fluoride may be determined by first treating specimens with an equal volume of 1 mol/L perchloric acid and heating at 100°C. for 15 min prior to following this procedure.

References:

1. L. Singer and R.H. Ophaug. Concentrations of ionic, total, and bound fluoride in plasma. Clin. Chem. 25: 523–525, 1979.
2. A.A. Cernik, J.A. Cooke and R.J. Hall. Specific ion electrode in the determination of urinary fluoride. Nature 227: 1260–1261, 1970.

Plasma and Urine Fluoride by Gas Chromatography

Principle:

Trimethylchlorosilane reacts with water and inorganic fluoride to form trimethylfluorosilane. This organic fluoride compound is extracted into benzene and measured by flame-ionization gas chromatography, using isopentane as internal standard.

Reagents:

Stock solution – 1 mg/mL fluoride in water (2.21 g NaF/L)
Aqueous standards – 0.01, 0.05, 0.10 and 0.20 mg/L for plasma determinations; 0.1, 0.5, 1.0, and 2.0 mg/L for urine determinations
25% Hydrochloric acid
Extraction solvent – 100 mL benzene containing approximately 60 mg trimethychlorosilane and approximately 0.35 mg isopentane

Instrumental Conditions:

Gas chromatograph with flame-ionization detector
2 m × 2 mm i.d. glass column containing 20% DC 200/50 on Chromosorb P
Injector, 130°C.; column, 75°C.; detector, 130°C.
Nitrogen flow rate, 20 mL/min

Procedure:

1. Transfer 2 mL plasma or urine to a stoppered polyethylene centrifuge tube. Add 1 mL 25% HCl and 1 mL extraction solvent and shake mechanically for 30 seconds.
2. Allow layers to settle (centrifuge if necessary) and inject 1–3 µL of the upper organic layer into the gas chromatograph. Wait 10–15 min after each injection for the recorder pen to return to baseline following the elution of the solvent (benzene).

	Retention time (min)
fluoride (as trimethylfluorosilane)	65
internal standard (isopentane)	90
solvent (benzene)	120

Calculation:

Calculation is based on a response factor derived from a standard curve. Aqueous standards of the proper concentration range, as well as aqueous blanks, must be analyzed with each set of specimens.

Evaluation:

Sensitivity: 0.01 mg/L
Linearity: 0.01–10 mg/L
C.V.: 3.4% within-run
Relative recovery: not established

Interferences:

No interferences have been observed. The use of glassware is avoided during the extraction to minimize contamination by fluoride.

Reference:

J.A. Fresen, F.H. Cox and M.J. Witter. The determination of fluoride in biological materials by means of gas chromatography. Pharm. Weekblad 103: 909–914, 1968.

FLUOROCARBONS

| | Fluorocarbon Blood Concentrations (mg/L) | |
	After Asthmatic Inhaler Use	Fatalities
fluorocarbon 11	0.5–4.5	1.2–32
fluorocarbon 12	0.2–4.7	0.6–12

The fluorocarbons have found widespread usage as refrigerants and aerosol propellants. The latter application has diminished due to legislation intended to restrict the release of these materials into the atmosphere. A number of hygienic and pharmaceutical products, such as bronchodilator drugs, are administered as fluorocarbon-propelled aerosols and thus many persons are exposed to relatively high concentrations of the chemicals. Episodes of toxicity caused by exposure to fluorocarbons, however, almost always are a result of the deliberate inhalation of commercial products by teenagers seeking a euphoric response.

Due to the high volatility and the short biologic half-life of the compounds (90% of a dose is exhaled within one hour), specimens for analysis must be drawn quickly after exposure and stored properly. A gas chromatographic method is presented that has adequate sensitivity for determination of blood concentrations of fluorocarbons at the levels shown above.

Blood Fluorocarbons by Gas Chromatography

Principle:
A sample of blood is placed into a sealed vessel at room temperature. After equilibration, a headspace sample is analyzed by flame-ionization gas chromatography.

Reagents:
Stock solution – bubble a small amount (10–30 mg) of fluorocarbon 11 or 12 (DuPont) through 10.0 mL of cyclohexane that has been preweighed in a 10 mL volumetric flask. Reweigh to calculate the concentration of the stock solution (prepare fresh)

Aqueous standards – add sufficient cyclohexane stock solution to 5 mL of water in a 30 mL serum bottle to produce fluorocarbon concentrations of 0.1, 0.5, 2.0 and 5.0 mg/L

Instrumental Conditions:
Gas chromatograph with flame-ionization detector
6′ × 1/8″ o.d. stainless steel column containing 0.2% Carbowax 1500 on Carbopack C
Injector, 200°C.; column, 125°C.; detector, 200°C.
Nitrogen flow rate, 17 mL/min

Procedure:

1. Introduce 5.0 mL of whole blood into a 30 mL serum bottle. Cap using aluminum foil over rubber septum.
2. Allow samples to equilibrate for 30 min at room temperature and then inject 1.0 mL headspace into the gas chromatograph using a 2 mL glass syringe and a 23 gauge metal needle.

	Retention time (min)
fluorocarbon 12 (CCl_2F_2)	0.7
fluorocarbon 11 (CCl_3F)	1.3
cyclohexane	3.2

Calculation:

Prepare a standard curve of peak height versus concentration of the aqueous standards. Determine the specimen concentration from this curve.

Evaluation:

Sensitivity: 0.1 mg/L
Linearity: 0.1–5.0 mg/L
C.V.: not established
Relative recovery: not established

Interferences:

Normal blood components do not interfere in the assay. To avoid losses of the volatile fluorocarbons, analyze specimens as soon as possible (or maintain in a frozen state prior to analysis), minimize contact with plastic and rubber, and keep containers tightly capped during sample manipulations.

References:

1. J.C. Standefer. Death associated with fluorocarbon inhalation: report of a case. J. For. Sci. 20: 548–551, 1975.
2. R.C. Baselt and R.H. Cravey. A fatal case involving trichloromonofluoromethane and dichlorodifluoromethane. J. For. Sci. 13: 407–410, 1968.

GENTAMICIN

Plasma Concentrations (mg/L)		
Therapeutic	Toxic	T½
3–8	>10	2 h

Gentamicin is a frequently used and a frequently assayed aminoglycoside antibiotic. Reagents are commercially available for determination of the drug in plasma by radioimmunoassay, EMIT and fluorescence immunochemical detection, but occasionally it may be necessary to use a technique with more specificity for the individual gentamicin components. The following liquid chromatographic method allows separation of the gentamicin complex and quantitation of individual components.

Serum Gentamicin by Liquid Chromatography

Principle:
The gentamicin complex is isolated from serum using an ion-exchange column. The eluate is analyzed by reversed-phase ion-pair liquid chromatography. Post-column derivatization is performed and detection is by fluorescent emission.

Reagents:
Stock solution – 1 mg/mL gentamicin in 0.1 mol/L pH 8.0 phosphate buffer (stored at −20°C.)

Serum standards – 1, 2, 5 and 10 mg/L (prepared fresh)

Sephadex column – 1.5 cm column (bed volume of 1 mL) containing CM-Sephadex (C-25)

Eluting buffer – 0.01 mol/L NaOH in 0.2 mol/L Na_2SO_4

Mobile phase – 97:3 water/methanol mixture containing 0.2 mol/L Na_2SO_4, 0.02 mol/L sodium pentanesulfonate and 0.1% acetic acid

Borate buffer – dissolve 24.7 g boric acid in 900 mL water, add conc. KOH to pH 10.4 and dilute to 1000 mL with water

OPA solution – dissolve 60 mg o-phthalaldehyde in 1 mL methanol, add 0.2 mL 2-mercaptoethanol and mix until decolorization occurs; add 100 mL borate buffer with vigorous stirring (use within 2 days)

Instrumental Conditions:
Liquid chromatograph with 418 nm fluorescence detector (excitation at 340 nm)

30 cm × 3.9 mm i.d. stainless steel μBondapak C_{18} column (Waters Associates)

4.3 cm × 4.2 mm i.d. 5 μm Micropart C_{18} precolumn (Applied Science Labs)

Solvent flow rate, 2 mL/min

Postcolumn derivatization performed via a mixing tee and a 2 m × 0.6 mm i.d. Teflon delay tube inserted between the column and the detector; OPA solution is delivered to the mixing tee from a pressurized glass vessel at a rate of 0.5 mL/min

Procedure:

1. Apply 400 μL serum to the Sephadex column. Add 1 mL and then 4 mL 0.2 mol/L Na_2SO_4.
2. Add 600 μL of the eluting buffer and allow column to drain. Add an additional 400 μL of the eluting buffer and collect the eluate. Inject 15 μL of this fraction into the chromatograph.

Gentamicin component	Retention time (min)
C_{1a}	3.0
C_2	4.4
C_1	6.0

Calculation:

Perform duplicate injections of the serum standards and calculate the average of the sum of the component peak heights for each. Prepare a standard curve of peak heights versus concentration and determine the specimen concentration from this curve.

Evaluation:

Sensitivity: 1 mg/1
Linearity: 1–10 mg/L
C.V.: not established
Relative recovery: 95–104%

Interferences:

Normal serum was free of interfering substances. Other aminoglycoside antibiotics may also be detected by this procedure and should be checked for interference.

Reference:

J.P. Anhalt. Assay of gentamicin in serum by high-pressure liquid chromatography. Animicrob. Agents Chemother. 11: 651–655, 1977.

GOLD

Therapeutic Serum Concentrations (mg/L)	T½
3–8	5–6 days

Monovalent gold compounds, such as aurothiomalate and aurothioglucose, are administered by intramuscular injection for the treatment of rheumatoid arthritis. Doses are generally given every one to four weeks, and the best therapeutic results are obtained when serum concentrations of gold exceed 3 mg/L.

A flame atomic absorption spectrophotometric technique is described that is based on direct introduction of diluted serum into the instrument.

Serum Gold by Atomic Absorption Spectrometry

Principle:
Serum is diluted fourfold with water and analyzed by flame atomic absorption spectrometry, with detection at 242.8 nm.

Reagents:
Stock solution – 1 mg/mL gold ion in water
Serum standards – 1, 2, 5 and 10 mg/L

Instrumental Conditions:
Atomic absorption spectrometer with air-acetylene reducing flame
Gold hollow cathode lamp
Measure absorption at 242.8 nm

Procedure:
1. Dilute 1 mL serum to 4 mL with water and vortex. Treat serum standards and a negative control serum in the same manner.
2. Aspirate the solution into the flame of the atomic absorption spectrometer.

Calculation:
Calculation is based on a response factor derived from a standard curve. A quality control specimen containing 4 mg/L gold ion is analyzed daily.

Evaluation:
Sensitivity: 0.1 mg/L
Linearity: 1–10 mg/L

C.V.: 3.2% day-to-day
Relative recovery: not established

Interferences:

None observed. Normal serum does not contain detectable amounts of gold by this technique.

Reference:

J.V. Dunckley. Estimation of gold in serum by atomic absorption spectroscopy. Clin. Chem. 17: 992–993, 1971.

HALOPERIDOL

Therapeutic Plasma Concentrations (mg/L)	T½
0.006–0.245	14–41 hr

Haloperidol is a butyrophenone derivative that is used as an antipsychotic drug. Therapeutic plasma concentrations are quite low and very sensitive techniques must be used for assay of the drug. Radioimmunoassay has been used experimentally but is not commercially available. The following procedure employs gas chromatography with nitrogen-specific detection for the analysis of this drug.

Plasma Haloperidol by Nitrogen-Specific Gas Chromatography

Principle:
Haloperidol and an internal standard are extracted from alkalinized plasma with ether. After several purification steps, the drugs are analyzed by gas chromatography using nitrogen-selective detection.

Reagents:
Stock solution – 1 mg/mL haloperidol in methanol
Plasma standards – 1, 5, 10, 20 and 50 μg/L
Internal standard – 1 mg/L azaperone (Janssen Pharmaceuticals) in acetone
2 mol/L Sodium hydroxide
Ether
0.2 mol/L Hydrochloric acid
Acetone

Instrumental Conditions:
Gas chromatograph with nitrogen-phosphorus detector
2 m × 4 mm i.d. glass column containing 3% OV-17 on 80/100 mesh Chromosorb W
Injector, 300°C.; column, 285°C.; detector, 300°C.
Flow rates: helium carrier, 60 mL/min; air, 60 mL/min; hydrogen, 3 mL/min

Procedure:
1. Transfer 2 mL plasma to a 15 mL screw-cap tube. Add 10 μL internal standard, 2 mL water and 200 μL 2 mol/L NaOH.
2. Extract with 5 mL ether by shaking for 10 seconds. Centrifuge and transfer the ether phase to a clean tube.

132

3. Add 2.5 mL 0.2 mol/L HCl and shake for 10 seconds. Centrifuge and discard the ether phase.
4. Add 300 μL 2 mol/L NaOH to the aqueous layer. Extract with 5 mL ether by shaking for 10 seconds.
5. Centrifuge and transfer the ether layer to a 5 mL conical centrifuge tube. Evaporate to dryness at 40°C. under a stream of nitrogen.
6. Dissolve the residue in 300 μL acetone, vortex and evaporate to a volume of 5–10 μL under a stream of nitrogen.
7. Inject the entire extract into the gas chromatograph.

	Retention time (min)
internal standard	4
haloperidol	7

Calculation:

Calculation is based on a response factor derived from a standard curve. A quality control specimen containing 20 μg/L haloperidol is analyzed daily.

Evaluation:

Sensitivity: 1 μg/L
Linearity: 2.5–50 μg/L
C.V.: 3–6%
Relative recovery: 94–104%

Interferences:

Normal plasma components did not interfere with the assay. Other drugs such as the tricyclic antidepressants, phenothiazines and benzodiazepines were found not to interfere.

Reference:

G. Bianchetti and P.L. Morselli. Rapid and sensitive method for determination of haloperidol in human samples using nitrogen-phosphorus selective detection. J. Chromatog. 153: 203–209, 1978.

HEXACHLOROPHENE

Blood Concentrations (mg/L)

Normal Adults	Users of Hexachlorophene Soap
0–0.089	0.100–0.655

Hexachlorophene is a contact antibacterial agent that has been used extensively in various commercial cosmetic and hygienic products. Many of the consumer porducts have been removed from the market following awareness of the accumulation of the chemical in chronic users. Hexachlorophene soaps and antiseptic solutions remain in use in hospitals, however, and toxicity may occur when these substances are applied frequently to burned or abraded skin.

A gas chromatographic procedure utilizing electron-capture detection is described for the measurement of trace amount of hexachlorophene in blood.

Blood Hexachlorophene by Electron-Capture Gas Chromatography

Principle:
Hexachlorophene and an internal standard are extracted from blood with an organic solvent and derivatized with acetic anhydride. The acetyl esters are analyzed by electron-capture gas chromatography.

Reagents:
Stock solution – 1 mg/mL hexachlorophene in methanol
Blood standards – 0.05, 0.10, 0.20 and 0.50 mg/L
Internal standard – 4 mg/L dichlorophene (Aldrich Chemical Co.) in methanol
Extraction solvent – ether/ethanol, 3:1 by volume
Hexane
Derivatization mixture – acetic anhydride, 1:1 by volume

Instrumental Conditions:
Gas chromatograph with electron-capture detector
0.5 m × 2 mm i.d. glass column containing 3% OV-225 on 80/100 mesh Supelcoport
Injector, 275°C.; detector, 300°C.
Nitrogen flow rate, 35 mL/min

Procedure:
1. Transfer 2 mL blood to a 15 mL screw-cap tube. Add 100 µL internal standard and 2 mL water and vortex.

2. Add 10 mL extraction solvent and shake for 3 min. Centrifuge and transfer the upper solvent layer to a 15 mL centrifuge tube.
3. Evaporate the solvent to dryness under a stream of air at 40°C.
4. Add 200 µL hexane and 30 µL derivatization mixture to the residue and heat for 10 min at 60°C.
5. Adjust the volume to approximately 300 µL with hexane, vortex and inject 3 µL into the gas chromatograph.

	Retention time (min)
internal standard diacetate	1.8
hexachlorophene diacetate	4.0

Calculation:

Calculation is based on a response factor derived from a standard curve.

Evaluation:

Sensitivity: 0.010 mg/L
Linearity: 0.05–0.50 mg/L
C.V.: not established
Relative recovery: not established

Interferences:

Blood from unexposed subjects was shown to be free of interfering substances. Other drugs and chemicals have not been studied for possible interference.

References:

1. B. Calesnick, C.H. Costello, J.P. Ryan and G.J. DiGregorio. Percutaneous absorption of hexachlorophene following daily whole body washings. Tox. Appl. Pharm. 32: 204–211, 1975.
2. W.E. Dodson, E.E. Tyrala and R.E. Hillman. Micromethod for measuring hexachlorophene in whole blood by gas-liquid chromatography. Clin. Chem. 23: 944–947, 1977.

IBUPROFEN

Ibuprofen is a nonnarcotic analgesic that is structurally related to fenoprofen. Doses of 300–400 mg are administered orally three or four times daily. A gas chromatographic procedure is described that allows determination of ibuprofen following its derivatization to a less polar compound. A less demanding liquid chromatographic method, applicable as well to some analogues of ibuprofen, is also presented.

Plasma Ibuprofen by Gas Chromatography

Principle:
Ibuprofen is extracted from acidified plasma with benzene. Following conversion to a methyl ester via imidazole formation, the drug is analyzed by flame-ionization gas chromatography. Naphthalene is used as internal standard.

Reagents:
Stock solution – 1 mg/mL ibuprofen in methanol
Plasma standards – 10, 20, 40 and 60 mg/L
1 mol/L Hydrochloric acid
Benzene
Chloroform (hydrocarbon-stabilized)
Imidazole reagent – 65 mg/mL 1,1'-carbonyldiimidazole (Aldrich) and 100 µg/mL naphthalene in chloroform (stable for 2 days)
Derivatization reagent – 10% triethylamine in methanol (v/v)
1 mol/L Sodium hydroxide

Instrumental Conditions:
Gas chromatograph with flame-ionization detector
1.8 m × 2 mm i.d. glass column containing 6% diethylene glycol succinate on 80/100 mesh Diatoport S (or Gas Chrom Q)
Injector, 190°C.; column, 150°C.; detector, 210°C.
Helium flow rate, 60 mL/min

Procedure:
1. Transfer 1 mL plasma to a 15 mL screw-cap tube. Add 0.25 1 mol/L HCl and 5 mL benzene and extract for 10 min.

2. Centrifuge and transfer 4 mL of the benzene layer to a 5 mL glass-stoppered centrifuge tube. Evaporate to dryness under a stream of nitrogen.
3. Wash down the walls of the tube with 0.5 mL chloroform and evaporate to dryness. Add 100 μL imidazole reagent, vortex and allow to stand for 1 min.
4. Add 100 μL derivatizing reagent, vortex and allow to stand for 5 min. Add 1 mL 1 mol/L NaOH and shake vigorously.
5. Centrifuge and inject 1 μL of the organic layer into the gas chromatograph.

	Retention time (min)
internal standard	3.4
ibuprofen methyl ester	6.8

Calculation:

Calculation is based on a response factor derived from a standard curve. A quality control specimen containing 40 mg/L ibuprofen is analyzed daily.

Evaluation:

Sensitivity: 0.5 mg/L
Linearity: 1–80 mg/L
C.V.: not established
Relative recovery: 88–107%

Interferences:

Normal plasma components do not interfere. Other drugs were not studied for possible interference.

Reference:

D.G. Kaiser and G.J. Van Giessen. GLC determination of ibuprofen [(±)-2-(p-isobutylphenyl)propionic acid] in plasma. J. Pharm. Sci. 63: 219–221, 1974.

Serum Ibuprofen and Analogues by Liquid Chromatography

Principle:

The drugs and an internal standard, phenolphthalein, are extracted from acidified serum with dichloromethane. The evaporated solvent extract is reconstituted in acetonitrile and analyzed by liquid chromatography with ultraviolet detection at 240 nm.

Reagents:

Stock solutions – 1 mg/mL methanol solutions of fenoprofen, ibuprofen, naproxen and tolmetin
Serum standards – 10, 25, 50 and 100 mg/L for each drug
Internal standard – 250 mg/L phenolphthalein in water
1 mol/L Hydrochloric acid
Dichloromethane

Acetonitrile
Mobile phase – acetonitrile/water/glacial acetic acid, 450:550:3.2 by volume

Instrumental Conditions:

Liquid chromatograph with 240 nm absorbance detector
15 cm × 4.6 mm i.d. 5 micron C-18 column (Altex)
Solvent flow rate, 2.0 mL/min
Column temperature, ambient

Procedure:

1. Transfer 0.5 mL serum to a 15 mL screw-cap tube. Add 50 µl internal standard and 0.5 mL 1 mol/L HCl and vortex. Add 10 mL dichloromethane and place on a rotator for 10 minutes.
2. Centrifuge to separate layers and discard the upper aqueous phase. Filter the organic layer through Whatman #1 filter paper into a 12 mL conical centrifuge tube.
3. Evaporate the solvent to dryness at 40°C under a stream of nitrogen. Dissolve the residue in 200 µL of acetonitrile and inject 20 µL into the chromatograph.

	Retention time (min)
internal standard	2.0
tolmetin	2.8
naproxen	3.4
fenoprofen	5.4
ibuprofen	8.9

Calculation:

Calculation is based on a response factor derived from a standard curve. A quality control specimen containing 50 mg/L of each drug is analyzed daily.

Evaluation:

Sensitivity: 5–10 mg/L
Linearity: 10–200 mg/L
C.V.: 1.8–5.2% within-day
Relative recovery: not established

Interferences:

Some other anti-inflammatory agents are isolated by this procedure and may interfere with the analysis; they include salicylate (1.5 min), oxyphenbutazone (3.3 min), indomethacin (7.5 min) and phenylbutazone (9.4 min). Salicylate does not normally interfere with measurement of the internal standard peak unless it is present at toxic concentrations, in which case changing the detection wavelength to 250 nm may alleviate the problem.

Reference:

B. Levine and Y.H. Caplan. Simultaneous liquid-chromatographic determination of five nonsteroidal anti-inflammatory drugs in plasma or blood. Clin. Chem. 31: 346–347, 1985.

INHALATION ANESTHESTICS

	Anesthetic Blood Conc. (mg/L)
chloroform	20–230
cyclopropane	80–180
enflurane	50–100
ether	500–1500
halothane	80–260
methoxyflurane	125–200
trichloroethylene	30–90

Anesthetic agents that are administered by inhalation include several gases and a number of volatile liquids. If it is necessary to monitor the blood concentrations of one of these drugs during general anesthesia, a rapid and convenient technique must be available. A gas chromatographic procedure is described that allows the rapid quantitative determination of any one of these substances by direct sample injection. Nitrous oxide cannot be measured by this method and is covered separately (see Index).

Blood Inhalation Anesthetics by Gas Chromatography

Principle:
The common inhalation anesthetic agents are analyzed by direct injection of whole blood into a gas chromatograph equipped with a flame-ionization detector and a molecular sieve column. The method is rapid and applicable to the measurement of anesthetic concentrations of these agents.

Reagents:
Blood standards – 80, 160 and 240 mg/L for cyclopropane, halothane and methoxyflurane; 500, 1000 and 1500 mg/L for ether (add measured volumes of each, representing the appropriate weights, to control blood specimens in full, sealed Vacutainer tubes)

Instrumental Conditions:
Gas chromatograph with replaceable glass injector sleeve and flame-ionization detector
0.75 m × 3 mm i.d. stainless steel column containing 0.3% diethylene glycol succinate on 60/80 mesh molecular sieve type 5A (liquid phase may be omitted with little effect on peak shape)
Injector, 200°C.; column, 120°C.; detector, 150°C.
Nitrogen flow rate, 90 mL/min

Procedure:

1. Blood is drawn anaerobically into a heparinized syringe, the needle removed and the syringe tip sealed with a rubber cap.
2. With a 5 μL direct-injection syringe (Hamilton #7105 N) draw up 0.5 μL of water. Then penetrate the rubber cap and draw up exactly 1 μL of blood.
3. Wipe off the needle of the 5 μL syringe and inject the contents into the gas chromatograph. Withdraw the needle and immediately rinse the syringe with water.

	Retention time (sce)
cyclopropane	17
halothane	23
methoxyflurane	35
ether	73

Calculation:

Calculation is based on a standard curve of peak height versus concentration of the blood standards. This procedure cannot be controlled by the usual methods due to difficulty in storage of quality control specimens containing these volatile substances.

Evaluation:

Sensitivity: 40 mg/L
Linearity: 80–240 mg/L
C.V.: 3–5% within-run
Relative recovery: 96–100%

Interferences:

The injection technique must be practiced and standardized in order to obtain consistent results. The glass insert for the injector should be replaced with a clean insert (used injectors may be cleaned by soaking in chromic acid solution overnight) after every 15–20 injections, replacing the septum at the same time. After several months of usage it may be necessary to replace the column packing in the first 1–2 cm of the column. The molecular sieve column should be reactivated by heating to 200°C. overnight after several months of use to remove absorbed water.

This procedure may be used for all of the common inhalation anesthetics. Specificity is not a problem unless several agents are being used in combination.

References:

1. T. Yokota, Y. Hitomi, K. Ohta and F. Kosaka. Direct injection method for gas chromatographic measurement of inhalation anesthetics in whole blood and tissues. Anesthesiol. 28: 1064–1073, 1967.
2. R. Baselt and C. Stewart. Unpublished results, 1976.

IRON

	Serum Concentrations (mg/L)		
	Normal Adults	Intoxicated Children	Fatally Poisoned Children
iron	0.5–1.6	2.8–25.5	18.8–50
iron-binding capacity	2.5–4.3		

Ferrous sulfate is one of the most frequently encountered agents in accidental childhood poisoning. Due to the desirability of confirming a diagnosis of iron intoxication prior to the institution of chelation therapy, a rapid means of determining the serum iron level is a necessity in clinical laboratories. Such a measurement need not be highly accurate (a serum iron of 3 mg/L or higher in a young child following ingestion of an iron salt is usually considered an indication for vigorous therapy), and the following colorimetric method offers the convenience and rapidity to fill this need, especially for smaller laboratories.

When monitoring iron status in both emergency and routine situations, it is preferable to have an accurate determination made of both total serum iron and total serum iron-binding capacity (TIBC), as an indirect means of assessing the degree of saturation of serum transferrin by iron. Two procedures are presented that are capable of these measurements, one involving visible spectrophotometry and the other, atomic absorption spectrometry.

Serum Iron by Colorimetry

Principle:
Serum iron is measured semi-quantitatively by direct addition of a chromoagenic reagent to the specimen and determination of absorbance of the purple-blue complex in a visible spectrophotometer.

Reagents:
Stock solution – 1 mg/mL iron (1 g iron wire dissolved in 10 mL conc. HC1 and diluted to 1 L with water)
Aqueous standards – 1, 2, 5 and 10 mg/L
Quality control specimen – 3 mg/L iron in water
TPT solution – 100 mg 2,4,6-tripyridyltriazine in 10 mL of 95% ethanol (stable for 6 months)
Thioglycolic acid

Instrumental Conditions:
Visible spectrophotometer set to 593 nm

Procedure:

1. Transfer 1 mL of unhemolyzed serum or plasma to an iron-free graduated centrifuge tube.
2. Add 1 drop TPT solution, 1 drop thioglycolic acid and dilute to 3 mL with water.
3. Transfer to a cuvette and read against a reagent blank at 593 nm in a visible spectrophotometer.

Evaluation:

Sensitivity: 0.5 mg/L
Linearity: 1–10 mg/L
C.V.: not established
Relative recovery: not established

Interferences:

This is a semi-quantitative procedure that is designed for emergency diagnosis only. Estimation of serum iron levels has also been performed by comparison of the treated specimen to a visual color chart to further reduce the time required, and the method has been used as a qualitative test of gastric aspirate and urine specimens. Moderate to extensive hemolysis may interfere by causing a falsely high reading.

References:

1. H.A. Cooper, M.D. Ekblad and V.F. Fairbanks. Emergency semi-quantitative estimation of plasma iron concentration. Am. J. Dis. Child. 122: 19–21, 1971.
2. D.S. Fischer and D.C. Price, A simple serum iron method using the new sensitive chromogen tripyridyl-s-triazine. Clin. Chem. 10: 21–31, 1964.

Serum Iron and TIBC by Visible Spectrophotometry

Principle:

Serum iron is allowed to react with ferrozine and the colored complex is determined by spectrophotometry. A second aliquot of serum is saturated with iron and the unbound iron is reacted with ferrozine. Iron-binding capacity is then calculated as the difference between the amount of iron added and the amount remaining unbound.

Reagents:

Stock solution – 1 mg/mL iron (Fisher reference standard)
Aqueous standards – 0.2, 0.5, 1.0, 2.0 and 4.0 mg/L
Acetate buffer – 43 g sodium acetate, 29 mL glacial acetic acid and 10 g ascorbic acid per L of water
Ferrozine reagent – 25 mg ferrozine in 10 mL water
Tris buffer – 2.423 g trishydroxymethylaminomethane and 1 g ascorbic acid per 100 mL of water
Ferrous iron solution – 52.6 mg $(NH)_4Fe(SO_4)_2.6H_2O$ per L of 0.025 mol/L acetic acid

Instrumental Conditions:

Visible spectrophotometer set to 562 nm

Procedure:

Serum iron:

1. Transfer 0.2 mL serum and 1.5 mL acetate buffer to a 1 cm cuvette. Determine the absorbance of this serum blank at 562 nm.
2. Add 0.2 mL ferrozine reagent and incubate at 45°C. for 20 min. Determine the absorbance of this solution at 562 nm and subtract the value for the serum blank.

Total iron-binding capacity:

3. Transfer 0.2 mL serum, 1.5 mL tris buffer and 0.2 mL ferrous iron solution to a 1 cm cuvette.
4. Incubate at 45°C. for 10 min and determine the absorbance of this reagent blank at nm.
5. Add 0.2 mL ferrozine reagent and incubate at 45°C. for 20 min. Determine the absorbance of this solution at 562 nm and subtract the value for the serum blank.

Calculation:

Calculation is based on a response factor derived from a standard curve for the aqueous standards. The total iron-binding capacity is determined by subtracting the concentration of unbound iron in the specimen (as measured in step 5) from the amount of iron added (7.5 mg/L). A quality control specimen consisting of pooled serum is analyzed daily.

Evaluation:

Sensitivity: 0.1 mg/L
Linearity: 0.2–4.0 mg/L
C.V.: 2.2% for serum iron, 1.2% for TIBC (within-run)
Relative recovery: 99–101%

Interferences:

Water and reagents should be free of iron contamination. Extensive hemolysis may cause inaccuracies in the determination.

References:

1. E. Horak and F.W. Sunderman, Jr. Direct spectrophotometric method for measurements of serum iron and latent iron-binding capacity. Amer. J. Clin. Path. 62: 133–134, 1974.
2. J.P. Persijin, W. van der Silk and A. Riethorst. Determination of serum iron and latent iron-binding capacity (LIBC). Clin. Chim. Acta 35: 91–98, 1971.

Serum Iron and TIBC by Atomic Absorption Spectrometry

Principle:

Serum iron is determined by flame atomic absorption spectrometry after protein precipitation with trichloroacetic acid. For the determination of total iron-binding capacity, a second aliquot of serum is saturated with ferric chloride, the excess is precipitated with magnesium carbonate, and the iron content is again assayed in a similar manner.

Reagents:

Stock solution – 1 mg/mL iron (Fisher reference standard)
Aqueous standards – 0.2, 0.5, 1.0, 2.0 and 4.0 mg/L
20% Trichloroacetic acid
Ferric chloride solution – 2.42 mg $FeCl_3.6H_2O$ in 100 mL water
Magnesium carbonate – solid $4MgCO_3.Mg(OH)_2.nH_2O$

Instrumental Conditions:

Atomic absorption spectrometer with an oxidizing air-acetylene flame
Iron hollow cathode lamp
Measure absorption at 248.3 nm

Procedure:

Serum iron:

1. Transfer 1 mL serum to a 12 × 75 mm plastic tube and add 1 mL 20% trichloroacetic acid.
2. Cool, centrifuge and aspirate the supernatant into the spectrometer. Compare to aqueous standards analyzed in the same manner.

Total iron-binding capacity:

3. Transfer 2 mL serum to a 12 × 75 mm plastic tube, add 2 mL ferric chloride solution, vortex and let stand 5 min. Treat aqueous standards in a similar manner but substitute 2 mL water for 2 mL ferric chloride.
4. Add 200 mg solid magnesium carbonate. Vortex four times during the next 30 min and centrifuge.
5. Transfer 2 mL supernatant to a clean plastic tube and add 2 mL 20% trichloroacetic acid. Heat at 90°C. for 15 min.
6. Cool, centrifuge and aspirate the supernatant into the spectrometer. Compare to aqueous standards analyzed in a like manner (substitute water for ferric chloride solution).

Calculation:

Calculation is based on a response factor derived from a standard curve for the aqueous standards. A quality control specimen consisting of pooled serum is analyzed daily.

Evaluation:

Sensitivity: 0.1 mg/L
Linearity: 0.2–4.0 mg/L
C.V.: 3.4% for serum iron, 1.9% for TIBC (day-to-day)
Relative recovery: 89–107%

Interferences:

Hemolysis to the extent of 300 mg hemoglobin per L does not significantly interfere with this procedure. Other metals do not interfere.

Reference:

A.D. Olson and W.B. Hamlin. A new method for serum iron and total iron-binding capacity by atomic absorption spectrophotometry. Clin. Chem. 15: 438–444, 1969.

ISONIAZID

Plasma Concentrations (mg/L)

Therapeutic	Toxic	T½
1–7	20–710	1–4 hr

Isoniazid (INH) is an antituberculin drug that is frequently involved in accidental and intentional poisoning. In overdosage the drug causes metabolic acidosis, hyperglycemia and severe convulsions, the latter effect being due to inhibition of gamma-aminobutyric acid (GABA) synthesis in the brain. Pyridoxine (vitamin B6) administration by intravenous injection is recognized as specific therapy for isoniazid poisoning and appears to act by stimulating GABA synthesis.

The drug is metabolized by N-acetylation and its rate of disappearance has been used as an indicator of acetylator status in man. Fast acetylators demonstrate an average isoniazid plasma half-life of 3 hours, while slow acetylators average 5 hours. The following colorimetric procedure is appropriate for the determination of toxic plasma levels of this drug.

Plasma Isoniazid by Colorimetry

Principle:
Plasma is deproteinized with metaphosphoric acid and a chromogenic reagent, nitritopentacyanoferroate, is added directly to the supernatant. The resulting color is measured at 440 nm in a visible spectrophotometer.

Reagents:
Stock solution – 1 mg/mL isoniazid in methanol
Plasma standards – 10, 20 and 50 mg/L
20% Metaphosphoric acid
2 mol/L Acetic acid
2% Sodium nitroprusside
4 mol/L Sodium hydroxide
Chromogenic reagent – equal volumes of 2% sodium nitroprusside and 4 mol/L NaOH
    (prepare fresh)

Instrumental Conditions:
Visible spectrophotometer set at 440 nm

145

Procedure:

1. Transfer 2 mL plasma to a 12 mL centrifuge tube. Add 4 mL water and 2 mL 20% metaphosphoric acid and vortex.
2. Allow to stand for 10 min. Centrifuge and transfer 4 mL of the supernatant to a clean tube.
3. Add 2 mL 2 mol/L acetic acid and 2 mL of the chromogenic reagent and vortex. After exactly 2 min, measure the absorbance against a plasma blank at 440 nm in the spectrophotometer.

Calculation:

Calculation is based on a response factor derived from a standard curve. A quality control specimen containing 20 mg/L isoniazid is analyzed daily.

Evaluation:

Sensitivity: 5 mg/L
Linearity: 10–50 mg/L
C.V.: not established
Relative recovery: not established

Interferences:

Normal plasma specimens yield an apparent isoniazid concentration of 1–2 mg/L. Other related drugs, such as iproniazid and pyrazinamide, will interfere if present. p-Aminosalicylic acid interferes only if present in very high concentrations.

Reference:

K.B. Bjornesjo and B. Jarnulf. Determination of isonicotinic acid hydrazide in blood serum. Scand. J. Clin. Lab. Invest. 20: 39–40, 1967.

KETAMINE

Anesthetic Plasma Conc. (mg/L)	T½
0.5–6.5	2–4 hr

Ketamine is an intravenous anesthetic inducing agent that is given in bolus injections of 2–4 mg/kg of body weight. Two metabolites, norketamine and dehydronorketamine, achieve lower plasma concentrations than the parent drug and their contribution to the anesthetic effects of ketamine remains to be elucidated. A gas chromatographic method is presented for the determination of ketamine in plasma, using flame-ionization detection.

Plasma Ketamine by Gas Chromatography

Principle:

Ketamine and an internal standard are extracted from alkalinized plasma into heptane. Two further extractions are performed to purify the drugs and an aliquot of the final extract is analyzed by flame-ionization gas chromatography.

Reagents:

Stock solution – 1 mg/mL ketamine in methanol
Plasma standards – 0.5, 1.0, 2.0, 4.0 and 8.0 mg/L
Internal standard – 4 mg/100 mL CL-392 (Parke-Davis) in water
Borate buffer – 2 g sodium borate dissolved in 10 mL 10 mol/L NaOH and diluted to 25 mL with water
Heptane
0.1 mol/L Hydrochloric acid
1,2-Dichloroethane

Instrumental Conditions:

Gas chromatograph with flame-ionization detector
2 m × 2 mm i.d. glass column containing 1% OV-101 on 100/120 mesh Gas Chrom Q
Injector, 210°C.; column, 158°C.; detector, 220°C.
Nitrogen flow rate, 20 mL/min

Procedure:

1. Transfer 2 mL plasma to a 15 mL screw-cap tube and add 100 µL internal standard. Vortex.
2. Add 0.3 mL borate buffer and 6 mL heptane and shake to extract. Centrifuge and transfer 5 mL of the organic layer to a 5 mL glass-stoppered centrifuge tube.

147

3. Add 0.3 mL 0.1 mol/L HCl and shake to extract. Centrifuge (after removing stopper) and discard heptane layer.
4. Add 25 μL borate buffer and 20 μL 1,2-dichloroethane. Vortex for 30 seconds and centrifuge.
5. Inject 2 μL of the lower organic layer into the gas chromatograph.

	Retention time (min)
internal standard	1.5
ketamine	3.0

Calculation:

Calculation is based on a response factor derived from a standard curve. A quality control specimen containing 2.0 mg/L ketamine is analyzed daily.

Evaluation:

Sensitivity: 0.5 mg/L
Linearity: 0.5–10 mg/L
C.V.: 3.7%
Relative recovery: not established

Interferences:

Normal plasma components do not interfere with this assay. Other drugs or ketamine metabolites were not studied for potential interference.

Reference:

B.J. Hodshon, T. Ferrer-Allado, V.L. Brechner and A.K. Cho. A gas chromatographic assay procedure for ketamine in plasma. Anesthesiol. 35: 506–508, 1972.

LEAD

Blood Concentrations (mg/L)		
Normal Adults	Intoxicated Adults	Fatal Poisoning
0.07–0.22	0.90–1.40	1.10–3.50

Humans are in a state of positive lead balance from the day of birth; a slow accumulation of this element occurs until a total body burden of up to 350 mg exists by age 60. The lead that is found in healthy adults is largely a result of environmental exposure to automobile exhaust, paints, plastics, ceramic glazes and other sources. Intoxication may occur accidentally after acute or chronic exposure to paint pigments, water from lead pipes, certain non-prescription medications or to contaminated industrial environments.

The effects of lead on heme biosynthesis form the basis for several diagnostic tests for lead poisoning, but blood lead determinations remain one of the more reliable and frequently requested assays. Chelation therapy is usually indicated when the blood lead concentration exceeds 0.80 mg/L. Two atomic absorption spectrometric techniques are included for blood lead measurement; the first is a flame technique and requires chelation and extraction of the lead, while the second, utilizing a graphite furnace, allows direct introduction of a hemolyzed specimen.

Blood Lead by Flame Atomic Absorption Spectrometry

Principle:
Lead is extracted from hemolyzed whole blood by chelation with diethyldithiocarbamate. The chelate is partitioned into methylisobutyl ketone and assayed by flame atomic absorption spectrometry.

Reagents:
Stock solution – 1 mg/mL lead (Fisher reference standard)
Aqueous standards – 0.10, 0.20, 0.40 and 0.80 mg/L (prepare fresh)
10% Trichloroacetic acid
5% Trichloroacetic acid
Bromphenol blue solution – 0.1% bromphenol blue in 95% ethanol
2.5 mol/L Sodium hydroxide
DDC solution – 1% sodium diethyldithiocarbamate in water
MIBK – methylisobutyl ketone

All glassware used in this procedure should be soaked overnight in 50% nitric acid and rinsed in distilled-deionized water

Instrumental Conditions:

Atomic absorption spectrometer with an oxidizing air-acetylene flame
Lead hollow cathode lamp
Measure absorption at 283.3 nm

Procedure:

1. Transfer 250 µL of heparinized whole blood to a 10 × 75 mm tube containing 1 mL water. Add 1 mL 10% trichloroacetic acid, vortex and let stand 45–60 min.
2. Centrifuge and decant into a 13 × 100 mm tube. Wash precipitate with 1 mL 5% trichloroacetic acid containing 1 drop bromphenol blue solution, centrifuge and add supernatant to the 13 × 100 mm tube.
3. Adjust pH of supernatant to 6.5–7.0 with approximately 0.2 mL 2.5 mol/L NaOH.
4. Add 0.2 mL DDC solution and 1 mL MIBK and vortex for 30 seconds. Centrifuge and aspirate upper MIBK layer into the flame of the spectrometer.

Calculation:

Calculation is based on a standard curve prepared each time a specimen is analyzed. This procedure cannot be controlled by the usual methods due to the difficulty in storage of whole blood lead solutions.

Evaluation:

Sensitivity: 0.05 mg/L
Linearity: 0.10–3.00 mg/L
C.V.: 1.9–9.5%
Relative recovery: 95–105%

Interferences:

Glassware and reagents should be carefully checked for lead contamination by analyzing reagent blanks. Addition of anticoagulants or preservatives other than heparin to blood specimens may cause reduced recoveries. Storage of whole blood specimens beyond several days usually results in poor recovery of lead.

Reference:

E. Berman, V. Valavanis and A. Dubin. A micromethod for determination of lead in blood. Clin. Chem. 14: 239–242, 1968.

Blood Lead by Graphite Furnace Atomic Absorption Spectrometry

Principle:

Whole blood is diluted with a surfactant and injected directly into the graphite furnace of an atomic absorption spectrometer.

Reagents:

Stock solution – 1 mg/mL lead (Fisher reference standard)

Aqueous standards – 0.10, 0.20, 0.40 and 0.80 mg/L (prepare fresh)
Surfactant solution – 0.1% Triton X-100 in water

All glassware used in this procedure should be soaked overnight in 50% nitric acid and rinsed in distilled-deionized water.

Instrumental Conditions:

Atomic absorption spectrometer with graphite furnace and deuterium background corrector
Lead hollow cathode lamp (or electrodeless discharge lamp)
Furnace program: dry 30 sec at 125°C.
                          char 40 sec at 525°C.
                          atomize 13 sec at 2000°C.
Nitrogen purge gas, 15 mL/min
Measure absorption at 283.3 nm

Procedure:

1. Transfer 50 μL heparinized whole blood to a 12 × 75 mm tube containing 200 μL surfactant solution. Rinse the pipet tip several times in the solution. Vortex.
2. Inject 15 μL of the solution into the graphite furnace and begin analysis program.

Calculation:

Calculation is based on a standard curve prepared each time a specimen is analyzed. This procedure cannot be controlled by the usual methods due to the difficulty in storage of whole blood lead solutions.

Evaluation:

Sensitivity: 0.05 mg/L
Linearity: 0.10–0.80 mg/L
C.V.: 2.4–4.1% within run
Relative recovery: 94–104%

Interferences:

Glassware and reagents should be carefully checked for lead contamination by analyzing reagent blanks. Anticoagulants other than oxalate do not interfere. Storage of whole blood specimens beyond several days usually results in poor recovery of lead.

Reference:

F.J. Fernandez. Micromethod for lead determination in whole blood by atomic absorption, with use of the graphite furnace. Clin. Chem. 21: 558–561, 1975.

LIDOCAINE

	Plasma Concentrations (mg/L)		
	Antiarrhythmic Therapy	Toxicity	T½
lidocaine	1–6	>8	44–107 min
MEGX	0.5–2	?	?

Lidocaine was originally developed as a local anesthetic, but has achieved popularity for the control of cardiac arrhythmias. The compound is often administered by constant intravenous infusion in acute situations. The primary metabolite, monoethylglycinexylidide (MEGX), has antiarrhythmic properties and may contribute to the effects of lidocaine, but is not routinely assayed in plasma.

To monitor intravenous lidocaine therapy, a procedure with a relatively short turn-around-time must be available. Such a procedure is described using flame-ionization gas chromatography. A more sensitive but more time-consuming gas chromatographic technique applicable to lidocaine assay is presented under Local Anesthetics (p. 157). Reagents are also available commercially for determination of unchanged lidocaine by EMIT and fluorescence immunoassay.

Plasma Lidocaine by Gas Chromatography

Principle:
Lidocaine and an internal standard are extracted from deproteinized plasma with a small volume of organic solvent. The extract is analyzed by flame-ionization gas chromatography.

Reagents:
Stock solution – 1 mg/mL lidocaine in methanol
Plasma standards – 1, 2, 4, 8 and 16 mg/L
Internal standard – 2 mg/L mepivacaine HCl in water
30% Trichloroacetic acid
5 mol/L Sodium hydroxide
Carbon disulfide

Instrumental Conditions:
Gas chromatograph with flame-ionization detector
1.8 m × 2 mm i.d. glass column containing 3% OV-17 on 100/120 mesh Gas Chrom Q
Injector, 240°C.; column, 210°C.; detector, 280°C.
Nitrogen flow rate, 30 mL/min

Procedure:

1. Transfer 1 mL plasma to a 12 mL centrifuge tube. Add 2 mL internal standard and 1 mL 30% trichloroacetic acid and vortex.
2. Centrifuge and transfer the supernatant to a clean tube. Add 1 mL 5 mol/L NaOH and vortex.
3. Add 100 μL carbon disulfide and vortex for 45 seconds. Centrifuge and inject 3 μL of the lower organic layer into the gas chromatograph.

	Retention time (min)
lidocaine	1.5
internal standard	3.5

Calculation:

Calculation is based on a response factor derived from a standard curve. A quality control specimen containing 4 mg/L lidocaine is analyzed daily.

Evaluation:

Sensitivity: 0.25 mg/L
Linearity: 0.5–6 mg/L
C.V.: 5.7% within-run
Relative recovery: not established

Interferences:

Normal plasma components do not interfere, although an occasional patient specimen produces a large peak eluting just after the internal standard. The lidocaine metabolites do not interfere. Other drugs have not been studied for potential interference. The internal standard, mepivacaine, is a widely used local anesthetic and will interfere if present in the patient specimen.

Reference:

B.J. Kline and M.F. Martin. Simplified GLC assay for lidocaine in plasma. J. Pharm. Sci. 67: 887–888, 1978.

LITHIUM

	Lithium Concentrations (mol/L)		
	Therapeutic	Toxic	T½
serum	0.5–1.3	>2	14–24 hr
erythrocytes	0.2–0.8	>0.8	?

Lithium carbonate is extensively used for the treatment of the manic phase of manic-depressive psychosis. The low therapeutic index of the compound requires frequent serum level monitoring. Specimens are best drawn in early morning, approximately 12 hours after the last dose.

Two convenient techniques for determination of lithium in serum involve flame photometry and atomic absorption spectrometry. The choice of one procedure over the other is primarily dependent on instrument availability. Occasionally an erythrocyte lithium determination is requested as a means of diagnosing toxicity in individuals who may accumulate lithium intracellularly. This assay may be performed by either technique on a hemolysate prepared by vortexing and centrifuging 0.5 mL of erythrocytes with 0.5 mL water and 0.1 mL chloroform.

Serum Lithium by Flame Photometry

Principle:
Serum is deproteinized with trichloroacetic acid and the supernatant is introduced into the flame photometer. The lithium signal is measured at 670.8 nm.

Reagents:
Stock solution – 1 mg/mL lithium ion (Fisher reference standard)
Serum standards – 0.2, 0.5, 1.0 and 2.0 mmol/L
20% Trichloroacetic acid

Instrumental Conditions:
Emission photometer with air-propane flame
Read emission at 670.8 nm

Procedure:
1. Transfer 2 mL serum to a 15 mL centrifuge tube. Add 4 mL water and 4 mL 20% trichloroacetic acid and vortex.
2. Allow to stand 10 min. Centrifuge and analyze the supernatant in the flame photometer.

Calculation:

Calculation is based on a response factor derived from a standard curve. A quality control specimen containing 1.0 mmol/L lithium is analyzed daily.

Evaluation:

Sensitivity: 0.04 mmol/L
Linearity: 0.2–2.0 mmol/L
C.V.: <1% within-run
Relative recovery: not established

Interferences:

Greater than physiological amounts of sodium and potassium will interfere, and thus anticoagulants containing these elements must be avoided. Standards must be prepared in pooled serum rather than water to duplicate the quenching effect of the serum specimen.

Reference:

H.J. van der Helm and D. Andriesse. The determination of lithium in serum during therapy with lithium salts. Clin. Chim. Acta 6: 747–748, 1961.

Serum and Urine Lithium by Atomic Absorption Spectrometry

Principle:

Serum and urine are diluted with water and directly analyzed by flame atomic absorption spectrometry.

Reagents:

Stock solution – 1 mg/mL lithium ion (Fisher reference standard)
Serum standards – 0.2, 0.5, 1.0 and 2.0 mmol/L
Urine standards – 1.0, 2.5, 5.0 and 10.0 mmol/L (in pooled urine or in water)

Instrumental Conditions:

Atomic absorption spectrometer with air-acetylene oxidizing flame and three slot burner
    head
Lithium hollow cathode lamp
Measure absorption at 670.8 nm

Procedure:

1. Serum: dilute 0.2 mL to 5.0 mL with water.
    Urine: dilute 0.2 mL to 25.0 mL with water
2. Aspirate diluted specimen into flame atomic absorption spectrometer.

Calculation:

Calculation is based on a response factor derived from a standard curve. A quality control specimen containing 1.0 mmol/L lithium (serum) or 5.0 mmol/L lithium (urine) is analyzed daily.

Evaluation:

Sensitivity: 0.1 mmol/L for serum and 0.5 mmol/L for urine
Linearity: 0.2–4.0 mmol/L for serum and 1–20 mmol/L for urine
C.V.: 5.3% within-run
Relative recovery: 89–112%

Interferences:

Sodium and potassium at concentrations of up to 180 and 8.0 mmol/L, respectively, did not interfere in this procedure. Clogging of the burner head by serum protein does not occur if a three slot burner head is used.

Reference:

J.L. Hansen. The measurement of serum and urine lithium by atomic absorption spectrophotometry. Amer. J. Med. Tech. 34: 1–9, 1968.

LOCAL ANESTHETICS

	Plasma Conc. (mg/L)		
	Therapeutic	Toxic	T½
bupivacaine	1–4	0138	2.6 hr
lidocaine	0.2–4	>8	0.7–1.8 hr
mepivacaine	0.2–5	>8	?
prilocaine	1–5	>8	?

The anilide local anesthetics are used in numerous minor surgical procedures, frequently in obstetrical practice. Monitoring of plasma levels may be desirable to determine the rate of absorption from the site of administration or the degree of exposure of newborn children following paracervical administration of the drugs to their mothers.

Lidocaine is also used as an antiarrhythmic agent and has been dealt with separately in a previous method (p. 152). The ester anesthetics are generally too short-lived in plasma for routine determination. A sensitive gas chromatographic procedure for measurement of low levels of four anilide local anesthetics is presented.

Plasma Local Anesthetics by Gas Chromatography

Principle:
The anilide local anesthetics are extracted from alkalinized plasma into ether. After several clean-up steps the final residue is analyzed by flame-ionization gas chromatography.

Reagents:
Stock solutions – 1 mg/mL methanol solutions of bupivacaine, lidocaine, mepivacaine and prilocaine
Plasma standards – 0.2, 0.5, 1.0, 2.0 and 4.0 mg/L of the appropriate drug
0.5 mol/L Sodium hydroxide
Ether
0.1 mol/L Hydrochloric acid
Carbon disulfide

Instrumental Conditions:
Gas chromatograph with flame-ionization detector
2 m × 2 mm i.d. glass column containing 3% OV-17 on 100/120 mesh Gas Chrom Q
Injector, 250°C.; column, 215°C.; detector, 250°C.
Nitrogen flow rate, 30 mL/min

Procedure:

1. Transfer 1 mL plasma to a 15 mL glass-stoppered centrifuge tube. Add 2 mL internal standard and 0.5 mL 0.5 mol/L NaOH and vortex.
2. Extract with 8 mL ether. Centrifuge (freeze if necessary to break emulsion) and transfer ether to a clean tube.
3. Add 1 mL 0.1 mol/L HCl and shake for 1 min. Centrifuge and discard ether layer.
4. Add 0.5 mL 0.5 mol/L NaOH and extract with 6 mL ether. Centrifuge and transfer ether to a 12 mL centrifuge tube.
5. Evaporate solvent to dryness under a stream of nitrogen at 43°C. Dissolve residue in 10–20 μL carbon disulfide and inject 5 μL into the gas chromatograph.

	Retention time (min)
prilocaine	2.6
lidocaine	2.9
internal standard	4.8
mepivacaine	6.5
bupivacaine	11.5

Calculation:

Calculation is based on a response factor derived from a standard curve. A quality control specimen containing 1 mg/L of the appropriate drug is analyzed daily.

Evaluation:

Sensitivity: 0.02 mg/L
Linearity: 0.02–20 mg/L
C.V.: 4% within-run
Relative recovery: 100–112%

Interferences:

Normal plasma components do not interfere with the assay, nor does meperidine, commonly used in conjunction with these drugs. Cyclizine, the internal standard, is an antihistamine that is used clinically; it will interfere if present in patient specimens.

Reference:

G.T. Tucker. Determination of bupivacaine (Marcaine) and other anilide-type local anesthetics in human blood and plasma by gas chromatography. Anesthesiol. 32: 255–260, 1970.

MAGNESIUM

Magnesium is an essential trace element whose dietary deficiency may result in irritability, neuromuscular abnormalities and cardiac and renal damage. Magnesium salts are taken internally as antacids and cathartics and are applied externally to relieve inflammation. Magnesium intoxication is rare, but there is an occasional need to assess magnesium levels in total parenteral nutrition patients. A convenient and specific procedure relies on flame atomic absorption spectrometry.

Serum Magnesium by Atomic Absorption Spectrometry

Principle:
Serum is diluted 1:50 with water and analyzed by flame atomic absorption spectrometry. Comparison is made to aqueous standards analyzed in the same manner.

Reagents:
Stock solution – 1 mg/mL magnesium ion (Fisher reference standard)
Aqueous standards – 0.5, 1 and 2 mmol/L

Instrumental Conditions:
Atomic absorption spectrometer with air-acetylene oxidizing flame
Magnesium hollow cathode lamp
Measure absorption at 285.2 nm

Procedure:
1. Transfer 200 μL serum to a 10 mL volumetric flask and dilute with water to 10 mL.
2. Mix and aspirate solution into the flame of the spectrometer.

Calculation:
Calculation is based on a response factor derived from a standard curve. A quality control specimen consisting of pooled serum is analyzed daily.

Evaluation:
Sensitivity: 0.2 mmol/L
Linearity: 0.5–2 mmol/L
C.V.: 2.4% within-run
Relative recovery: 95–104%

Interferences:

Sodium, potassium, calcium and phosphorus at low to high physiological concentrations had little or no effect on magnesium concentrations. Neither protein concentration nor EDTA had any apparent effect.

Reference:

J.L. Hansen and E.F. Freier. The measurement of serum magnesium by atomic absorption spectrophotometry. Amer. J. Med. Tech. 33: 1–9, 1967.

MEFENAMIC ACID

Serum Concentrations (mg/L)

Therapeutic	Toxic	T½
2–20	25–110	2 hr

Mefenamic acid is a non-narcotic analgesic and anti-inflammatory agent commonly administered in oral doses of 250–500 mg. The following gas chromatographic procedure is suitable for estimation of the drug in serum at therapeutic concentrations and in cases of overdosage. A liquid chromatographic method that does not require derivatization is also presented.

Serum Mefenamic Acid by Gas Chromatography

Principle:

Mefenamic acid is extracted from acidified serum with an organic solvent. An internal standard is added to the extract and the solution is evaporated to dryness. Formation of the butyl derivatives of both substances is accomplished with iodobutane and analysis is performed by flame-ionization gas chromatography.

Reagents:

Stock solution – 1 mg/mL mefenamic acid in methanol
Serum standards – 2, 5, 10 and 20 mg/L
Internal standard – 1 mg/mL 5-(p-methylphenyl)-5-phenylhydantoin (Aldrich) in ethanol
1 mol/L Hydrochloric acid
Dichloromethane
N,N-Dimethylacetamide
TMAH – 20% tetramethylammonium hydroxide in methanol (Aldrich)
1-Iodobutane

Instrumental Conditions:

Gas chromatograph with flame-ionization detector
1.5 m × 4 mm i.d. glass column containing 3% SP-2250 DA on 100/120 mesh Supelcoport (Supelco)
Injector, 285°C.; column, 250°C.; detector, 290°C.
Nitrogen flow rate, 60 mL/min

Procedure:

1. Transfer 2 mL serum to a 35 mL screw-cap tube. Add 0.5 mL 1 mol/L HCl and 15 mL dichloromethane and shake to extract.

2. Centrifuge and filter 12 mL of the organic layer through Whatman #54 filter paper into a 15 mL centrifuge tube. Add 50 μL internal standard and evaporate mixture to dryness at 50°C. under a stream of nitrogen.
3. Add 80 μL N,N-dimethylacetamide, 10 μL TMAH and 20 μL 1-iodobutane and vortex. Allow to stand for 5 min.
4. Centrifuge and inject 2 μL of the supernatant into the gas chromatograph.

	Retention time (min)
mefenamic acid derivative	1.8
internal standard derivative	4.1

Calculation:

Calculation in based on a response factor derived from a standard curve. A quality control specimen containing 5 mg/L mefenamic acid is analyzed daily.

Evaluation:

Sensitivity: 1 mg/L
Linearity: 1–25 mg/L
C.V.: not established
Relative recovery: not established

Interferences:

Normal serum constituents do not interfere, nor do other common analgesic and anti-inflammatory drugs.

Reference:

L.J. Dusci and L.P. Hackett. Gas-liquid chromatographic determination of mefenamic acid in human serum. J. Chromatog. 161: 340–342, 1978.

Serum Mefenamic Acid by Liquid Chromatography

Principle:

Serum is treated directly with acetonitrile to precipitate proteins. The supernatant is evaporated to dryness, reconstituted in the mobile phase and analyzed by liquid chromatography with ultraviolet detection at 282 nm.

Reagents:

Stock solution – 1 mg/mL mefenamic acid in methanol
Serum standards – 2, 5, 10 and 20 mg/L
Acetonitrile
Mobile phase – acetonitrile/45 mmol/L KH_2PO_4, 60:40 (adjusted to pH 3.0 with H_3PO_4)

Instrumental Conditions:

Liquid chromatograph with 282 nm absorbance detector
30 cm × 3.9 mm i.d. μBondapak C_{18} column (Waters Associates)

Solvent flow rate, 2.0 mL/min
Column temperature, ambient

Procedure:

1. Transfer 100 μL serum to a 12 mL conical centrifuge tube and add 1 mL acetonitrile. Vortex for 2 min and centrifuge to precipitate proteins.
2. Transfer 0.5 mL of the supernatant to a clear tube and evaporate to dryness at 50°C. under a stream of nitrogen. Dissolve the residue in 100 μL of mobile phase and inject 20 μL into the chromatograph.

	Retention time (min)
mefenamic acid	4.1

Calculation:

Calculation is based on a response factor derived from a standard curve. A quality control specimen containing 10 mg/L mefenamic acid is analyzed daily.

Evaluation:

Sensitivity: 1 mg/L
Linearity: 1–30 mg/L
C.V.: not established
Relative recovery: not established

Interferences:

Normal serum constituents do not interfere. Other anti-inflammatory drugs, including ibuprofen, indomethacin, naproxen, oxyphenbutazone and phenylbutazone, elute earlier than mefenamic acid and do not interfere. Flufenamic acid, a related drug, elutes just after mefenamic acid and may cause interference; changing the mobile phase to acetonitrile/0.7%. NH_4Cl, 35:65 (adjusted to pH 7.8 with NH_4OH) allows adequate separation of these two drugs.

Reference:

L.J. Dusci and L.P. Hackett. Determination of some anti-inflammatory drugs in serum by high-performance liquid chromatography. J. Chrom. 172: 516–519, 1979.

MEPERIDINE

Plasma Concentrations (mg/L)

	Therapeutic	Fatal Intoxication	T½
meperidine	0.07–0.50	1–20	2.4–4.0 hr
normeperidine	0.00–0.48	0–30	>4 hr

Meperidine (pethidine) is a synthetic narcotic analgesic which has about one-eighth the potency of morphine. It may be administered orally or by intravenous or intramuscular injection and is commonly used during obstetrical procedures for the relief of pain. Normeperidine, an active metabolite, may not appear in plasma until after several doses have been given. For emergency toxicology purposes, meperidine may be determined by either the Urine Basic Drug Screen by Thin-Layer Chromatography (p. 41) or the Serum Basic Drug Screen by Gas Chromatography (p. 43). In order to monitor therapeutic levels of meperidine and normeperidine, the following sensitive assay by flame-ionization gas chromatography is included.

Plasma Meperidine and Normeperidine by Gas Chromatography

Principle:

Meperidine, normeperidine and an internal standard (a minor methadone metabolite) are extracted from alkalinzed plasma with ether. After partitioning into aqueous acid and finally back into ether, normeperidine is converted to a heptafluorobutyryl derivative to reduce polarity. The drugs are analyzed by flame-ionization gas chromatography.

Reagents:

Stock solutions –
    1 mg/mL meperidine in methanol
    1 mg/mL normeperidine in methanol
Plasma standards – 0.05, 0.10, 0.20 and 0.50 mg/L for both drugs
Internal standard – 4 mg/L 2-ethyl-5-methyl-3,3-diphenyl-1-pyrroline (Eli Lilly) in water
2.5 mol/L Sodium hydroxide
Octyl alchohol
Ether
0.2 mol/L Hydrochloric acid
Hexane
50% Sodium hydroxide
Derivatizing reagent – 3% heptafluorobutyrylimidazole in ethyl acetate
Cyclohexane

Instrumental Conditions:

Gas chromatograph with flame-ionization detector
2 m × 2 mm i.d. glass column containing 3% OV-17 on 80/100 mesh Gas Chrom Q
Injector, 250°C.; column, 175°C.; detector, 275°C.
Helium flow rate, 34 mL/min

Procedure:

1. Transfer 1 mL plasma to a 15 mL screw-cap tube. Add 100 µL internal standard, 250 µL 2.5 mol/L NaOH and 2 drops octyl alcohol.
2. Extract with 10 mL ether by shaking for 1 min. Centrifuge and transfer ether to a clean tube.
3. Extract ether with 5 mL 0.2 mol/L HCl. Centrifuge and discard ether layer.
4. Wash acid layer with 5 mL hexane, centrifuge and discard hexane phase.
5. Add 3 drops 50% NaOH to the aqueous phase and extract with 7 mL ether. Centrifuge transfer ether to a 12 mL centrifuge tube.
6. Evaporate ether to dryness under a stream of nitrogen at 40–45°C. Add 40 µL derivatizing reagent and allow to stand in the dark for 30 min.
7. Evaporate mixture to dryness and dissolve residue in 30 µL cyclohexane. Inject 2 µL into the gas chromatograph.

	Retention time (min)
meperidine	1.8
normeperidine derivative	2.8
internal standard	4.2

Calculation:

Calculation is based on a response factor derived from a standard curve. A quality control specimen containing 0.20 mg/L of each drug is analyzed daily.

Evaluation:

Sensitivity: 0.02 mg/L
Linearity: 0.04–1.0 mg/L
C.V.: not established
Relative recovery: not established

Interferences:

Extracts of normal plasma are free of interfering peaks. Other drugs were not studied for potential interference. The derivatization reaction for normeperidine is light sensitive and not reproducible unless carried out in a dark environment.

Reference:

H.H. Szeto and C.E. Inturrisi. Simultaneous determination of meperidine and normeperidine in biofluids. J. Chromatog. 125: 503–510, 1976.

MERCURY

	Mercury Concentrations (mg/L)		
	Normal Adults	Symptomatic Patients	Fatalities
blood	<0.05	>0.20	>0.60
urine	<0.01	>0.10	>0.80

Mercury is a nonessential trace element that is present in human tissues as a result of its natural and man-made presence in the environment. We are exposed to elemental and inorganic mercury by way of commercial products and industrial processes. Organic forms of mercury are used as preservatives and insecticides, and both freshwater and marine fish may accumulate substantial concentrations of methylmercury. Whole blood is the preferred specimen for diagnosing intoxication due to any of the various forms of mercury, while urine is acceptable for the determination of exposure to elemental or inorganic mercury.

The following procedure for measurement of total mercury in blood or urine is based on the cold vapor atomic absorption technique and requires specialized equipment. An alternative method that is specific for methylmercury in blood relies on electron-capture gas chromatography.

Blood and Urine Mercury by Atomic Absorption Spectrometry

Principle:
Inorganic and organic mercury in blood or urine is reduced to elemental mercury by reaction with sodium borohydride in a sealed vessel. The released mercury vapor is flushed through the absorption cell of an atomic absorption spectrometer.

Reagents:
Stock solution – 1 mg/mL mercury ion (Fisher reference standard)
Aqueous standards – 0.01, 0.05, 0.10 and 0.20 mg/L (prepare fresh)
Antifoam – tri-n-butyl phosphate
Borohydride reagent – 50 g/L sodium borohydride in 1 mol/L NaOH (prepare fresh)
Apparatus – 1 reaction vessel and washing vessel are connected in series to the spectrometer absorption cell by means of polyvinyl chloride tubing; the vessels are made of 15 × 2.5 cm test tubes and each inlet tube comes to within 0.5 cm of the bottom of the vessel and ends in a fine tip; the first vessel is initially empty and the second contains 10 mL water and 3 drops antifoam and is immersed in ice water; an air source capable of delivering a constant 3 L/min flow is connected to the inlet of the reaction vessel

Instrumental Conditions:

Atomic absorption spectrometer with flow-through quartz absorption cell
Mercury hollow cathode lamp
Measure absorption at 253.7 nm

Procedure:

1. With the air flow off, transfer 2 mL blood or urine to the reaction vessel. Add 3 mL water and 1 drop of antifoam and close the vessel with the stopper containing the inlet and outlet tubes.
2. Inject 1 mL borohydride reagent through the rubber stopper of the reaction vessel using a hypodermic syringe. Vortex the vessel for 2 min.
3. Turn on the air supply and read the absorbance peak of the mercury vapor as it passes through the absorption cell of the spectrometer. Clean the reaction vessel and flush the system with air before analyzing the next sample.

Calculation:

Calculation is based on a standard curve prepared each time an analysis is performed. Quality control urine specimens containing known amounts of mercury are available commercially and should be analyzed with each patient specimen.

Evaluation:

Sensitivity: <0.001 mg/L
Linearity: 0.01–0.05 mg/L
C.V.: 5–7%
Relative recovery: 97–124% for inorganic mercury, 89–117% for methylmercury

Interferences:

Reagent blanks should be analyzed frequently to monitor contamination from reagents, glassware and residual mercury in the analytical apparatus. The method is highly specific for mercury.

References:

1. D.C. Sharma and P.S. Davis. Direct determination of mercury in blood by use of sodium borohydride reduction and atomic absorption spectrophotometry. Clin Chem. 25: 769–772, 1979.
2. T.W. Clarkson, M.R. Greenwood and L. Magos. Atomic absorption determination of total, inorganic, and organic mercury in biological fluids. In Clinical Chemistry and Chemical Toxicology of Metals (S.S. Brown, ed.), Elsevier, New York, 1977, pp. 201–208.

Blood Methylmercury by Electron-Capture Gas Chromatography

Principle:

Methylmercury is extracted from blood as the iodide into benzene. Following several clean-up steps, the extract is analyzed by electron-capture gas chromatography. The procedure is also applicable to the determination of ethylmercury.

Reagents:

Stock solution – 1 mg/mL methylmercury in methanol (as the choride salt)
Aqueous standards – 0.01, 0.02, 0.05 and 0.10 mg/L (prepare fresh)
8 mol/L Urea
1 mol/L Oxalic acid
1 mol/L Potassium iodide
Benzene
0.1 mol/L Sodium hydroxide
Cysteine solution – 1.5% cysteine in water, adjust to pH 10 with ammonium hydroxide

Instrumental Conditions:

Gas chromatograph with electron-capture detector
1.2 m × 4 mm i.d. glass column containing 2% ethylene glycol succinate on 60/80 mesh
    Chromosorb G
Injector, 180°C.; column, 150°C.; detector 180°C.
Nitrogen flow rate, 120 mL/min

Procedure:

1. Transfer 1 mL heparinized whole blood to a 50 mL polypropylene tube. Add 8 mL 8 mol/L urea, 2 mL 1 mol/L oxalic acid and 1 mL 1 mol/L KI and vortex.
2. Add 15 mL benzene and shake to extract. Centrifuge and transfer the benzene to a clean tube. Repeat the extraction with a second 15 mL aliquot of benzene and combine this extract with the first.
3. Add 1 mL 0.1 mol/L NaOH to the benzene. Shake, centrifuge and discard the lower aqueous layer.
4. Add 1 mL cysteine solution to the benzene and extract. Centrifuge and transfer the cysteine solution to a 15 mL screw-cap tube.
5. Add 1 mL 1 mol/L oxalic acid, 1 mL 1 mol/L KI and 1 mL benzene to the cysteine solution. Vortex for several minutes and centrifuge.
6. Transfer the benzene layer to a clean tube. Inject 10 μL into the gas chromatograph.

	Retention time (min)
methylmercuric iodide	0.6
ethylmercuric iodide	1.6

Calculation:

Calculation is based on a standard curve prepared each time a specimen is analyzed.

Evaluation:

Sensitivity: 0.001 mg/L
Linearity: 0.01–0.10 mg/L
C.V.: not established
Relative recovery: not established

Interferences:

Recovery of methylmercury from blood averages only 60–70% and so it is preferable, if sample volume allows, to use the method of standard additions for accurate calibration rather than to rely on aqueous standards. The original methods required addition to each specimen of radioactive methylmercury as an internal standard to calculate absolute recovery. Reagents and glassware should be checked for interfering peaks on the gas chromatogram by analyzing reagent blanks.

References:

1. R. Von Burg, F. Farris and J.C. Smith. Determination of methylmercury in blood by gas chromatography. J. Chromatogr. 97: 65–70, 1974.
2. C.J. Cappon and J.C. Smith. A simple and rapid procedure for the gas-chromatographic determination of methylmercury in biological specimens. Bull. Env. Cont. Tox. 19: 600–607, 1978.

METHADONE

| | Drug or Metabolite Concentration (mg/L) | | | | |
| | Single 10–15 mg Dose | | Maintenance Subjects | | |
	Plasma	Urine	Plasma	Urine	T½
Methadone	0.03–0.08	0.2–2.0	0.20–1.10	1–50	15–25 hr
EDDP	0	0.2–2.0	<0.1	1–50	?

Methadone is a synthetic narcotic analgesic that is approximately as potent as morphine on a weight basis. The drug is given in large daily oral doses to heroin addicts in narcotic maintenance programs who become quite tolerant to its toxic effects. The primary metabolite, 2-ethylidene-1,5-dimethyl-3,3-diphenylpyrrolidine (EDDP), is inactive and does not accumulate in plasma, but its presence in urine may be employed as an indication of methadone usage. A gas chromatographic procedure is presented for the quantitative determination of methadone and EDDP in plasma and urine. Methadone may also be assayed for emergency toxicology purposes using the Urine Basic Drug Screen by Thin-Layer Chromatography or the Serum Basic Drug Screen by Gas Chromatography. Reagents are commercially available for detection of methadone in urine by radioimmunoassay and EMIT.

Plasma and Urine Methadone and EDDP by Gas Chromatography

Principle:
Methadone, its primary metabolite and an internal standard are extracted from alkalinized plasma or urine with an organic solvent. Plasma extracts are subjected to several clean-up steps. The final residue is analyzed by flame-ionization gas chromatography.

Reagents:
Stock solutions –
    1 mg/mL methadone in methanol
    1 mg/mL EDDP in methanol
Plasma standards – 0.05, 0.10, 0.20 and 0.50 mg/L methadone
Urine standards – 0.5, 1.0, 2.0 and 5.0 mg/L for methadone and EDDP
Internal standard – 20 mg/L SKF-525A (Smith, Kline and French) in water
Ammonium hydroxide – conc. NH₄OH
1-Chlorobutane
0.2 mol/L Hydrochloric acid
Hexane

170

60% Sodium hydroxide
Chloroform

Instrumental Conditions:

Gas chromatograph with flame-ionization detector
2 m × 2 mm i.d. glass column containing 3% OV-1 on 80/100 mesh Gas Chrom Q
Injector, 230°C.; column 180°C.; detector, 230°C.
Helium flow rate, 32 mL/min

Procedure:

Plasma:

1. Transfer 4 mL plasma to a 15 mL screw-cap tube. Add 50 μL internal standard and 2 drops conc. NH_4OH and vortex.
2. Extract with 10 mL chlorobutane by shaking for 1 min. Centrifuge and transfer organic layer to a clean tube.
3. Extract organic phase with 5 ml 0.2 mol/L HCl. Centrifuge and discard organic layer.
4. Wash aqueous phase with 5 mL hexane, centrifuge and discard hexane. Add 3 drops 60% NaOH to aqueous layer and vortex.
5. Extract aqueous layer with 8 mL chloroform. Centrifuge and discard upper aqueous layer.
6. Transfer chloroform to a 12 mL centrifuge tube and evaporate to dryness at 50°C. under a stream of nitrogen. Rinse sides of tube with 200 μL chloroform and evaporate to dryness.
7. Dissolve residue in 20 μL chloroform and inject 4 μL into the gas chromatograph.

Urine:

1. Transfer 2 mL urine to a 15 mL screw-cap tube. Add 250 μL internal standard and 1 drop 60% NaOH and vortex.
2. Extract with 8 mL chloroform. Centrifuge and transfer chloroform to a 12 mL centrifuge tube.
3. Evaporate chloroform to dryness at 50°C. under a stream of nitrogen. Dissolve residue in 100 μL chloroform and inject 4 μL into the gas chromatograph.

	Retention time (min)
EDDP	3.2
methadone	4.7
internal standard	8.8

Calculation:

Calculation is based on a response factor derived from a standard curve. A quality control specimen containing 0.20 mg/L methadone in plasma or 2.0 mg/L methadone and EDDP in urine is analyzed daily.

Evaluation:

Sensitivity: 0.02 mg/L
Linearity: 0.05–0.50 mg/L for plasma and 0.5–5.0 mg/L for urine

C.V.: not established
Relative recovery: not established

Interferences:

Normal plasma and urine components do not interfere. Other drugs were not studied for potential interference.

Reference:

C.E. Inturrisi and K. Verebely. A gas-liquid chromatographic method for the quantitative determination of methadone in human plasma and urine. J. Chromatog. 65: 361–369, 1972.

METHAQUALONE

Plasma Concentrations (mg/L)		
Therapeutic	Toxic	T½
1–5	2–200	33–38 hr

Methaqualone is a weakly basic sedative-hypnotic drug that has been popularized as a drug of abuse. The compound may be determined qualitatively using the Urine Basic Drug Screen by Thin-Layer Chromatography or quantitatively with the Serum Basic Drug Screen by Gas Chromatography. For laboratories without access to gas chromatography, however, the following ultraviolet spectrophotometric technique is a convenient quantitative means of confirming a diagnosis of methaqualone intoxication. Reagents are also available for determination of methaqualone in urine by radioimmunoassay.

Serum Methaqualone by Ultraviolet Spectrophotometry

Principle:

Methaqualone is extracted from alkalinized serum into hexane. After evaporation of the hexane, the residue is dissolved in dilute acid and analyzed at 234 nm in the ultraviolet spectrophotometer.

Reagents:

Stock solution – 1 mg/mL methaqualone in methanol
Serum standards – 2, 5, 10 and 20 mg/L
1 mol/L Sodium hydroxide
Hexane
0.1 mol/L Hydrochloric acid

Instrumental Conditions:

Ultraviolet recording spectrophotometer

Procedure:

1. Transfer 2 mL serum to a 60 mL separatory funnel and add 1 mL 1 mol/L NaOH.
2. Extract with 20 mL hexane by shaking for 1 min. Allow layers to separate and discard lower aqueous layer.
3. Pour hexane layer through Whatman #31 filter paper into a 50 mL beaker. Evaporate hexane to dryness on a 56°C. hot plate.
4. Dissolve residue in 4 mL of 0.1 mol/L HCl. Transfer solution to a quartz cuvette.
5. Read against a serum blank from 320–220 nm in the ultraviolet spectrophotometer.

Subtract the absorbance at 320 nm from the maximum absorbance at 234 nm for each specimen.

Calculation:

Calculation is based on a response factor derived from a standard curve. A quality control serum containing 10 mg/L methaqualone is analyzed daily.

Evaluation:

Sensitivity: 2 mg/L
Linearity: 2–20 mg/L
C.V.: not established
Relative recovery: not established

Interferences:

Chlordiazepoxide and diazepam, if present in substantial concentrations in serum, will interfere with the quantitation of methaqualone. The presence of these drugs may be detected by a shift in the 234 nm maximum to a higher wavelength.

Reference:

C.B. Walberg. Presented at the California Association of Toxicologists meeting, Los Angeles, California, May 5, 1973.

METHOTREXATE

48 Hour Plasma Concentrations (μmol/L)

Therapeutic	Toxic
<0.5	>0.9

Methotrexate is a folic acid antagonist that is frequently utilized as an antineoplastic agent by intravenous infusion. Plasma concentrations are generally monitored 48 hours following the end of the infusion, at which time they should be less than 0.5 μmol/L. Higher concentrations may require postponement of additional doses or continued administration of the antidote leucovorin. A method is presented for methotrexate plasma level monitoring by high-pressure liquid chromatography. Reagents are also commercially available for determination of the compound by radioimmunoassay and EMIT.

Plasma Methotrexate by Liquid Chromatography

Principle:

Methotrexate and an internal standard (a methotrexate analogue) are isolated from plasma by ion-pair extraction into an organic solvent. The evaporated extract is dissolved in water and analyzed by liquid chromatography with ultraviolet detection at 254 nm or 315 nm. The 7-hydroxy metabolite of methotrexate may also be assayed by this technique.

Reagents:

Stock solution – 1 mg/mL methotrexate in water (stable at 4°C. for 3 months)
Plasma standards – 0.2, 0.5, 1.0 and 2.0 μmol/L (91, 227, 455 and 909 μg/L)
Internal standard – 4 mg/10 mL N-[4[[(2,4-diamino-6-quinazolinyl) methylamino]benzoyl]] aspartic acid (Developmental Therapeutic Program, National Cancer Institute) in water
2 mol/L Perchloric acid
Ammonium sulfate – solid $(NH_4)_2SO_4$
Extraction solvent – ethyl acetate/isopropanol, 10:1 by volume
Mobile solvent – pH 7.0 0.025 mol/L sodium phosphate buffer

Instrumental Conditions:

Liquid chromatograph with 354 nm ultraviolet detector (sensitivity is improved slightly at 315 nm)
25 cm × 4.6 mm i.d. stainless steel column containing Partisil 10/SAX (Whatman)
Solvent flow rate, 1.2 mL/min
Column temperature, ambient

Procedure:

1. Transfer 1 mL plasma to a 12 mL centrifuge tube. Add 10 μL internal standard, 1 mL water and 1.5 mL 2 mol/L $HClO_4$. Vortex and centrifuge.
2. Transfer supernatant to a 10 mL screw-cap tube. Add 5 g solid $(NH_4)_2SO_4$ and 2 mL extraction solvent and shake for 1 min.
3. Centrifuge and transfer organic layer to a 5 mL conical centrifuge tube. Evaporate to dryness under a stream of nitrogen.
4. Dissolve residue in 100 μL water and inject 10 μL into the chromatograph.

	Retention time (min)
methotrexate	7.3
7-hydroxymethotrexate	8.9
internal standard	11.3

Calculation:

Calculation is based on a response factor derived from a standard curve. A quality control specimen containing 0.5 μmol/L methotrexate is analyzed daily.

Evaluation:

Sensitivity: 0.2 μmol/L
Linearity: 0.2–20 μmol/L
C.V.: 3%
Relative recovery: not established

Interferences:

Normal plasma components did not interfere with the assay. Other drugs were not studied for potential interference.

Reference:

E. Watson, J.L. Cohen and K.K. Chan. High-pressure liquid chromatographic determination of methotrexate and its major metabolite, 7-hydroxymethotrexate, in human plasma. Cancer Treatment Reports 62: 381–387, 1978.

METHYLDOPA

Therapeutic	Toxic	T½
1–5	>7	4–14 hr

Methyldopa is a synthetic antihypertensive agent that may be administered orally or by intravenous infusion. Sedation is present after therapeutic doses and coma may occur during intoxication. A sulfate conjugate of methyldopa accumulates in plasma during chronic therapy and may reach concentrations as high as 67 mg/L. The following fluorometric procedure is specific for the unchanged drug.

Plasma Methyldopa by Fluorescence Spectrophotometry

Principle:
Methyldopa is assayed in deproteinized serum by oxidation to a highly fluorescent trihydroxyindole derivative. Fluorescent emission is measured at 500 nm after excitation at 400 nm.

Reagents:
Stock solution – 1 mg/mL methyldopa in methanol
Plasma standards – 1, 2, 4 and 8 mg/L
1 mol/L Perchloric acid
10% Potassium carbonate
pH 6.0 Phosphate buffer
0.25% Potassium ferricyanide
Sodium hydroxide-ascorbic acid mixture – 5 mol/L NaOH and 2% ascorbic acid, 9:2 (prepare fresh)

Instrumental Conditions:
Fluorescence spectrophotometer set to excite at 400 nm
Measure fluorescence at 500 nm

Procedure:
1. Transfer 1 mL plasma to a 12 mL centrifuge tube. Add 2 mL water and 0.5 mL cold 1 mol/L $HClO_4$, vortex and place in an ice bath for 30 min.
2. Centrifuge and transfer 2 mL of the supernatant to a 12 mL centrifuge tube. Neutralize the solution with 10% K_2CO_3.
3. Add 1 mL pH 6.0 phosphate buffer, 4 mL water and 200 μL 0.25% potassium ferricyanide. Vortex and let stand exactly 5 min.

4. Add 1 mL sodium hydroxide/ascorbic acid mixture, vortex and let stand 1.75 hr with occasional shaking. Transfer to a cuvette and determine emission at 500 nm.

Calculation:

Calculation is based on a response factor derived from a standard curve. A quality control specimen containing 4 mg/L methyldopa is analyzed daily.

Evaluation:

Sensitivity: 0.1 mg/L
Linearity: 1–8 mg/L
C.V.: not established
Relative recovery: 93–105%

Interferences:

Normal plasma components do not interfere with this assay. Other drugs were not studied for potential interference.

Reference:

E. Myhre, E.K. Brodwall, O. Stenbaek and T. Hansen. Plasma turnover of methydopa in advanced renal failure. Acta Med. Scand. 191: 343–347, 1972.

METHYLPHENIDATE

Methylphenidate is a phenethylamine derivative that is widely used in the treatment of depression, narcolepsy and childhood behavioral disorders. It is normally administered orally in doses of 5–20 mg, although when abused it may be injected intravenously. The major metabolite, ritalinic acid, achieves higher plasma and urine concentrations than the parent drug but is probably inactive. A sensitive electron-capture gas chromatographic procedure is described for the determination of methylphenidate in plasma.

Plasma Methylphenidate by Electron-Capture Gas Chromatography

Principle:

Methylphenidate is extracted from alkalinized plasma into cyclohexane. A halogenated derivative is prepared and the extract is analyzed by electron-capture gas chromatography.

Reagents:

Stock solution – 1 mg/mL methylphenidate in methanol
Plasma standards – 0.010, 0.020, 0.040 and 0.080 mg/L
Borate buffer – saturated sodium borate
Cyclohexane
Trichloroacetyl chloride
Pyridine
1 mol/L Sodium hydroxide

Instrumental Conditions:

Gas chromatograph with electron-capture detector
1.8 m × 2 mm i.d. glass column containing 3% OV-1 on 80/100 mesh Chromosorb G-HP
Injector, 270°C.; column, 250°C.; detector, 320°C.
Helium flow rate, 45 mL/min

Procedure:

1. Transfer 2 mL plasma to a 15 mL screw-cap tube. Add 1 mL borate buffer and 4 mL cyclohexane and shake to extract.
2. Centrifuge and transfer 3 mL of the organic phase to a clean tube. Add 50 µL trichloroacetyl chloride and 50 µL pyridine, vortex and allow to stand 20 min.

3. Add 2 mL 1 mol/L NaOH and shake the tube. Centrifuge and transfer 2.5 mL of the organic phase to a 5 mL conical centrifuge tube.
4. Evaporate the organic phase to dryness under a stream of nitrogen at 40°C. Dissolve the residue in 100 μL cyclohexane and inject 4 μL into the gas chromatograph.

	Retention time (min)
methylphenidate derivative	3

Calculation:

Calculation is based on a response factor derived from a standard curve. A quality control specimen containing 0.020 mg/L methylphenidate is analyzed daily.

Evaluation:

Sensitivity: 0.009 mg/L
Linearity: 0.010–0.080 mg/L
C.V.: 6.7% within-run
Relative recovery: not established

Interferences:

Instrument sensitivity may decline after a period of time due to column deterioration. Response can be restored by repacking the first 6–10 cm of the column. Other drugs have not been studied for potential interference.

Reference:

R.S. Ray, J.S. Noonan, P.W. Murdick and V.L. Tharp. Detection of methylphenidate and methamphetamine in equine body fluids by gas chromatographic analysis of an electron-capturing derivative. Amer. J. Vet. Res. 33: 27–31, 1972.

NICKEL

Nickel Concentrations (µg/L)					
Normal Subjects		Refinery Workers		Nickel Carbonyl Poisoning	
Plasma	Urine	Plasma	Urine	Plasma	Urine
1–4	0.3–10	3–11	8–800	?	100–2500

Nickel is an essential trace element that is present in very low concentrations in all body fluids. Measurement of nickel in plasma or urine may be useful in the diagnosis of acute myocardial infarction, the management of nickel hypersensitivity or the monitoring of exposure to nickel in metal workers. Acute intoxication is rare, although isolated incidents of exposure to the highly toxic nickel carbonyl vapor occur each year. Chelation therapy is usually indicated when urine nickel concentrations exceed 100 µg/L.

An electrothermal atomic absorption procedure is described for the analysis of nickel in plasma and urine that requires minimal sample preparation.

Plasma and Urine Nickel by Graphite Furnace Atomic Absorption Spectrometry

Principle:
Nickel is extracted from the deproteinized specimen as a chelate into an organic solvent. The extract is analyzed by electrothermal atomic absorption spectrometry.

Reagents:
Stock solution – 1 mg/mL nickel ion (Fisher reference standard)
Aqueous standards – 1, 2, 5, 10 and 20 µg/L (prepare fresh)
3 mol/L Trichloroacetic acid (ultra-pure)
Sulfuric acid – conc. H_2SO_4 (ultra-pure)
APDC solution – 0.12 mol/L ammonium pyrrolidinedithiocarbamate in water (prepare fresh and extract 4 times with MIBK before use)
pH Indicator – 1 g/L m-cresol
Ammonium hydroxide – conc. NH_4OH (ultra-pure)
Methylisobutyl ketone

All glassware is soaked overnight in 50% nitric acid and rinsed before use; all water for reagent preparation and rinsing is deionized-distilled.

Instrumental Conditions:
Atomic absorption spectrometer with graphite furnace
Nickel hollow cathode lamp

182

Furnace program: dry 20 sec at 140°C.
　　　　　　　　char 10 sec at 420°C.
　　　　　　　　ash 10 sec at 1060°C.
　　　　　　　　atomize 15 sec at 2600°C.
Argon purge gas in interrupt mode
Measure absorption at 232 nm

Procedure:

1. Transfer 3 mL plasma or urine to a 12 mL centrifuge tube. Add 1 mL 3 mol/L trichloroacetic acid and 1 mL conc. H_2SO_4 and vortex.
2. Centrifuge to separate proteins and decant supernatant to a 12 mL glass-stoppered centrifuge tube. Add 0.3 mL APDC solution and 1 drop pH indicator and vortex.
3. Adjust solution to pH 9 with conc. NH_4OH. Add 1 mL methylisobutyl ketone and shake for 2 min.
4. Centrifuge and transfer a portion of the upper organic layer to a 3 mL test tube. Inject 20 μL into the furnace and begin temperature program. Determine the average peak absorbance of 3–5 injections for each specimen.

Calculation:

Calculation is based on a response factor derived from a standard curve. A quality control specimen consisting of pooled plasma or urine is analyzed daily.

Evaluation:

Sensitivity: <1 μg/L
Linearity: 1–20 μg/L
C.V.: 12%
Relative recovery: not established

Interferences:

Nickel contamination of reagents and glassware will always be present. Reagent blanks must be run frequently and their average value substracted from that of the aqueous standards and specimens. A deuterium background corrector is not necessary when the 10 second ashing step at 1060°C. is performed.

Reference:

I. Anderson, W. Torjussen and H. Zachariasen. Analysis for nickel in plasma and urine by electrothermal atomic absorption spectrometry, with sample preparation by protein precipitation. Clin. Chem. 24: 1198–1202, 1978.

NICOTINE

	Nicotine Concentrations (mg/L)		
	Nonsmokers	Smokers	Fatal Intoxication
plasma	0.006	0.010–0.050	11–63
urine	0.07	0.1–3.0	17–58

Nicotine is a toxic alkaloid that causes stimulation of autonomic ganglia and the central nervous system. Cigarettes contain an average of 1.5% nicotine and a smoker may receive a dose of 1–4 mg of the drug for each cigarette smoked. Even nonsmokers show traces of nicotine in their body fluids due to exposure to cigarette smoke. Nicotine is also used as an insecticide and poisoning occasionally results from ingestion of the commercially available form. A gas chromatographic method is presented that is sufficiently sensitive to measure plasma nicotine concentrations attained during smoking.

Plasma Nicotine by Nitrogen-Specific Gas Chromatography

Principle:
Nicotine is extracted from alkalinized plasma with ether, back extracted into aqueous acid and finally returned to an organic solvent. The extract is analyzed by nitrogen-specific gas chromatography, using quinoline as internal standard.

Reagents:
Stock solution – 1 mg/mL nicotine in methanol
Plasma standards – 0.005, 0.010, 0.020 and 0.040 mg/L
5 mol/L Sodium hydroxide
Ether
2 mol/L Hydrochloric acid
Internal standard – 0.5 mg/L quinoline in water
Heptane

Instrumental Conditions:
Gas chromatograph with nitrogen-phosphorus detector
2 m × 2 mm i.d. glass column containing 10% Apiezon L and 10% KOH on 80/100 mesh
    Chromosorb W (or 3% SP-2250 DB on 100/120 mesh Supelcoport)
Injector, 210% C.; column, 170°C.; detector, 250°C.
Helium flow rate, 60 mL/min.

Procedure:

1. Transfer 3 mL plasma to a 15 mL screw-cap tube. Add 2 mL 5 mol/L NaOH and 8 mL ether and shake to extract.
2. Centrifuge and transfer ether to a 12 mL centrifuge tube. Evaporate to low volume (0.2–0.5 mL) under a stream of nitrogen at room temperature.
3. Add 100 µL 2 mol/L HCl to the ether and vortex. Centrifuge and discard ether layer.
4. Wash aqueous phase with 0.5 mL ether, centrifuge and discard ether. Evaporate remaining traces of ether under a stream of nitrogen.
5. Add 100 µL internal standard and vortex. Transfer the solution to a 3 mL conical centrifuge tube with a narrow tapered end.
6. Add 400 µL 5 mol/L NaOH and 50 µL heptane and vortex for 1 min. Centrifuge and inject 5 µL of the heptane into the gas chromatograph.

	Retention time (min)
internal standard	2.8
nicotine	3.6

Calculation:

Calculation is based on a response factor derived from a standard curve. A quality control specimen containing 0.020 mg/L nicotine is analyzed daily.

Evaluation:

Sensitivity: 0.0001 mg/L
Linearity: 0.001–0.100 mg/L
C.V.: 6.5%
Relative recovery: 99–107%

Interferences:

Apparent nicotine concentrations of 0.0005–0.0040 mg/L were found in plasma from non-smokers who deliberately avoided exposure to cigarette smoking; it is believed that contamination may occur during the extraction process if smoking occurs in or near the laboratory. Fifteen other drugs were found not to interfere with the analysis.

References:

1. C. Feyerabend, T. Levitt and M.A.H. Russell. A rapid gas-liquid chromatographic estimation of nicotine in biological fluids. J. Pharm. Pharmacol. 27: 434–436, 1975.
2. N. Hengen and M. Hengen. Gas-liquid chromatographic determination of nicotine and cotinine in plasma. Clin. Chem. 24: 50–53, 1978.

NITRITE

Inorganic and organic nitrites are used therapeutically as antihypertensive agents and as antidotes for cyanide poisoning. Sodium nitrite is also used commercially as a curing agent for processed meats. Accidental poisoning occurs occasionally as a result of exposure to nitrites. Although the nitrite ion disappears rapidly from the plasma, urinary concentrations of nitrite may be used to assess exposure. A colorimetric procedure is described for this purpose. One of the primary toxic effects of nitrites is the production of methemoglobinemia, and thus the measurement of the methemoglobin level represents an alternative means of monitoring nitrite exposure.

Urine Nitrite by Colorimetry

Principle:
Nitrite is reacted with sulfanilic acid and naphthylamine to produce a red color, which is measured in a spectrophotometer at 510 nm.

Reagents:
Stock solution – 1 mg/mL nitrite ion in water
Aqueous standards – 10, 20, 50 and 100 mg/L
Sulfanilic acid solution – dissolve 0.6 g sulfanilic acid in 100 mL 20% HCl
Naphthylamine solution – 0.48 g α-naphthylamine in 100 mL 20% HCl
Sodium acetate solution – 16.4 g sodium acetate/100 mL water

Instrumental Conditions:
Visible spectrophotometer set to 510 nm

Procedure:
1. Transfer 1 mL urine to a 50 mL volumetric flask. Add 1 mL sulfanilic acid solution, mix and let stand 10 min.
2. Add 1 mL naphthylamine solution and 1 mL sodium acetate solution and dilute to 50 mL with water. Mix and let stand 10 min.
3. Read in the spectrophotometer at 510 nm against a reagent blank.

Calculation:
Calculation is based on a standard curve prepared each time a specimen is analyzed.

Evaluation:
Sensitivity: 5 mg/L
Linearity: 10–50 mg/L

C.V.: not established
Relative recovery: not established

Interferences:

None are known.

Reference:

A.I. Vogel. Quantitative Inorganic Analysis, 3rd ed., Longmans, Green and Co., London, 1961, pp. 784–785.

NITROUS OXIDE

Anesthetic Blood Concentrations (vol.%)
17–22

Nitrous oxide is frequently used as the sole anesthetic agent for minor surgical procedures or as an adjunct to other more potent agents for major surgery. Induction and recovery are quite rapid due to the insolubility of the gas in tissues, and there is no evidence that the compound undergoes biotransformation. The gas is subject to abuse, and deaths have occurred as a result of asphyxiation. A convenient method for its determination in blood involves gas chromatography with thermal conductivity detection.

Blood Nitrous Oxide by Thermal-Conductivity Gas Chromatography

Principle:
A sample of whole blood, preferably collected in a Vacutainer without exposure to air, is transferred to a 10 mL Vacutainer and allowed to equilibrate with helium. A volume of head-space gas is analyzed by gas chromatography on a molecular sieve column with thermal conductivity detection.

Reagents:
Nitrous oxide lecture bottle

Instrumental Conditions:
Gas chromatograph with thermal conductivity detector
6' × 1/8" stainless steel column containing 45/60 mesh molecular sieve type 5A
Injector, 220°C.; column, 200°C.; detector, 220°C.
Helium flow rate, 26 mL/min

Procedure:
1. Using a 5 mL glass syringe and a 20 gauge needle, introduce into 10 mL Vacutainer tubes 5 mL of blood for the following samples: negative control, 5, 10 and 20 vol. % nitrous oxide standards, patient specimen.
2. Using a 3 mL gas-tight plastic syringe and a 25 gauge needle, introduce 0.25, 0.5 or 1.0 mL of pure nitrous oxide into the 5, 10 and 20 vol. % standards, respectively.
3. Fill a dry 5 mL glass syringe equipped with a 25 gauge needle with helium from the injection port of the gas chromatograph. With each of the above tubes, penetrate the stopper with the needle and allow the helium in the syringe to enter the tube. After pressure equilibrium is reached, inject an additional 1.0 mL of helium into the tube.

4. Shake each tube vigorously for 30 seconds and allow to stand at room temperature for 10 minutes. Withdraw 1.0 mL of headspace gas using a 3 mL gastight plastic syringe with a 26 gauge needle and inject into the gas chromatograph.

	Retention time (min)
oxygen	0.3
nitrogen	0.6
nitrous oxide	4.0
carbon dioxide	5.6

Calculation:

Plot a graph of peak height versus concentration for the blank and three standards. Using this graph, which should be linear, determine the concentration of the unknown.

Evaluation:

Sensitivity: 2 vol. %
Linearity: 5–20 vol. %
C.V.: not established
Relative recovery: not established

Interferences:

None are known. This is a semi-quantitative procedure. A more accurate means of calibration is described in reference 1.

References:

1. T. Yokota, Y. Hitomi, K. Ohta and F. Kosaka. Direct injection method for gas chromatographic measurement of inhalation anesthetics in whole blood and tissues. Anesthesiol. 28: 1064–1073, 1967.
2. R. Baselt. Unpublished results, 1976.

OPIATES

	Therapeutic Conc. (mg/L)		Toxic Conc. (mg/L)	
	Plasma	Urine	Plasma	Urine
codeine	0.01–0.10	5–30	0.2–5.0	25–250
hydromorphone	0.001–0.030	0.1–1.0	0.1–2.0	1–5
levorphanol	?	?	0.1–3	1–5
morphine	0.01–0.07	0.5–10	0.1–1.0	0.5–25
oxycodone	0.01–0.10	0.2–2	0.2–5	1–5

The term opiates refers primarily to morphine and codeine, but is loosely used to describe a group of narcotic analgesics that includes these two drugs and their semi-synthetic derivatives. Most of these drugs achieve relatively low plasma concentrations but tend to concentrate in the urine, often as glucuronide conjugates. Acid hydrolysis of urine may be performed to release the conjugated drug so that it may be assayed by chromatographic techniques. A flame-ionization gas chromatographic method is presented that is suitable for quantitation of the opiates in urine, while the electron-capture method that follows is appropriate for the quantitative analysis of plasma specimens. Opiates in both blood and urine may be analyzed by the more specific gas chromatography-mass spectrometry procedure.

A qualitative means of assaying these drugs was described in the Urine Basic Drug Screen by Thin-Layer Chromatography (p. 41), and toxic serum concentrations of codeine can often be detected using the Serum Basic Drug Screen by Gas Chromatography (p. 43). Reagents are available commercially for determination of the opiates in urine by radioimmunoassay and EMIT; these procedures show similar cross-reactivity with morphine, morphine glucuronide and codeine.

Urine Opiates by Gas Chromatography

Principle:

Urine is spiked with an internal standard, nalorphine, before any manipulations are begun. The specimen must be acid hydrolyzed before extraction in order to free any conjugated drugs in the sample. After solvent extraction and clean-up, the drugs are acetylated for more efficient chromatography using acetic anhydride and pyridine. Injection is made onto the OV-17 column, with OV-1 for confirmation, and detection is by flame-ionization.

Reagents:

Stock solutions – 1 mg/mL methanol solutions of codeine, morphine or other drugs as needed.

Urine standards – 0.5, 2.0 and 5.0 mg/L of each of the above drugs
Internal standard – 50 mg nalorphine HCl/200 mL H_2O
Hydrochloric acid – conc. HCl
0.2 mol/L Hydrochloric acid – 8.6 mL conc. HCl/500 mL H_2O
Extraction solvent – ethyl acetate/isopropanol, 9:1
pH 9.2 Buffer – K_2HPO_4, 40% (200 g/500 mL H_2O)
10 mol/L Sodium hydroxide – 200 g NaOH/500 mL H_2O
Derivatizing reagent – acetic anhydride/pyridine, 1:1 (prepare fresh)
Hexane
Methanol
Chloroform

Instrumental Conditions:

Gas chromatograph with flame-ionization detector
6′ × 2 mm i.d. glass columns containing 2% OV-1 or 2% OV-17 on 100/120 mesh
   Chromosorb G-HP
Column temperature: 230°C. (OV-1) or 270°C. (OV-17)
Injector, 250°C.; detector, 300°C.
Nitrogen flow rate, 33 mL/min

Procedure:

1. Pipet into a 30 mL siliconized screw-cap centrifuge tube, 5 mL urine, 0.5 mL conc. HCl and 100 µL internal standard.
2. Hydrolyze for 1 hour in a boiling water bath. Cool and adjust the pH of the solution to about 7 using 10 mol/L NaOH dropwise. Add 4 mL pH 9.2 buffer and vortex.
3. Add 16 mL extraction solvent and shake for 1 minute. Centrifuge, then filter solvent through Whatman #1 paper into a clean 30 mL tube.
4. Add 4 mL 0.2 mol/L HCl and shake for 1 minute. Centrifuge and discard upper solvent layer. Wash aqueous layer with 10 mL hexane, centrifuge, and discard hexane.
5. Transfer aqueous layer to 50 mL beaker and leave in hood overnight to evaporate to dryness.
6. Transfer residue using 1–2 mL methanol to a 15 mL graduated centrifuge tube and evaporate to dryness under air in a 40°C. water bath.
7. Add 100 µL derivatizing reagent and vortex to dissolve residue. Incubate 30 min in an 80°C. water bath. Evaporate to dryness under a stream of dry air and dissolve the residue in 50 µL of $CHCl_3$. Inject 2 µL onto the OV-17 column at 270°C., using OV-1 at 230° for confirmation.

	Retention time (min)	
	OV-1	OV-17
levorphanol derivative	2.1	1.6
codeine derivative	2.8	3.7
morphine derivative	3.9	5.3
internal standard derivative	5.6	7.0

Calculation:

Calculation is based on a response factor derived from a standard curve. A quality control specimen containing 2.0 mg/L of each drug is analyze daily.

Evaluation:

Sensitivity: 0.05 mg/L
Linearity: 0.5–5.0 mg/L
C.V.: not established
Relative recovery: not established

Interferences:

Other basic drugs or extraneous materials may occasionally produce gas chromatographic peaks that conincide with one of the opiates. The use of both OV-17 and OV-1 columns helps to eliminate these interferences.

References:

1. J. Wright and R. Baselt. Unpublished results, 1974.
2. N.C. Jain, T.S. Sneath, R.D. Budd and W.J. Leung. Gas chromatographic/thin-layer chromatographic analysis of acetylated codeine and morphine in urine. Clin. Chem. 21: 1486–1489, 1975.

Plasma Opiates by Electron-Capture Gas Chromatography

Principle:

Morphine and codeine are extracted from alkalinized plasma with ethyl acetate. The solvent is evaporated to dryness and the drugs are converted to halogenated derivatives prior to analysis by electron-capture gas chromatography. Sensitivity is adequate for measurement of therapeutic plasma concentrations.

Reagents:

Stock solutions – 1 mg/mL codeine and morphine in methanol
Plasma standards – 0.01, 0.05, 0.10 and 0.20 mg/L for both drugs
2 mol/L Sodium hydroxide
Ethyl acetate
Benzene/methanol, 4:1 by volume
Heptafluorobutyric anhydride

Instrumental Conditions:

Gas chromatograph with electron-capture detector
1.2 m × 4 mm i.d. glass column containing 3% OV-17 on 100/120 mesh Gas Chrom Q
Injector, 250°C.; column, 230°C.; detector, 300°C.
5% Methane in argon flow rate, 30 mL/min

Procedure:

1. Transfer 2 mL plasma to a 15 mL screw-cap tube. Add 0.2 mL 2 mol/L NaOH and 10 mL ethyl acetate and shake to extract.

2. Centrifuge and transfer 9 mL of the organic layer to a 12 mL centrifuge tube. Evaporate to dryness under a stream of nitrogen.
3. Wash the walls of the tube with 1 mL benzene/methanol and again evaporate to dryness.
4. Add 200 μL heptafluorobutyric anhydride, vortex and allow to stand for 45 min.
5. Evaporate to dryness under a stream of nitrogen. Dissolve residue in 100 μL ethyl acetate and inject 2 μL into the gas chromatograph.

	Retention time (min)
morphine derivative	1.7
codeine derivative	2.7

Calculation:

Calculation is based on a response factor derived from a standard curve. A quality control specimen containing 0.10 mg/L of each drug is analyzed daily.

Evaluation:

Sensitivity: 0.0001 mg/L for morphine
Linearity: 0.0001–0.2 mg/L
C.V.: 9% day-to-day
Relative recovery: not established

Interferences:

Other drugs of abuse did not interfere. Codeine may be used as an internal standard (add 20 μL of the stock solution in step 1) when it is known that codeine is not present in the specimen. The sensitivity for codeine is substantially lower than for morphine since the codeine derivative has only one heptafluorobutyryl residue per molecule, compared to two for morphine.

Reference:

G. Nicolau, G.V. Lear, B. Kaul and B. Davidow. Determination of morphine by electron capture gas-liquid chromatography. Clin. Chem. 23: 1640–1643, 1977.

Blood and Urine Opiates by Gas Chromatography-Mass Spectrometry

Principle:

Morphine, codeine and an internal standard, nalorphine, are extracted from alkalinized blood or urine (urine is first treated with beta-glucuronidase to hydrolyze drug conjugates) with an organic solvent mixture. The solvent is evaporated to dryness and the residue reconstituted in dilute acid. After being washed with solvent, the acid layer is made basic and extracted with a solvent mixture. This extract is evaporated to dryness, the residue reacted with trifluoroacetic anhydride and the reaction mixture analyzed by gas chromatography-mass spectrometry with selected ion monitoring.

Reagents:

Stock solutions – 1 mg/mL methanol solutions of codeine, morphine or other drugs as needed

Blood standards – 0.01, 0.05, 0.10 and 0.20 mg/L for each of the above drugs

Urine standards – 0.5, 2.0 and 5.0 mg/L of each of the above drugs

Internal standard – 2 mg/L nalorphine HCl

50% Potassium hydrogen phosphate – 50 g K_2HPO_4/100 mL H_2O

Sodium chloride

Extraction solvent – chloroform/isopropanol, 9:1

0.1 mol/L Hydrochloric acid

Wash solvent – toluene/heptane/isoamyl alcohol, 70:20:10

Buffer powder – 2.1 mixture of solid $NaHCO_3$ and Na_2CO_3

Trifluoroacetic anhydride

Chloroform

Instrumental Conditions:

Gas chromatograph with mass selective detector (Hewlett-Packard 5970B MSD or equivalent)

12 m × 0.20 mm i.d. methylsilicone capillary column (Hewlett-Packard)

Injector, 300°C.; transfer line, 250°C.

Column temperature program: initial, 150°C. (1 min)
                            20°C./min. increase
                            final, 300°C. (4 min)

Helium flow rate, 1 mL/min

Splitless on time, 0.7 min

Solvent delay time, 2.0 min

Electron multiplier voltage, 1800

Ions monitored, 282.20, 364.10, 380.10, 390.15, 395.15, 477.10

Procedure:

1. Transfer 3 mL blood or 1 mL urine to a 50 mL screw-cap tube and add 100 μL or 1 mL internal standard, respectively. Hydrolyze urine by adding 1 mL of pH 5 0.2 mol/L acetate buffer containing 2000 IU/mL beta-glucuronidase (Sigma no. G-0751) and incubating at 37°C overnight.

2. Add 1 mL 50% K_2HOP_4 and enough solid NaCl to saturate the solution. Add 30 mL extraction solvent and place on a rotator for 30 min. Centrifuge.

3. Discard the aqueous layer and transfer the organic layer to a clean tube. Evaporate to dryness at 50°C. under a stream of dry air. Dissolve the residue in 2 mL 0.1 mol/L HCl and transfer to a 15 mL screw-cap tube.

4. Add 5 mL wash solvent and place on a rotator for 30 min. Centrifuge and discard the upper organic phase.

5. Saturate the aqueous layer with buffer powder and add 10 mL extraction solvent. Place on a rotator for 30 min. Centrifuge and discard the aqueous layer.

6. Transfer the organic layer to a 12 mL glass-stoppered conical centrifuge tube and evaporate to dryness at 50°C. under a stream of dry air. Add 20 μL trifluoroacetic

anhydride and 20 μL chloroform and heat for 30 min at 70°C. Cool and inject 1 μL into the chromatograph.

	Retention time (min)	Principle ions (m/z)
hydromorphone-TFA	5.7	380, 477
morphine-TFA	6.0	364, 477
codeine-TFA	6.2	282, 395
internal standard-TFA	6.5	390

Calculation:

Calculation is based on a response factor derived from a standard curve of ion chromatogram peak height ratio (i.e., 364/390 ratio for morphine/internal standard) versus drug concentration. A quality control specimen containing a mid-level concentration of the appropriate drug is analyzed daily. Ion intensity ratios (364/477 for morphine and 282/395 for codeine) should compare well between standards and unknown to further confirm drug identification in the unknown specimens.

Evaluation:

Sensitivity: 0.01 mg/L
Linearity: 0.01–5 mg/L
C.V.: 8–10 % day-to-day
Relative recovery: not established

Interferences:

Normal blood or urine components do not interfere with the assay. Other commonly used or abused drugs have not been found to interfere.

References:

1. D. Pearce, S. Wiersema, M. Kuo and C. Emery. Simultaneous determination of morphine and codeine in blood by use of select ion monitoring and deuterated internal standards. Clin. Tox. 14: 161–168, 1979.
2. M.A. Peat. Unpublished results, 1985.

ORAL HYPOGLYCEMIC AGENTS

	Plasma Concentrations (mg/L)		
	Therapeutic	Toxic	T½
acetohexamide	20–70	?	1 hr
chlorpropamide	75–250	200–750	33 hr
metformin	0.5–2.0	?	?
phenformin	0.1–0.5	3–4	13 hr
tolbutamide	40–100	640	7 hr

The oral hypoglycemic agents, used for the treatment of maturity-onset diabetes, are synthetic drugs that are classified chemically as either sulfonylurea derivatives (acetohex-amide, chlorpropamide, tolbutamide, etc.) or biguanide derivatives (metformin, phenfor-min, etc.). The sulfonylureas tend to develop relatively high plasma concentrations and thus are amenable to determination by a variety of techniques, including colorimetry, gas chromatography and liquid chromatography. The latter procedure is preferred for its higher degree of accuracy and precision. The biguanides result in much lower plasma levels and so it is necessary to use more sensitive methods; these drugs may be effectively assayed at therapeutic concentrations in plasma by either electron-capture gas chromatography or by ion-pair liquid chromatography.

Plasma Sulfonylurea Derivatives by Colorimetry

Principle:

The sulfonylurea drugs are extracted from acidified plasma with isoamyl acetate. At an elevated temperature the drugs degrade to amine derivatives and react with fluorodinitro-benzene. The resulting colored complex is measured spectrophotometrically.

Reagents:

Stock solutions – 1 mg/mL methanol solutions of acetohexamide, chlorpropamide and tolbutamide
Plasma standards – 20, 50, 100 and 200 mg/L of the appropriate drug
0.02 mol/L Hydrochloric acid
Isoamyl acetate
FDNB reagent – 0.1% 1-fluoro-2,4-dinitrobenzene in isoamyl acetate (prepare fresh)

Instrumental Conditions:

Visible spectrophotometer set to 346 nm (400 nm may be used as an alternative)

Procedure:

1. Transfer 0.5 mL plasma to a 15 mL screw-cap tube. Add 2.5 mL 0.02 mol/L HCl and 10 mL isoamyl acetate and shake to extract.
2. Centrifuge and transfer 6 mL of the upper organic layer to a 15 mL centrifuge tube. Add 1 mL FDNB reagent and vortex.
3. Place a marble on the top of the tube and heat at 125°C. for 10 min. Allow to stand at room temperature for an additional 30 min.
4. Read in the spectrophotometer at 346 nm against a plasma blank (color is stable for 24 hours).

Calculation:

Calculation is based on a response factor derived from a standard curve. A quality control specimen containing the appropriate drug at a mid-range concentration is analyzed daily.

Evaluation:

Sensitivity: 20 mg/L
Linearity: 20–200 mg/L
C.V.: not established
Relative recovery: not established

Interferences:

This a nonspecific procedure; the chromogenic reagent will react with all primary and secondary amines as well as with other functional groups. It is quantitative if the identity of the drug being assayed is known. Hemolysis will result in false positive readings.

References:

1. R.H. Carmichael. A method for the routine determination of chlorpropamide in plasma. Clin. Chem. 5: 597–602, 1959.
2. H. Spingler. Ueber einer Moeglichkeit zur Colorimetrischen Bestimmung von N-(4-Methyl-benzolsufonyl)-N'-butyl-harnstoff in Serum. Klin. Wochenschr. 35: 533–535, 1957.

Plasma Sulfonylurea Derivatives by Gas Chromatography

Principle:

Chlorpropamide and tolbutamide are extracted from acidified plasma with chloroform. Each drug is used as the internal standard for the other. Formation of methyl derivatives is accomplished with dimethyl sulfate and determination is by flame-ionization gas chromatography, with on-column decomposition to the corresponding sulfonamides.

Reagents:

Stock solutions – 1 mg/mL methanol solutions of chlorpropamide and tolbutamide
Plasma standards – 20, 50, 100 and 200 mg/L of the appropriate drug
Internal standard – use appropriate stock solution above
Saturated sodium dihydrogen phosphate
Chloroform

Methanolic potassium carbonate – 1 mL 10% aqueous K_2CO_3 plus 9 mL methanol
Dimethyl sulfate
pH 5.6 Acetate buffer – 4.8 mL 0.2 mol/L acetic acid and 45.2 mL 0.2 mol/L sodium
    acetate diluted to 1 L
Heptane

Instrumental Conditions:

Gas chromatograph with flame-ionization detector
2 m × 2 mm i.d. glass column containing 3% OV-17 on 100/200 mesh Chromosorb W-HP
Injector, 285°C.; column, 190°C.; detector, 285°C.
Nitrogen flow rate, 50 mL/min

Procedure:

1. Transfer 1 mL plasma to a 15 mL screw-cap tube. Add 100 µL of the stock solution of
   either chlorpropamide or tolbutamide as internal standard. Add 1 mL saturated
   NaH_2PO_4 and 10 mL chloroform an shake to extract.
2. Centrifuge and discard the upper aqueous layer. Transfer the chloroform to a 15 mL
   centrifuge tube and evaporate to dryness under a stream of nitrogen at 40°C.
3. Add 1 mL methanolic K_2CO_3 and 100 µL dimethyl sulfate and heat at 70°C. for 5 min.
   Evaporate the methanol to dryness at 70°C. under a stream of nitrogen.
4. Add 1 mL pH 5.6 acetate buffer and 5 mL heptane and vortex for 1 min. Centrifuge and
   transfer heptane to a clean tube.
5. Evaporate heptane to dryness at 40°C. under a stream of nitrogen. Dissolve the residue
   in 100 µL chloroform and inject 2 µL into the gas chromatograph.

	Retention time (min)
chlorpropamide derivative	2.5
tolbutamide derivative	4.5

Calculation:

Calculation is based on a response factor derived from a standard curve. A quality control
specimen containing the appropriate drug at a mid-range concentration is analyzed daily.

Evaluation:

Sensitivity: 1 mg/L
Linearity: 1–50 mg/L
C.V.: not established
Relative recovery: not established

Interferences:

Several commonly used sedative-hypnotic drugs were shown not to interfere with this assay.
Plasma lipids sometimes interfere and may be removed by washing the residue in step 2
with a small volume of hexane.

198

References:

1. D.L. Simmons, R.J. Ranz and P. Picotte. Determination of serum tolbutamide by gas chromatography. J. Chromatog. 71: 421–426, 1972.
2. K. Sabih and K. Sabih. Gas chromatographic method for determination of tolbutamide and chlorpropamide. J. Pharm. Sci. 59: 782–784, 1970.

Plasma Sulfonylurea Derivatives by Liquid Chromatography

Principle:

Chlorpropamide and tolbutamide are extracted from plasma with a solvent containing internal standard. The concentrated extract is directly analyzed by reversed-phase liquid chromatography, with detection at 254 nm.

Reagents:

Stock solutions – 1 mg/mL methanol solutions of chlorpropamide and tolbutamide
Plasma standards – 20, 50, 100 and 200 mg/L of the appropriate drug
Internal standard solution – 2.5 mg/L 1-isopentyl-3-(p-tolylsulfonyl)urea (Aldrich) in chloroform
Sodium chloride – solid NaCl
Acetonitrile
Mobile phase – 72 parts 1% acetic acid adjusted to pH 5.5 with 2 mol/L NaOH and 28 parts acetonitrile, by volume

Instrumental Conditions:

Liquid chromatograph with 254 nm ultraviolet detector
30 cm × 4 mm i.d. stainless-steel column containing μBondapak C_{18} (Waters Associates)
Column temperature, ambient
Solvent flow rate, 2.2 mL/min

Procedure:

1. Transfer 200 μL plasma to a 15 mL screw-cap tube. Add 10 mL internal standard solution and about 1 g NaCl and shake to extract.
2. Centrifuge and discard the aqueous layer. Transfer the chloroform to a 15 mL centrifuge tube and evaporate to dryness at 40°C. under a stream of nitrogen.
3. Dissolve the residue in 40 μL acetonitrile and inject 25 μL into the chromatograph.

	Retention time (min)
chlorpropamide	3
tolbutamide	6
internal standard	9

Calculation:

Calculation is based on a response factor derived from a standard curve. A quality control specimen containing the appropriate drug at a mid-range concentration is analyzed daily.

Evaluation:

Sensitivity: 7 mg/L
Linearity: 10–200 mg/L
C.V.: 5.4–6.7% between-run
Relative recovery: 93–109%

Interferences:

Endogenous plasma components do not interfere. Other drugs were not studied for potential interference.

Reference:

R.E. Hill and J. Crechiolo. Determination of serum tolbutamide and chlorpropamide by high-performance liquid chromatography. J. Chromatog. 145: 165–168, 1978.

Plasma Biguanide Derivatives by Electron-Capture Gas Chromatography

Principle:

Acetonitrile is used to precipitate proteins and extract the drugs from plasma. Halogenated derivatives are prepared using monochlorodifluoroacetic anhydride and the derivatives are analyzed by electron-capture gas chromatography.

Reagents:

Stock solutions – 1 mg/mL methanol solutions of buformin, metformin and phenformin
Plasma standards – 0.1, 0.2, 0.5 and 1.0 mg/L of the appropriate drug
Internal standard – appropriate stock solution above diluted 1:50 with methanol
Acetonitrile
Amyl acetate
Monochlorodifluoroacetic anhydride
4 mol/L Sodium hydroxide

Instrumental Conditions:

Gas chromatograph with electron-capture detector
2 m × 4 mm i.d. glass column containing 3% OV-17 on 100/200 mesh Gas Chrom Q
Injector, 225°C.; column, 210°C.; detector, 325°C.
Nitrogen flow rate, 50 mL/min

Procedure:

1. Transfer 200 μL plasma to a 15 mL centrifuge tube. Add 10 μL internal standard and 5 mL acetonitrile and vortex.
2. Centrifuge and transfer supernatant to a 5 mL conical centrifuge tube. Evaporate to dryness under a stream of nitrogen at 40°C.
3. Dissolve the residue in 100 μL amyl acetate. Add 10 μL monochlorodifluoroacetic anhydride, vortex and let stand 1–2 min.

4. Add 0.5 mL 4 mol/L NaOH and vortex. Centrifuge and inject 1 μL of the upper organic layer into the gas chromatograph.

	Retention time (min)
metformin derivative	1.7
buformin derivative	3.2
phenformin derivative	3.5

Calculation:

Calculation is based on a response factor derived from a standard curve. A quality control specimen containing the appropriate drug at a concentration of 0.5 mg/L is analyzed daily.

Evaluation:

Sensitivity: 0.01 mg/L
Linearity: 0.1–1.0 mg/L
C.V.: 5–9% within-run, 6–14% day-to-day
Relative recovery: not established

Interferences:

Normal plasma components do not interfere. Other drugs were not studied for potential interference. Metformin may be used as an internal standard for buformin and phenformin assay, while either of the latter drugs may be used for metformin analysis.

References:

1. M.S. Lennard, C. Casey, G.T. Tucker and H.F. Woods. Determination of metformin in biological samples. Brit. J. Clin. Pharm. 6: 183–185, 1978.
2. S.B. Martin, J.H. Karam and P.H. Forsham. Simple electron capture gas chromatographic method for the determination of oral hypoglycemic biguanides in biological fluids. Anal. Chem. 47: 545–548, 1975.

Plasma Biguanide Derivatives by Liquid Chromatography

Principle:

Phenformin is extracted from deproteinized plasma at an alkaline pH with dichloromethane. The concentrated extract is analyzed by ion-pair liquid chromatography with detection at 235 nm. Other biguanide derivatives may be measured with this procedure.

Reagents:

Stock solution – 1 mg/mL phenformin
Plasma standards – 0.1, 0.2, 0.5 and 1.0 mg/L
1 mol/L Acetic acid
Methanol
3 mol/L Sodium hydroxide
Dichloromethane
Injection solvent – 0.1 mol/L acetic acid/methanol, 1:1 by volume

Mobile phase – 1:1 methanol/water solution containing 0.2% acetic acid and 0.005 mol/L heptanesulfonic acid

Instrumental Conditions:

Liquid chromatograph with 235 nm ultraviolet detector
30 cm × 4 mm i.d. stainless-stell column containing µBondapak C_{18} (Waters Associates)
Column temperature, ambient
Solvent flow rate, 1 mL/min

Procedure:

1. Transfer 1 mL plasma to a 15 mL centrifuge tube. Add 100 µL 1 mol/L acetic acid and 2 mL methanol and vortex.
2. Centrifuge and decant supernatant into a 15 mL screw-cap tube. Add 1 mL 3 mol/L NaOH and 12 mL dichloromethane and shake to extract.
3. Centrifuge and discard upper aqueous layer. Transfer 10 mL of the organic phase to a 12 mL centrifuge tube and add 100 µL 1 mol/L acetic acid.
4. Evaporate to dryness under a stream of nitrogen at 40°C. Dissolve the residue in 50 µL of the injection solvent. Inject 25 µL into the chromatograph.

	Retention time (min)
phenformin	6

Calculation:

Calculation is based on a response factor derived from a standard curve. A quality control specimen containing 0.5 mg/L phenformin is analyzed daily.

Evaluation:

Sensitivity: 0.02 mg/L
Linearity: 0.1–1.0 mg/L
C.V.: not established
Relative recovery: not established

Interferences:

Endogenous plasma components do not interfere with the assay. Other drugs were not studied for potential interference. The method is applicable to determination of the other biguanide derivatives as well.

Reference:

H.M. Hill and J. Chamberlain. Determination of oral anti-diabetic agents in human body fluids using high performance liquid chromatography. J. Chromatog. 149: 349–358, 1978.

ORGANOCHLORINE PESTICIDES

	Plasma Concentrations (mg/L)	
	Healthy Adults	Intoxication
aldrin	0.0001–0.003	>0.03
chlordane	<0.001	1–4
DDT	0.002–0.011	?
dieldrin	0.0001–0.003	0.15–0.30
endrin	<0.003	0.01–0.05
lindane	<0.001	0.3–0.8

Although the chlorinated insecticides have been banned from widespread commercial usage in the United States, most of the agents continue to be found in trace amounts in human tissues. Several of the agents remain available in small quantities to the private consumer and thus the potential exists for acute or chronic intoxication. The following electron-capture gas chromatograph technique is sufficiently sensitive for the monitoring of background blood concentrations of the chlorinated hydrocarbons in healthy individuals. The four major isomers of technical lindane (benzene hexachloride) are detected separately, as are the major metabolites of DDT and its isomers. A related agent, pentachlorophenol, is dealt with in a separate section (see Index).

Plasma Organochlorine Pesticides by Electron-Capture Gas Chromatography

Principle:
The chlorinated hydrocarbon insecticides and their metabolites are extracted from plasma with hexane. The concentrated extract is analyzed by electron-capture gas chromatography on 10% DEGS, using a second column for confirmation of positive results.

Reagents:
Stock solutions – 1 mg/L hexane solutions of the appropriate agents
Plasma standards – 0.001, 0.005, 0.010, 0.050, and 0.100 mg/L of the appropriate agent
Hexane (nanograde)
Sodium sulfate – anhydrous Na_2SO_4

Instrumental Conditions:
Gas chromatograph with election-capture detector
2 m × 2 mm i.d. aluminum column containing 10% diethylene glycol succinate on 60/80 mesh Chromosorb G
1.2 m × 2 mm i.d. aluminum column containing 5% Dow 200 on 60/80 mesh Chromosorb G

Injector, 224°C.; column, 180°C.; detector, 224°C.
Nitrogen flow rate, 80 mL/min

Procedure:

1. Transfer 2 mL plasma to a 15 mL glass-stoppered centrifuge tube. Add 5 mL hexane and shake to extract.
2. Centrifuge and discard the lower aqueous phase with the aid of a disposable pipet. Add a small amount of solid Na_2SO_4 and vortex.
3. Transfer 4 mL of the hexane to a 15 mL centrifuge tube and evaporate to dryness under a stream of nitrogen at 40°C.
4. Dissolve the residue in 50 μL hexane and inject 10 μL into the gas chromatograph, using either column.

	Retention time (min)	
	10% DEGS	5% Dow 200
aldrin	3.1	11.3
α-BHC	4.4	4.2
γ-BHC (lindane)	7.0	5.2
o,p′-DDE	8.4	17.8
heptachlor epoxide	9.6	14.4
p,p-DDE	11.3	22.0
dieldrin	14.4	22.0
o,p′-DDT	16.0	28.7
δ-BHC	21.0	5.2
β-BHC	23.8	4.6
p,p′-DDT	30.3	38.2
p,p′-DDD	38.3	28.7

Calculation:

Calculation is based on a response factor derived from a standard curve. A quality control specimen containing the appropriate agent at a mid-range concentration is analyzed daily.

Evaluation:

Sensitivity: 0.0001 mg/L
Linearity: 0.001–0.100 mg/L
C.V.: not established
Relative recovery: not established

Interferences:

In order to prevent contamination from reagents and glassware, reagent blanks must be frequently analyzed. The use of two chromatographic columns to confirm positive results increases the specificity of the method.

Reference:

W.E. Dale, A. Curley and C. Cueto, Jr. Hexane extractable chlorinated insecticides in human blood. Life Sci. 5: 47–54, 1966.

ORGANOPHOSPHATE PESTICIDES

	Urinary Metabolites of Organophosphate Pesticides After Toxic Exposure (mg/L)	
	Organic Phosphates	p-Nitrophenol
diazinon	>0.1	—
dichlorvos	>0.1	—
malathion	>0.2	—
methylparathion	>0.2	1–15
parathion	>0.2	1–15

The rapid metabolism of the organophosphate pesticides by man requires that analytical techniques designed to demonstrate exposure to these substances be sensitive to their metabolites. The table above shows the amounts of urinary biotransformation products likely to be present following a potentially toxic exposure to the commonly used agents. A nonspecific method is described for the colorimetric determination of the organic phosphate residues that are present in urine after exposure to any of these compounds, while a more specific gas chromatographic procedure is presented for measurement of urinary p-nitrophenol, a metabolite of parathion and methylparathion. A rapid and possibly more clinically useful test is the measurement of the plasma or erythrocyte cholinesterase level; this procedure is available in most clinical laboratories.

Urine Organic Phosphates by Colorimetry

Principle:

The organic phosphate metabolites of the organophosphate pesticides are extracted from acidified urine with ether. Following evaporation of the solvent and oxidation of the organic matter, a chromogenic reagent is added and the resulting color is measured at 820 nm.

Reagents:

Stock solution – 1 mg/mL diethylphosphoric acid in methanol
Urine standards – 0.5, 1, 2 and 4 mg/L
Hydrochloric acid – conc. HCl
Ether
Sodium sulfate – anhydrous Na_2SO_4
0.1 mol/L Hydrochloric acid
Ethanol (absolute)
0.1 mol/L Potassium hydroxide
60% Perchloric acid

Ascorbic acid reagent – 10 mL 6 mol/L H_2SO_4, 20 mL water and 10 mL 2.5% ammonium molybdate are mixed together; add 10 mL 10% ascorbic acid and mix (prepare fresh)

Instrumental Conditions:

Visible spectrophotometer set to 820 nm

Procedure:

1. Transfer 20 mL urine to a 125 mL separatory funnel. Adjust pH to about 2 with conc. HCl and extract with 40 mL ether.
2. Discard lower aqueous layer. Add sufficient Na_2SO_4 to ether to break any emulsion and shake vigorously.
3. Filter the ether through a glass wool plug inserted in the funnel stem into a clean separatory funnel. Wash ether with 1 mL 0.1 mol/L HCl.
4. Add sufficient Na_2SO_4 to absorb the aqueous layer, shake and filter ether as before into a 50 mL centrifuge tube. Add 5 mL ethanol and 0.5 mL 0.1 mol/L KOH.
5. Heat at 50°C. for 10 min and then evaporate to dryness under a stream of nitrogen. Dissolve the residue in 2 mL water.
6. Transfer the solution to a small test tube, add 0.5 mL 60% perchloric acid and heat at 190–210°C. until a colorless dry residue remains. Cool the tube.
7. Add 4 mL ascorbic acid reagent and incubate at 37°C. for 0.5–1 hour. Read against a negative urine control at 820 nm in the spectrophotometer.

Calculation:

Calculation is based on a response factor derived from a standard curve. A quality control specimen containing 1 mg/L diethylphosphoric acid is analyzed daily.

Evaluation:

Sensitivity: 0.2 mg/L
Linearity: 0.5–4 mg/L
C.V.: not established
Relative recovery: not established

Interferences:

Normal urine may contain small amounts of organic phosphorus compounds. The use of a control urine as a blank for the reference cell will help to eliminate false positive results. The phosphate metabolites of organophosphate pesticides are known to be unstable in stored specimens and therefore analysis should be conducted soon after sampling.

Reference:

A.M. Mattson and V.A. Sedlak. Ether-extractable urinary phosphates in man and rats derived from malathion and similar compounds. J. Agr. Food Chem. 8: 107–110, 1960.

Urine p-Nitrophenol by Electron-Capture Gas Chromatography

Principle:

Conjugated p-nitrophenol in urine is hydrolyzed by heating in the presence of acid. The released compound is extracted into an organic solvent. On-column derivatization to a less polar trimethysilyl ether is performed, and analysis is by electron-capture gas chromatography.

Reagents:

Stock solution – 1 mg/mL p-nitrophenol in methanol
Urine standards – 1, 2, 5 and 10 mg/L
Hydrochloric acid – conc. HCl
20% Sodium hydroxide
Extraction solvent – benzene/ether, 80:20 by volume
Sodium sulfate – anhydrous Na_2SO_4
Derivatization reagent – hexamethyldisilazane/hexane, 20:80 by volume

Instrumental Conditions:

Gas chromatograph with electron-capture detector
2 m × 2 mm i.d. glass column containing 5% DC-200 on 80/100 mesh Gas Chrom Q
Injector, 200°C.; column, 140°C.; detector, 250°C.

Procedure:

1. Transfer 3 mL urine to a 15 mL screw-cap tube. Add 0.3 mL conc. HCl, cap the tube and heat in a boiling water bath for 1 hour.
2. Cool and adjust the pH to 11 or higher with approximately 0.4 mL 20% NaOH. Extract twice with 5 mL extraction solvent and discard the solvent.
3. Adjust the pH of the aqueous layer to 2 or lower with conc. HCl. Extract with 5 mL extraction solvent.
4. Centrifuge and transfer the organic layer to a 15 mL centrifuge tube. Add a small amount of anhydrous Na_2SO_4 and vortex.
5. Transfer 1 mL of the organic layer to a 5 mL glass-stoppered centrifuge tube. Add 1 mL of the derivatization reagent and vortex.
6. Inject 5 μL of the mixture into the gas chromatograph.

Calculation:

Calculation is based on a response factor derived from a standard curve. A quality control specimen containing 1 mg/L p-nitrophenol is analyzed daily.

Evaluation:

Sensitivity: 0.5 mg/L
Linearity: 0.1–10 mg/L
C.V.: 2–5% within-run
Relative recovery: 92–100%

Interferences:

The method is relatively specific for p-nitrophenol in urine. Some loss of p-nitrophenol may occur during the hydrolysis step if the tube is not tightly capped.

Reference:

M. Cranmer. Determination of p-nitrophenol in human urine. Bull. Env. Cont. Tox. 5: 329–332, 1970.

OXALATE

	Oxalate Concentrations (mg/L)		
	Normal Subjects	Ethylene Glycol Intoxication	Fatal Oxalic Acid Poisoning
Serum	1.0–2.4	>20	18–110
Urine	8–50	>150	>150

Oxalate is a natural component of serum and urine that derives primarily from dietary oxalic acid and from the metabolism of ascorbic acid and glycine. Primary hyperoxaluria is a genetic disorder that results in the excessive generation of oxalate, with associated increases in serum and urine oxalate levels. Poisoning with ethylene glycol or oxalic acid as well as severe renal failure also result in elevated oxalate concentrations in serum. A somewhat time-consuming gas chromatographic procedure is presented for oxalate determination in serum. A more convenient enzymatic method is available in some laboratories for oxalate measurement in both serum and urine.

Serum Oxalate by Gas Chromatography

Principle:

Oxalic acid is extracted from deproteinized serum with ether after salt saturation and acidification of the aqueous phase. A diethyl derivative is formed by reaction with ethanol in an acid medium, and analysis is performed by flame-ionization gas chromatography.

Reagents:

Stock solution – 1 mg/mL oxalate in water
Aqueous standards – 1, 2, 5 and 10 mg/L
Acetone
Internal standard – 13 mmol/L diethylmalonic acid in ethanol
Saturated sodium chloride
Hydrochloric acid – conc. HCl
Formic acid
Extraction solvent – 10% ethanol in ether
Sodium sulfate – anhydrous Na_2SO_4
Ethanolic sulfuric acid – conc. H_2SO_4/ethanol, 20:80 by volume

Instrumental Conditions:

Gas chromatograph with flame-ionization detector
3 m × 3 mm i.d. glass column containing 4% DEGS on 80/100 mesh Chromosorb G
Injector, 200°C.; detector, 200°C.

Column temperature: initial, 110°C (3 min)
                    5°C./min increase
                    final, 185°C. (3 min).
Nitrogen flow rate, 30 mL/min

Procedure:

1. Transfer 3 mL serum to a 15 mL centrifuge tube. Add 3 mL acetone and vortex.
2. Centrifuge and transfer the supernatant to a rotary evaporator. Evaporate to dryness at 40°C. under partial vacumn.
3. Dissolve the residue in 3 mL water. Add 100 µL internal standard, 3 mL saturated NaCl, 2 mL conc. HCl and 0.2 mL formic acid.
4. Transfer the solution to a 125 mL separatory funnel and extract with 50 mL of the extraction solvent. Allow layers to settle and discard the lower aqueous layer.
5. Add 1–2 g anhydrous Na_2SO_4 to the ether and shake. Filter the ether layer through a pledget of glass wool inserted in the funnel stem into a 50 mL centrifuge tube.
6. Evaporate the ether to a volume of about 0.5 mL under a stream of nitrogen at 30°C. add 1 drop ethanolic H_2SO_4, vortex and allow to stand at room temperature for 24 hr.
7. Inject 4 µL of the solution into the gas chromatograph.

	Retention time (min)
oxalic acid derivative	7
internal standard	9

Calculation:

Calculation is based on a response factor derived from a standard curve. A quality control specimen consisting of pooled serum is analyzed daily.

Evaluation:

Sensitivity: 0.8 mg/L
Linearity: 1–10 mg/L
C.V.: 8.7%
Relative recovery: not established

Interferences:

The method is relatively specific for oxalic acid. Other related substances, such as pyruvic acid, lactic acid, glycolic acid and succinic acid, are well-separated from both oxalic acid and the internal standard.

References:

1. P. Nuret and M. Offner. A new method for determination of oxalate is blood serum by gas chromatography. Clin. Chim. Acta 81: 9–12, 1978.
2. M.T. Duburque, J.M. Melon, J. Thomas et al. Dosage et identification de l'acide oxalique dans les milieux biologiques. Ann. Biol. Clin. 28: 95–101, 1970.

PANCURONIUM

Plasma Concentrations (mg/L)			
99% Paralysis	80% Paralysis	50% Paralysis	T½
0.22	0.17	0.09	2 hr

Pancuronium is a synthetic steroid-like quaternary ammonium compound used as a muscle relaxant during surgical procedures. It is a nondepolarizing neuromuscular blocking agent and is a popular alternative to d-tubocurarine. Pancuronium is administered intravenously in small doses and therapeutic plasma concentrations are relatively low. A sensitive fluorometric method is described for its assay in plasma; the procedure also measures the metabolities of pancuronium but since the major metabolite also has pharmacological activity this is not a serious disadvantage.

Plasma Pancuronium by Fluorescence Spectrophotometry

Principle:

Pancuronium in plasma is reacted with a rose bengal dye solution. The complex is extracted into chloroform and analyzed by fluorescence spectrophotometry.

Reagents:

Stock solution – 1 mg/mL pancuronium in methanol
Plasma standards – 0.10, 0.20, 0.50 and 1.00 mg/L
2.5% Phenol solution – 2.5 g phenol and 5 mL ethanol diluted to 100 mL with chloroform (stable for 1 hr in the dark)
pH 7.8 Phosphate buffer – 25 mL 0.2 mol/L KH_2PO_4 and 22.6 mL 0.2 mol/L NaOH diluted to 100 mL with water
Dye solution – 100 mg/L rose bengal in 0.05 mol/L K_2HPO_4 (stable for 6 hr in the dark)
Acetone

Instrumental Conditions:

Fluorescence spectrophotometer set to excite at 546 nm
Record emission at 570 nm

Procedure:

1. Transfer 1 mL plasma to a 15 mL screw-cap tube. Add 7 mL 2.5% phenol solution, 1 mL phosphate buffer and 0.5 mL dye solution and mix on a rotator for 30 min.
2. Centrifuge and discard upper aqueous phase. Transfer 0.5 mL of the organic layer to a 12 mL centrifuge tube.
3. Add 3.5 mL acetone and vortex for 10 seconds. Wait one min and repeat the vortexing. Read immediately in the fluorometer against a plasma blank.

Calculation:

Calculation is based on a response factor derived from a standard curve. A quality control specimen containing 0.2 mg/L pancuronium is analyzed daily.

Evaluation:

Sensitivity: 0.02 mg/L
Linearity: 0.1–1.0 mg/L
C.V.: 4% within-run
Relative recovery: not established

Interferences:

The deacetylated metabolites of pancuronium are measured with equivalent sensitivity by this procedure. Other neuromuscular blocking agents and other drugs used during general anesthesia, with the exception of d-tubocurarine, were found not to interfere.

Reference:

U.W. Kersten, D.K.F. Meijer and S. Agoston. Fluorometric and chromatographic determination of pancuronium bromide and its metabolites in biological materials. Clin. Chim. Acta 44; 59–66, 1973.

PARALDEHYDE

Plasma Concentrations (mg/L)			
Sedation	Anesthesia	Fatalities	T½
10–100	>200	500–1600	4–10 hr

Paraldehyde is a cyclic trimer of acetaldehyde that is administered in oral doses of 5–10 mL as a sedative. The compound is a liquid at room temperature and slowly oxidizes to acetic acid on exposure to air. Although in vivo paraldehyde is metabolized to acetaldehyde and then to acetic acid, acetaldehyde has not been detected in the plasma of subjects administered the parent drug. A convenient method for determination of paraldehyde in plasma involves depolymerization to acetaldehyde and measurement of this compound by headspace gas chromatography.

Plasma Paraldehyde by Gas Chromatography

Principle:
Plasma is mixed with an internal standard and concentrated hydrochloric acid and heated in a sealed vial. After conversion of any paraldehyde present to acetaldehyde, the head space gases are sampled and analyzed using a gas chromatograph with a flame-ionization detector.

Reagents:
Stock solution – 1 mg/mL paraldehyde in water
Plasma standards – 25, 50, 100 and 200 mg/L
Internal standard – 0.2% methyl ethyl ketone in water
Hydrochloric acid – conc. HCl

Instrumental Conditions:
Gas chromatograph with flame-ionization detector
6′ × ⅛″ stainless-steel column containing 0.2% carbowax on 60/80 mesh Carbopack C (Supelco, Inc.)
Injector, 150°C.; column, 125°C.; detector, 150°C.
Nitrogen flow rate, 17 mL/min

Procedure:
1. Pipet 3 mL plasma into a 10 mL serum bottle. Add 0.3 mL internal standard and 0.3 mL of concentrated HCl.
2. Seal the bottle with a rubber septum covered with aluminum foil and heat in boiling water for 5 minutes. Cool to room temperature before analysis (IMPORTANT!).

3. Withdraw 0.5 mL headspace gas into a 2 mL glass syringe equipped with a 23 gauge needle and inject this into the gas chromatograph.

	Retention time (min)
acetaldehyde	0.6
internal standard	2.3

Calculation:

Calculation is based on a response factor derived from a standard curve. A quality control specimen containing 50 mg/L paraldehyde is analyzed daily.

Evaluation:

Sensitivity: 20 mg/L
Linearity: 25–1000 mg/L
C.V.: 3–4% within-run
Relative recovery: 98–103%

Interferences:

The method is relatively specific for acetaldehyde. However, acetaldehyde may be present as an endogenous compound or as a metabolite of ethanol or paraldehyde, in a plasma concentration of 0.2–1.5 mg/L. Though the production of larger amounts is unlikely, this possibility may be excluded by performing the analysis without the acid-heat treatment to show the absence of acetaldehyde.

References:

1. R.H. Cravey. Personal communication, 1966.
2. R.C. Baselt. Unpublished results, 1976.
3. J.P. Hancock, J.C. Harrill and E.T. Solomons. Head space gas chromatographic analysis of paraldehyde in toxicologic specimens. J. Analyt. Tox. 1: 161–163, 1977.

PAPAVERINE

Therapeutic Plasma Concentrations (mg/L)	T½
0.2–4.0	0.8–1.5 hr

Papaverine is an opium alkaloid that is extensively employed as a peripheral vasodilator and antispasmodic drug. It is administered by intramuscular or intravenous injection of 30–120 mg or orally in daily doses of 300–600 mg. A flame-ionization gas chromatographic method is employed for the measurement of therapeutic plasma levels. This procedure may also be used to determine strychnine in plasma, using papaverine as internal standard, if the appropriate standards are employed.

Plasma Papaverine by Gas Chromatography

Principle:
Papaverine and an internal standard (strychnine) are extracted from plasma with toluene. Following several clean-up extractions, the drugs are analyzed by flame-ionization gas chromatography.

Reagents:
Stock solution – 1 mg/mL papaverine in methanol
Plasma standards – 0.1, 0.5, 1.0 and 2.0 mg/L
Internal standard – 10 mg/L solution of strychnine in methanol
9 mol/L Sodium hydroxide
Toluene
1 mol/L Hydrochloric acid
Ether
Sodium sulfate – anhydrous Na_2SO_4
Chloroform

Instrumental Conditions:
Gas chromatography with flame-ionization detector
1.2 m × 4 mm i.d. glass column containing 3% OV-17 on 80/100 mesh Gas-Chrom Q
Injector, 275°C. column; 265°C.; detector, 280°C.
Nitrogen flow rate, 80 mL/min

Procedure:
1. Transfer 3 mL plasma to a 125 mL screw-cap tube. Add 100 μL internal standard and vortex.

2. Add 1 mL 9 mol/L NaOH and 10 mL toluene and shake to extract. Centrifuge and transfer the toluene layer to a clean tube.
3. Extract the toluene with 3 mL 1 mol/L HCl. Centrifuge and discard the upper organic layer.
4. Add 1 mL 9 mol/L NaOH to the aqueous phase and extract with 4 mL ether. Centrifuge and transfer the ether layer to a 15 mL centrifuge tube.
5. Add 0.5 g Na_2SO_4 and vortex. Centrifuge and decant the supernatant into a clean tube.
6. Evaporate to dryness at 40°C. under a stream of nitrogen. Dissolve the residue in 25 µL chloroform and inject 3 µL into the chromatograph.

	Retention time (min)
papaverine	3.4
internal standard	7.6

Calculation:

Calculation is based on a response factor derived from a standard curve. A quality control specimen containing 0.2 mg/L papaverine is analyzed daily.

Evaluation:

Sensitivity: 0.01 mg/L
Linearity: 0.1–2.0 mg/L
C.V.: not established
Relative recovery: not established

Interferences:

Endogenous plasma materials do not interfere with the assay. Other drugs were not studied for potential interference.

References:

1. J.D. Arnold, J. Baldridge, B. Riley and G. Brody. Papaverine hydrochloride; the evaluation of two new dosage forms. Int. J. Clin. Pharm. 15: 230–233, 1977.
2. V. Bellia, J. Jacob and H.T. Smith. Determination of papaverine in blood samples by gas chromatography using a flame-ionization and a nitrogen-phosphorus detector. J. Chromatog. 161: 231–235, 1978.

PARAQUAT

	Paraquat Concentrations (mg/L)		
	Spray Operators	Intoxication	Fatalities
blood	?	0.1–1.6	0.1–63
urine	0–0.3	0.9–64	0.6–1766

Paraquat is a bis-quaternary ammonium compound that is extensively used as an herbicide. It is supplied as a 5% powder for domestic use or as a 20–30% aqueous concentrate for commercial agricultural purposes. Paraquat has recently been detected as a contaminant of marijuana grown in Mexico and smuggled into the United States. Clinical emergencies involving paraquat are almost always a result of accidental or intentional ingestion of a commercial product. The course of poisoning is often quite prolonged, and it has been found that both forced diuresis and hemodialysis may enhance the rate of elimination of the chemical. A rapid colorimetric technique is presented for the qualitative or semi-quantitative determination of paraquat in urine, while quantitative measurement of the substance in plasma may be performed by gas chromatography or liquid chromatography.

Urine Paraquat by Colorimetry

Principle:
Paraquat is reduced, by addition of sodium dithionite to urine, to a free radical that produces a blue color in alkaline solution. The concentration may be estimated visually or spectrophotometrically by comparison to standards.

Reagents:
Stock solution – 1 mg/mL paraquat in water (stable for several weeks at 4°C. in the dark)
Urine standards – 1, 2, 5 and 10 mg/L (prepare fresh)
Dithionite solution – 1% sodium dithionite in 1 mol/L NaOH (prepare fresh)

Instrumental Conditions:
Visible spectrophotometer set to 396 nm

Procedure:
1. Transfer 5 mL urine to a 12 mL centrifuge tube. Add 1 mL dithionite solution and vortex.
2. Within 5 min read in the spectrophotometer at 396 nm against a urine blank, or compare the color visually to standards prepared in the same manner.

216

Calculation:

Calculation is based on a response factor derived from a standard curve. This is a semi-quantitative procedure and results should be expressed as such.

Evaluation:

Sensitivity: 1 mg/L
Linearity: 1–10 mg/L
C.V.: not established
Relative recovery: not established

Interferences:

None reported.

References:

1. D.J. Berry and J. Grove. The determination of paraquat (1,1'-dimethyl-4,4'-bipyridylium cation) in urine. Clin. Chim. Acta 34: 5–11, 1971.
2. B. Widdop. Detection of paraquat in urine. Brit. Med. J. 2: 1135, 1976.

Plasma Paraquat by Nitrogen-Specific Gas Chromatography

Principle:

Paraquat and an internal standard, the ethyl analogue of paraquat, are converted to diene reduction products with sodium borohydride. These products are extracted into ether and the concentrated extract is analyzed by gas chromatography with nitrogen-specific detection.

Reagents:

Stock solution – 1 mg/mL paraquat in water (stable for several weeks at 4°C. in the dark)
Plasma standards – 0.1, 0.5, 2.0 and 5.0 mg/L (prepare fresh)
Internal standard – 10 mg/L ethyl viologen (Shell Oil Co.) in water (stable for several weeks at 4°C. in the dark)
25% Trichloroacetic acid.
4 mol/L Sodium hydroxide
Sodium borohydride
Ether
Methanol

Instrumental Conditions:

Gas chromatograph with nitrogen-phosphorus detector
2 m × 2 mm i.d. glass column containing 3% Poly A-135 on 80/100 mesh Supelcoport (Supelco, Inc.)
Injector, 200°C.; column, 190°C.; detector, 210°C.
Nitrogen flow rate, 35 mL/min

Procedure:

1. Transfer 3 mL plasma to a 12 mL centrifuge tube. Add 1 mL internal standard and vortex.
2. Add 1 mL 25% trichloroacetic acid, vortex for 30 seconds and centrifuge. Decant the supernatant into a 15 mL glass-stoppered centrifuge tube.
3. Add sufficient 4 mol/L NaOH until the pH of the solution exceeds 10 (about 1 mL). Add 200 mg sodium borohydride and vortex until dissolved.
4. Stopper the tube and incubate at 60°C. for 12.5 min. Cool, add 5 mL ether and shake for 1 min.
5. Centrifuge and transfer the ether layer to a 12 mL centrifuge tube. Repeat the ether extraction and combine the ehter layers.
6. Evaporate the ether to about 0.5 mL under a stream of nitrogen at room temperature. Transfer the concentrated extract to a 1 mL Reacti-vial (Pierce Chemical).
7. Evaporate ether to dryness. Dissolve the residue in 20–100 µL methanol and inject 1–3 µL into the gas chromatograph.

	Retention time (min)
paraquat derivative	4.5
internal standard derivative	8.0

Calculation:

Calculation is based on a response factor derived from a standard curve. This procedure cannot be controlled by the usual methods due to the instability of paraquat in aqueous solution.

Evaluation:

Sensitivity: 0.03 mg/L
Linearity: 0.1–5.0 mg/L
C.V.: 2% within-day
Relative recovery: 92–98%

Interferences:

Normal plasma components do not interfere with the assay. Other drugs or chemicals were not studied for potential interference. The monoene reduction products of paraquat and the internal standard elute at 2.5 and 3.5 min, respectively.

Reference:

A. van Dijk, R. Ebberink, G. de Groot et al. A rapid and sensitive assay for the determination of paraquat in plasma by gas-liquid chromatography. J. Analyt. Tox 1: 151–154, 1977.

Plasma Paraquat by Liquid Chromatography

Principle:

Plasma is deproteinized with an organic solvent mixture. An aliquot of the supernatant is analyzed by liquid chromatography on cation-exchange resin with detection to 254 nm.

Reagents:

Stock solution – 1 mg/mL paraquat in water (stable for several weeks at 4°C. in the dark)
Plasma standards – 0.2, 0.5, 1.0 and 2.0 mg/L (prepare fresh)
Chloroform/ethanol, 4:1 by volume
0.4% Uranyl acetate
Mobile phase – 0.025% ammonium hydroxide and 0.2 mol/L dimethylamine HCl in methanol
0.4 mol/L Phosphoric acid

Instrumental Conditions:

Liquid chromatograph with 254 nm ultraviolet detector
50 cm × 4.6 mm i.d. stainless-steel column containing 30–44 μm Vydac cation-exchange resin
Column temperature, ambient
Solvent flow rate, 6 mL/min
The column must be regenerated after every 12 determinations by washing with 0.4 mol/L phosphoric acid; the mobile phase must not be allowed to stand in contact with the column for any length of time.

Procedure:

1. Transfer 2 mL serum to a 12 mL centrifuge tube. Add 2 mL cold chloroform/ethanol and vortex for 1 min.
2. Centrifuge at 4°C. and transfer a portion of the upper aqueous phase to a clean tube. Add an equal volume of 0.4% uranyl acetate and vortex.
3. Centrifuge and inject 100 μL of the supernatant into the chromatograph.

	Retention time (min)
paraquat	3

Calculation:

Calculation is based on a response factor derived from a standard curve. This procedure cannot be controlled by the usual methods due to the instability of paraquat in aqueous solution.

Evaluation:

Sensitivity: 0.2 mg/L
Linearity: 0.2–2.5 mg/L
C.V.: not established
Relative recovery: not established

Interferences:

Normal plasma components do not interfere with the assay. Other drugs or chemicals were not studied for potential interference.

Reference:

J.J. Miller, E. Sanders and D. Webb. Measurement of paraquat in serum by high-performance liquid chromatography. J. Analyt. Tox 3: 1–3, 1979.

PENTACHLOROPHENOL

	Pentachlorophenol Concentrations (mg/L)			
	Normal Hawaiian Subjects	Exposed Workers	Nonfatal Intoxication	Fatalities
plasma	0.05–1.0	1–20	>30	39–173
urine	0.00–0.6	0–39	4–60	28–520

Pentachlorophenol is widely employed as a wood preservative, contact herbicide, disinfectant and mildew retardant. The compound is used domestically and commercially and is well-absorbed following oral, pulmonary or dermal exposure. Poisoning has occurred after careless usage of pentachlorophenol products and following oral, pulmonary or dermal exposure. Poisoning has occurred after careless usage of pentachlorophenol products and following accidental or intentional ingestion. Forced diuresis has been shown to be effective in enhancing the excretion of the chemical, which is metabolized to only a small extent. An electron-capture gas chromatographic method is presented for the determination of pentachlorophenol in plasma and urine.

Plasma and Urine Pentachlorophenol by Electron-Capture Gas Chromatography

Principle:

Pentachlorophenol is extracted from the acidified specimen with benzene. Diazomethane is used to form the methyl ether of pentachlorophenol and the derivative is analyzed by electron-capture gas chromatography.

Reagents:

Stock solution – 1 mg/mL pentachlorophenol in methanol
Plasma standards – 0.1, 1, 10 and 50 mg/L
Urine standards – 0.1, 1, 10 and 50 mg/L
Benzene
Sulfuric acid – conc. H_2SO_4
Diazomethane reagent – add 0.5 g N-methyl-N′-nitro-N-nitrosoguanidine slowly in small increments to a mixture of 25 mL hexane and 2 mL 20% NaOH in a flask; decant the hexane layer and store frozen for up to one week (prepare in well-ventilated hood)
Isooctane

Instrumental Conditions:

Gas chromatograph with electron-capture detector
1.8 m × 2 mm i.d. glass column containing 4% OV-1 and 6% QF-1 on 80/100 mesh Chromosorb W

Injector, 220°C.; column, 190°C.; detector, 280°C.
Nitrogen flow rate, 85 mL/min

Procedure:

1. Transfer 2 mL plasma or urine to a 15 mL screw-cap tube. Add 6 mL benzene and 2 drops conc. H_2SO_4 and place on a tilted rotator for 2 hours at 50 rpm.
2. Centrifuge and transfer 3 mL of the benzene layer to a 10 mL volumetric flask. Add 200 µL diazomethane reagent and allow to stand for 15 min.
3. Remove excess diazomethane by bubbling nitrogen through the solution until the yellow color disappears.
4. Dilute to 10 mL with isooctane and inject 2–8 µL into the gas chromatograph.

	Retention time (min)
pentachlorophenol derivative	2.2

Calculation:

Calculation is based on a response factor derived from a standard curve. A quality control specimen containing 10 mg/L pentachlorophenol is analyzed daily.

Evaluation:

Sensitivity: 0.01 mg/L
Linearity: 0.1–50 mg/L
C.V.: 1–7%
Relative recovery: 89–99%

Interferences:

Normal plasma and urine components do not interfere with the assay. The use of excess diazomethane solution can lead to interferences due to reagent impurities.

Reference:

J.B. Rivers. Gas chromatographic determination of pentachlorophenol in human blood and urine. Bull. Env. Cont. Tox. 8: 294–296, 1972.

PENTAZOCINE

	Pentazocine Concentrations (mg/L)		
	Therapeutic	Fatalities	T½
plasma	0.05–0.20	1–5	2 hr
urine	1–20	3–32	

Pentazocine is a synthetic narcotic analgestic that is about one-third to one-sixth as potent as morphine. It may be administered orally or by injection in doses of 30–100 mg and, since it is a weak antagonist, has a low potential for abuse. Overdosage is not uncommon, however, and usually occurs following intentional abuse. Therapeutic concentrations of the drug may be conveniently analyzed in plasma by fluorometry, although up to 25% of the apparent pentazocine by this technique may represent inactive metabolites. A flame-ionization gas chromatographic method offers higher specificity for the parent drug, but is more suitable for toxic concentrations of the drug in plasma and urine. Pentazocine may also be measured in urine using the Urine Opiates by Gas Chromatography procedure (p. 189), which involves the formation of an acetyl derivative. It should be noted that acid hydrolysis of urine specimens for the purpose of releasing conjugated pentazocine will result in partial conversion of the drug to a hydroxy derivative, formed by hydrolysis of the double bond in the side chain; for this reason enzymatic hydrolysis of pentazocine conjugates is indicated.

Plasma Pentazocine by Fluorescence Spectrophotometry

Principle:
Pentazocine is extracted from alkalinized plasma with benzene and re-extracted into dilute acid. The aqueous extract is analyzed directly by fluorescence spectrophotometry.

Reagents:
Stock solution – 1 mg/mL pentazocine in methanol
Plasma standards – 0.05, 0.10 and 0.20 mg/L
Carbonate buffer – 1:1 mixture of solid Na_2SO_3 and $NaHCO_3$
Benzene
0.2 mol/L Hydrochloric acid

Instrumental Conditions:
Fluorescence spectrophotometer set to excite at 278 nm
Record emission at 310 nm

Procedure:

1. Transfer 3 mL plasma into a 30 mL screw-cap tube. Add 6 mL water and 400 mg carbonate buffer.
2. Add 11.5 mL benzene and shake to extract. Centrifuge and transfer 10 mL benzene to a 15 mL screw-cap tube.
3. Extract the benzene with 1.5 mL 0.2 mol/L HCl. Centrifuge and discard the upper organic layer.
4. Transfer at least 1 mL of the aqueous phase to a quartz cuvette and read in the spectrophotometer against a plasma blank.

Calculation:

Calculation is based on a response factor derived from a standard curve. A quality control specimen containing 0.10 mg/L pentazocine is analyzed daily.

Evaluation:

Sensitivity: 0.03 mg/L
Linearity: 0.03–0.20 mg/L
C.V.: not established
Relative recovery: not established

Interferences:

The benzene used as a solvent, if not of spectrophotometric grade, may need to be washed with dilute acid, base and water prior to use to insure a low reagent blank. The hydroxylated pentazocine metabolites interfere in the assay and may constitute up to 25% of the total drug in plasma. Other drugs were not studied for potential interference.

Reference:

B.A. Berkowitz, J.H. Asling, S.H. Shnider and E.L. Way. Relationship of pentazocine plasma levels to pharmacological activity in man. Clin. Phar. Ther. 10: 320–328, 1969.

Plasma and Urine Pentazocine by Gas Chromatography

Principle:

Pentazocine and an internal standard are extracted from alkalinized plasma or urine with benzene. After several clean-up steps, the drugs are analyzed by flame-ionization gas chromatography.

Reagents:

Stock solution – 1 mg/mL pentazocine in methanol
Plasma standards – 0.2, 1, 2 and 5 mg/L
Urine standards – 1, 5, 10 and 20 mg/L
Internal standard – 5 mg/L α-methadol (Eli Lilly) in water
1 mol/L Ammonium hydroxide
Benzene

0.1 mol/L Hydrochloric acid
n-Butanol

Instrumental Conditions:

Gas chromatograph with flame-ionization detector
2 m × 2 mm i.d. glass colume containing 2.5% OV-1 on 80/100 mesh Chromosorb G
Injector, 250°C.; column, 200°C.; detector, 250°C.
Nitrogen flow rate, 60 mL/min

Procedure:

1. Transfer 0.5 mL urine and 2 mL water, or 2.5 mL plasma, to a 15 mL screw-cap tube.
2. Extract with 9 mL benzene. Centrifuge and transfer benzene layer to a clean tube.
3. Extract benzene with 2.5 mL 0.1 mol/L HCl. Centrifuge and discard upper solvent layer.
4. Add 1 mL 1 mol/L NH_4OH and extract with 7 mL benzene. Centrifuge and transfer benzene layer to a 15 mL conical centrifuge tube.
5. Evaporate solvent to dryness at 50°C. under a stream of nitrogen. Dissolve the residue in 20 μL n-butanol and inject 2 μL into the chromatograph.

	Retention time (min)
internal standard	3.7
pentazocine	5.3

Calculation:

Calculation is based on a response factor derived from a standard curve. A quality control specimen containing 1 mg/L (plasma) or 5 mg/L (urine) pentazocine is analyzed daily.

Evaluation:

Sensitivity: 0.05 mg/L
Linearity: 0.2–5 mg/L for plasma and 1–20 mg/L for urine
C.V.: 3–5%
Relative recovery: not established

Interferences:

Normal plasma and urine constituents did not interfere with the assay. Other drugs were not studied for potential interference.

Reference:

A.H. Beckett, J.F. Taylor and P. Kourounakis. The absorption, distribution and excretion of pentazocine in man after oral and intravenous administration. J. Pharm. Pharmac. 22: 123–128, 1970.

PHENACETIN

	Plasma Concentrations (mg/L)		
	Therapeutic	Toxic	T½
phenacetin	1–20	50–250	0.6 hr
acetaminophen	3–18	?	2 hr

Phenacetin is a nonnarcoic analgestic that is frequently found in nonprescription and prescription medications in combination with drugs such as acetaminophen, aspirin, caffeine, codeine and propoxyphene. The compound is metabolized by O-deethylation to acetaminophen, the major biotransformation product. Both substances have nearly equal activity as analgesic and antipyretic drugs in man. Two chromatographic methods are described for determination of phenacetin and acetaminophen in plasma; the first is a gas chromatographic procedure and requires derivatization of the drugs, while the second involves only a single extraction and analysis by liquid chromatography.

Plasma Phenacetin and Acetaminophen by Gas Chromatography

Principle:

Phenacetin and acetaminophen are extracted from plasma with an organic solvent containing the internal standard. The concentrated extract is treated with a derivatization reagent to form the N-trimethylsilyl derivative of phenacetin and the N,O-ditrimethylsilyl derivative of acetaminophen. Analysis is by flame-ionization gas chromatography.

Reagents:

Stock solutions –
   1 mg/mL phenacetin in methanol
   1 mg/mL acetaminophen in methanol
Plasma standards – 10, 50, 100 and 200 mg/L for each drug
Internal standard solution – 30 mg/L p-bromoacetanilide in ethyl acetate
pH 8.0 1 mol/L Phosphate buffer
Pyridine (anhydrous)
BSA – N,O-bis(trimethylsilyl)acetamide

Instrumental Conditions:

Gas chromatograph with flame-ionization detector
1.8 m × 2 mm i.d. glass column containing 5% OV-1 on 80/100 mesh Gas Chrom Q
Injector, 180°C.; column, 160°C.; detector, 200°C.
Nitrogen flow rate, 50 mL/min

Procedure:

1. Transfer 2 mL plasma to a 15 mL screw-cap tube. Add 1 mL phosphate buffer and 5 mL internal standard solution and shake to extract.
2. Centrifuge and transfer the upper organic layer to a 15 mL conical centrifuge tube. Evaporate to dryness at 30°C. under a stream of nitrogen.
3. Dissolve the residue in 15 μL pyridine and transfer to a 1 mL Reacti-vial (Pierce Chemical). Add 15 μL BSA, and let stand for 15–30 min at room temperature.
4. Inject 2 μL of the mixture into the chromatograph.

	Retention time (min)
internal standard derivative	10.8
phenacetin derivative	12.9
acetaminophen derivative	15.6

Calculation:

Calculation is based on a response factor derived from a standard curve. A quality control specimen containing phenacetin and acetaminophen at mid-range concentrations is analyzed daily.

Evaluation:

Sensitivity: 0.05 mg/L
Linearity: 1–100 mg/L
C.V.: not established
Relative recovery: 98–106%

Interferences:

Several related drugs were shown not to interfere with the determination of phenacetin and acetaminophen. The silyl derivatives of the drugs are readily hydrolyzed by moisture and should be chromatographed soon after their formation.

Reference:

L.F. Prescott. The gas-liquid chromatographic estimation of phenacetin and paracetamol in plasma and urine. J. Pharm. Pharmac. 23: 111–115, 1971.

Plasma Phenacetin and Acetaminophen by Liquid Chromatography

Principle:

The two drugs are extracted from plasma together with an internal standard into ethyl acetate. The concentrated extract is analyzed by reversed-phase liquid chromatography with detection at 254 nm.

Reagents:

Stock solutions –
  1 mg/mL phenacetin in methanol
  1 mg/mL acetaminophen in methanol
  1 mg/mL acetoacetanilide in methanol
Plasma standards – 1, 5, 10, 20 and 40 mg/L for each drug
Internal standard – 50 mg/L acetoacetanilide in water (dilution of stock solution)
pH 7.0 1 mol/L Phosphate buffer
Ethyl acetate
Methanol
pH 4.4 Phosphate buffer – 0.3 mL 1 mol/L KH_2PO_4 and 0.05 mL 4.4 mol/L phosphoric acid
  in 1800 mL water
Mobile phase – acetonitrile/pH 4.4 phosphate buffer, 19:81 by volume

Instrumental Conditions:

Liquid chromatograph with 254 nm ultraviolet detector
30 cm × 4 mm i.d. stainless-steel column containing, μBondapak C_{18} (Waters Associates)
Column temperature, 50°C.
Solvent flow rate, 3 mL/min

Procedure:

1. Transfer 0.5 mL plasma to a 15 mL screw-cap tube. Add 0.5 mL internal standard and 0.5 mL pH 7 phosphate buffer and vortex.
2. Extract with 7 mL ethyl acetate. Centrifuge and transfer the ethyl acetate to a 15 mL conical centrifuge tube.
3. Evaporate to dryness at 50°C. under a stream of nitrogen. Dissolve the residue in 50 μL methanol and inject 10 μL into the chromatograph.

	Retention time (min)
acetaminophen	1.5
internal standard	3.4
phenacetin	5.0

Calculation:

Calculation is based on a response factor derived from a standard curve. A quality control specimen containing phenacetin and acetaminophen at mid-range concentrations is analyzed daily.

Evaluation:

Sensitivity: 0.5 mg/L
Linearity: 0.2–40 mg/L for phenacetin and 0.5–400 mg/L for acetaminophen
C.V.: 2–5% within-run, 3–6% day-to-day
Relative recovery: 92–110%

Interferences:

Of 33 drugs tested for interference, only theophylline was found to interfere significantly by co-eluting with acetaminophen. A plasma theophylline concentration of 23 mg/L increased the apparent acetaminophen level by 7 mg/L.

Reference:

G.R. Gotelli, P.M. Kabra and L.J. Marton. Determination of acetaminophen and phenacetin in plasma by high-pressure liquid chromatography. Clin. Chem. 23: 957–959, 1977.

PHENCYCLIDINE

	Phencyclidine Concentrations (mg/L)			
	Casual Users	Nonfatal Intoxication	Fatalities	T½
plasma	0.01–0.24	0.09–0.80	0.5–4.0	11 hr
urine	0.04–4.0	0.4–340	5–120	

Phencyclidine is a veterinary tranquilizer that is widely abused for its euphoric and hallucinogenic properties. Doses of 1–6 mg are administered by smoking, injection, ingestion or insufflation. The plasma concentrations observed during clinical intoxication are often quite low, and therefore a sensitive procedure must be used to assay the drugs. The gas chromatographic procedure presented is sensitive to 0.01 mg/L of the drug in plasma when a nitrogen phosphorus detector is used, but a sensitivity of 0.10 mg/L is easily achieved using the same procedure with a flame-ionization detector. A more specific technique involving mass spectrometry is included for confirmation of positive results. Concentrations of 1 mg/L or higher may be detected in plasma or urine using the methods listed under Basic Drug Screen (p. 41). Reagents are commercially available for the determination of phencyclidine in urine by radioimmunoassay, fluorescence immunoassay and EMIT.

Plasma Phencyclidine by Nitrogen-Specific Gas Chromatography

Principle:
Phencyclidine and an internal standard are extracted from alkalinized plasma into an organic solvent. After several clean-up extractions, the residue is analyzed by nitrogen-specific gas chromatography. Flame-ionization detection may also be used with reasonably good sensitivity.

Reagents:
Stock solution – 1 mg/mL phencyclidine in methanol
Plasma standards – 0.1, 0.2, 0.5 and 1.0 mg/L
Internal standard – 20 mg/L ketamine in water
0.5 mol/L Sodium hydroxide
Extraction solvent – heptane/isoamyl alcohol, 98.3:1.7 by volume
0.1 mol/L Hydrochloric acid
pH 9.8 Buffer – 24.8 g Na_2CO_3 and 25.2 g $NaHCO_3$ dissolved in 500 mL water
Toluene

Instrumental Conditions:
Gas chromatograph with nitrogen-phosphorus detector
2 m × 2 mm i.d. glass column containing 2% OV-1 on 100/120 mesh Chromosorb G-HP

Injector, 250°C.; column, 175°C.; detector, 250°C.
Nitrogen flow rate, 33 mL/min

Procedure:

1. Transfer 2 ml plasma to a 15 mL screw-cap tube. Add 100 µL internal standard and 0.5 mL 0.5 mol/L NaOH and vortex.
2. Extract with 10 mL extraction solvent. Centrifuge and transfer the organic layer to a clean tube.
3. Extract with 1 mL 0.1 mol/L HCl. Centrifuge and discard upper organic layer.
4. Add 0.5 mL pH 9.8 buffer and vortex. Extract with 1 mL toluene.
5. Centrifuge and transfer the upper organic layer to a 15 mL conical centrifuge tube. Evaporate to a volume of approximately 100 µL under a stream of nitrogen at 40°C.
6. Inject 2 µL into the chromatograph.

	Retention time (min)
internal standard	3.9
phencyclidine	4.9

Calculation:

Calculation is based on a response factor derived from a standard curve. A quality control specimen containing 0.2 mg/L phencyclidine is analyzed daily.

Evaluation:

Sensitivity: 0.01 mg/L
Linearity: 0.01–1.00 mg/L
C.V.: not established
Relative recovery: not established

Interferences:

Normal plasma components and other common drugs of abuse do not interfere. Ketamine is an anesthetic induction agent and if present in the specimen would result in under estimation of the true phencyclidine concentration.

References:

1. R. Baselt and C. Stewart. Unpublished results, 1977.
2. D.N. Bailey, R.F. Shaw and J.J. Guba. Phencyclidine abuse: plasma levels and clinical findings in casual users and in phencyclidine-related deaths. J. Analyt. Tox. 2: 233–237, 1978.

Blood Phencyclidine by Gas Chromatography-Mass Spectrometry

Principle:

Phencyclidine and an internal standard, deuterated phencyclidine, are extracted from alkalinized blood with n-butyl chloride. The organic solvent is back-extracted with dilute acid and the aqueous acid fraction made basic and extracted with n-butyl chloride. The solvent is evaporated to dryness, reconstituted in ethyl acetate and analyzed by capillary column gas chromatography-mass spectrometry using selected ion monitoring.

Reagents:

Stock solution – 1 mg/mL phencyclidine in methanol

Blood standards – 5, 10, 25, 50 and 100 μg/L

Internal standard – 3 mg/L $^2H_5$-phencyclidine hydrochloride in water (Research Triangle Institute)

Saturated sodium tetraborate

n-Butyl chloride

0.5 mol/L Sulfuric acid

10 mol/L Sodium hydroxide

1% Hydrochloric acid in methanol

Ethyl acetate

Instrumental Conditions:

Gas chromatograph with mass selective detector (Hewlett-Packard 5970B MSD or equivalent)

12 m × 0.20 mm i.d. methylsilicone capillary column (Hewlett-Packard)

Injector, 300°C.; transfer line, 240°C.

Column temperature program: initial, 125°C. (1 min)
                              30°C./min increase
                              final, 300°C. (5 min)

Helium flow rate, 1 mL/min

Splitless on time, 0.7 min

Solvent delay time, 3.0 min

Election multiplier voltage, 1800

Ions monitored, 200.15, 205.15, 242.25, 243.25

Procedure:

1. Transfer 3 mL blood to a siliconized 15 mL screw-cap glass tube and add 100 μL internal standard. Add 2 mL saturated sodium tetraborate and 8 mL n-butyl chloride and place on a rotator for 15 min.
2. Centrifuge to separate layers. Transfer the organic layer into a clean tube and add 3 mL 0.5 mol/L H_2SO_4. Place on a rotator for 15 min.
3. Centrifuge to separate layers and discard the upper organic layer. Add 0.5 mL 10 mol/L NaOH to the aqueous fraction and vortex. Add 8 mL n-butyl chloride and place on a rotator for 15 min.
4. Centrifuge and transfer the upper organic layer to a siliconized 12 mL centrifuge tube. Add 50 μL 1% HCl in methanol and evaporate to dryness at 50°C. under a stream of dry air. Dissolve the residue in 50 μL ethyl acetate and inject 1 μL into the chromatograph.

	Retention time (min)	Base peak (m/z)
phencyclidine	4.51	200.15
internal standard	4.50	205.15

Calculation:

Calculation is based on a response factor derived from a standard curve of ion chromatogram peak height ratio (200/205) versus drug concentration. A quality control specimen containing 50 µg/L phencyclidine is analyzed daily. Ion intensity ratios (242/200 and 243/200) should compare well between standards and unknown to further confirm drug identification.

Evaluation:

Sensitivity: 2.5 µg/L
Linearity: 5–100 µg/L
C.V.: not established
Relative recovery: 95–105%

Interferences:

Endogenous blood components do not interfere in the assay. Chemical analogues of phencyclidine, such as phenylcyclohexylpiperidine and thienylcyclohexylpiperidine, may be distingushed on the basis of retention time or ion intensity differences.

References:

1. D.S. Pearce. Detection and quantitation of phencyclidine in blood by use of [^{2}H$_5$] phencyclidine and select ion monitoring applied to non-fatal cases of phencyclidine intoxication. Clin. Chem. 22: 1623–1626, 1976.
2. M.A. Peat. Unpublished results, 1985.

PHENOTHIAZINES

	Plasma Concentrations (mg/L)	
	Therapeutic	Fatalities
chlorpromazine	0.5–3.0	3–35
thioridazine	0.5–5.0	0.8–13
trifluoperazine	0.5–3.0	3–8

The phenothiazine drugs are administered in large daily doses for the treatment of psychotic disorders. While specific chromatographic procedures are described for chlor-promazine (p. 85) and thioridazine (p. 283), these techniques are time-consuming and require sophisticated equipment. A convenient fluorometric method is available that may be applied to the measurement of several of the more common phenothiazines in plasma. The method is somewhat nonspecific and will detect most of the non-conjugated metabolites of the drugs. The total value for the parent drug and its metabolite may be several times the concentration of the parent drug alone, but since many of the metabolites are pharmacologically active the result produced by the fluorometric method can be clinically useful. The concentrations presented above are representative of those measured by this technique.

Qualitative determination of the phenothiazines in urine may be performed using the Urine Basic Drug Screen by Thin-Layer Chromatography (p. 41).

Plasma Phenothiazines by Fluorescence Spectrophotometry

Principle:

The phenothiazines are extracted with heptane, reextracted into acetic acid and finally oxidized with hydrogen peroxide to form fluorophores. The procedure distinguishes between the common phenothiazines but does not distinguish between a drug and its metabolites.

Reagents:

Stock solutions –
  1 mg/mL chlorpromazine (11.15 mg HCl salt/10 mL methanol)
  1 mg/mL trifluorperazine (11.79 mg HCl salt/10 mL methanol)
  1 mg/mL thioridazine (10.99 mg HCl salt 10/mL methanol)
Plasma standards – 1, 2 and 5 mg/L for each of the above drugs (prepare fresh)
20% Ammonium hydroxide
Extraction solvent – heptane/isoamyl alcohol, 98.3:1.7 by volume
50% Acetic acid
30% Hydrogen peroxide

Instrumental Conditions:

Fluorescence spectrophotometer set to excite at the indicated wavelength
Record the emission spectrum over the indicated range

Procedure:

1. Pipet 4 mL plasma into a 15 mL screw-capped tube. Add 1.0 mL 20% NH_4OH and vortex.
2. Add 10.0 mL of the extraction solvent, cap the tube and place on a tilted rotator for 30 minutes.
3. Centrifuge for 2 minutes and transfer 8.0 mL of the upper organic layer to a clean tube.
4. Add 4.0 mL 50% acetic acid, cap the tube and place on the rotator for 30 minutes.
5. Centrifuge and discard the upper organic layer. Transfer 3.0 mL of the lower aqueous layer to a clean screw-capped tube.
6. Add 0.2 mL 30% H_2O_2, cap the tube and heat in a 100°C. water bath for 15 minutes.
7. Cool the sample and record the emission spectrum at the appropriate wavelengths. Subtract the value for the plasma blank.

	Excite	Analyze	Emission Peak
chlorpromazine	340	330–430	380
trifluoperazine	350	350–460	405
thioridazine	355	370–480	430

Calculation:

Calculation is based on a standard curve prepared each time a specimen is analyzed. This procedure cannot be controlled by the usual methods due to the instability of phenothiazine drugs in biological fluids.

Evaluation:

Sensitivity: 0.5 mg/L
Linearity: 1–10 mg/L
C.V.: not established
Relative recovery: not established

Interferences:

Many of the unconjugated phenothiazine metabolites present in plasma will be measured by this procedure. Other drugs have not been studied for potential inteference.

Reference:

J.B. Ragland, V.J. Kinross-Wright and R.S. Ragland. Determination of phenothiazines in biological samples. Anal. Biochem. 12: 60–69, 1965.

PHENYLBUTAZONE

	Therapeutic Plasma Conc. (mg/L)	T½
phenylbutazone	50–100	72 hr
oxyphenbutazone	20–50	72 hr

Phenylbutazone is a non-steroidal anti-inflammatory drug that is administered in daily oral doses of 100–400 mg. It is metabolized to oxyphenbutazone, an active compound that is also used as a drug and that accumulates in plasma during chronic phenylbutazone therapy. Toxicity is frequently associated with plasma phenylbutazone concentrations which exceed 100 mg/L. The following ultraviolet spectrophotometric method is not highly specific and responds to both phenylbutazone and oxyphenbutazone; since both substances are approximately equally active, the method is suitable for therapeutic monitoring purposes. A more specific gas chromatographic procedure, limited to the detection of the parent drug, may be used for single or multiple-dose kinetic studies.

Plasma Phenylbutazone by Ultraviolet Spectrophotometry

Principle:
Phenylbutazone is extracted from acidified plasma with heptane. After re-partitioning into dilute aqueous alkali, the drug is determined by ultraviolet spectrophotometry at 265 nm.

Reagents:
Stock solution – 1 mg/mL phenylbutazone in methanol
Plasma standards – 25, 50, 100 and 200 mg/L
3 mol/L Hydrochloric acid
Heptane
2.5 mol/L Sodium hydroxide

Instrumental Conditions:
Ultraviolet spectrophotometer set to 265 nm

Procedure:
1. Transfer 2 mL plasma to a 35 mL screw-cap tube. Add 0.5 mL 3 mol/L HCl.
2. Extract with 20 mL heptane and centrifuge. Transfer 15 mL of the heptane layer to a clean tube.
3. Extract with 4 mL 2.5 mol/L NaOH and centrifuge. Discard the upper heptane layer.
4. Transfer about 3 mL of the lower aqueous phase to a quartz cuvette and read against a plasma blank at 265 nm in the spectrophotometer.

Calculation:

Calculation is based on a response factor derived from a standard curve. A quality control specimen containing 75 mg/L phenylbutazone is analyzed daily.

Evaluation:

Sensitivity: 10 mg/L
Linearity: 20–200 mg/L
C.V.: not established
Relative recovery: not established

Interferences:

A major metabolite of phenylbutazone, oxyphenbutazone, will be detected by this procedure. Other basic drugs that absorb ultraviolet light in the region of 265 nm may interfere.

Reference:

J.J Burns, R.K. Rose, T. Chenkin et al. The physiological disposition of phenylbutazone (Butazolidin) in man and a method for its estimation in biological materials. J. Pharm. Exp. Ther. 109: 346–357, 1953.

Plasma Phenylbutazone by Gas Chromatography

Principle:

Phenylbutazone is extracted from acidified plasma with heptane. The residue after evaporation of the heptane is dissolved in an internal standard solution and analyzed by flame-ionization gas chromatography.

Reagents:

Stock solution – 1 mg/mL phenylbutazone in methanol
Plasma standards – 50, 100 and 200 mg/L
1 mol/L Hydrochloric acid
Heptane
Internal standard solution – 25 mg/mL diphenylphthalate in ethyl acetate

Instrumental Conditions:

Gas chromatograph with flame-ionization detector
1 m × 2 mm i.d. glass column containing 3% Apiezon L on 80/100 mesh Chromosorb W-HP
Injector, 310°C.; column, 230°C.; detector, 300°C.
Nitrogen flow rate, 120 mL/min

Procedure:

1. Transfer 1 mL plasma to a 15 mL screw-cap tube and add 1 mL 1 mol/L HCl. Extract with 6 mL heptane.
2. Centrifuge and transfer 2 mL of the heptane layer to a 5 mL conical centrifuge tube. Evaporate to dryness at 50°C. under a stream of nitrogen.

3. Dissolve the residue in 20 μL of the internal standard solution. Inject 1 μL into the chromatograph.

	Retention time (min)
phenylbutazone	3.6
internal standard	6.0

Calculation:

Calculation is based on a response factor derived from a standard curve. A quality control specimen containing 75 mg/L phenylbutazone is analyzed daily.

Evaluation:

Sensitivity: 0.5 mg/L
Linearity: 0.5–200 mg/L
C.V.: 4%
Relative recovery: not established

Interferences:

Normal plasma components do not interfere with the assay, nor do metabolites of phenylbutazone. Other drugs were not studied for potential interference.

Reference:

I.J. McGilveray, K.K. Midha, R. Brien and L. Wilson. The assay of phenylbutazone in human plasma by a specific and sensitive gas-liquid chromatographic procedure. J. Chromatog. 89: 17–22, 1974.

PLATINUM

Therapeutic Plasma Concentrations (mg/L)	T½
0.7 after 1 hour	58–73 hr
0.3 after 1 day	
0.1 after 12 days	

Cis-dichlorodiammine platinum (cisplatin) is in use as a drug for the treatment of certain forms of squamous cell carcinoma. The compound is administered by intravenous injection at a dose of 0.5–4 mg/kg. Plasma concentrations of platinum decline rapidly at first, with a distribution half-life of 25–49 minutes, and then slowly, with an elimination half-life of up to 73 hr. Determination of plasma concentrations may be useful in monitoring the course of therapy and in preventing toxicity due to drug accumulation. A very convenient technique involves electrothermal atomic absorption spectrometry performed directly on plasma specimens.

Plasma Platinum by Graphite Furnace Atomic Absorption Spectrometry

Principle:
Platinum is analyzed by direct injection of plasma into the graphite furnace of an atomic absorption spectrophotometer.

Reagents:
Stock solution – 1 mg/mL platinum ion
Plasma standards – 0.2, 0.5, 1.0 and 2.0 mg/L

Instrumental Conditions:
Atomic absorption spectrometer with graphite furnace and deuterium background corrector
Platinum program: dry 120 sec at 250°C.
char 240 sec at 650°C.
atomize 20 sec at 2700°C.
Measure absorption at 265.9 nm

Procedure:
1. Introduce 30 μL of plasma into the furnace of the atomic absorption spectrometer.
2. Begin temperature program and read peak absorbance at 265.9 nm.

Calculation:

Calculation is based on a response factor derived from a standard curve. A quality control specimen containing 0.5 mg/L platinum is analyzed daily.

Evaluation:

Sensitivity: 0.07 mg/L
Linearity: 0.2–2.0
C.V.: 8%
Relative recovery: not established

Interferences:

Smoke from destruction of the organic matter in the specimen may interfere with the analysis at lower concentrations of platinum. The use of the deuterium background corrector helps to neutralize this effect, but the best results are obtained when a temperature ramping device is used to reach the atomization temperature. Platinum is not contained in the plasma of normal subjects at concentrations measurable by this technique.

Reference:

A.F. LeRoy, M.L. Wehling, H.L. Sponseller et al. Analysis of platinum in biological materials by flameless atomic absorption spectrophotometry. Biochem. Med. 18: 184–191, 1977.

PROCAINAMIDE

	Plasma concentrations (mg/L)		
	Therapeutic	Toxic	$T\frac{1}{2}$
procainamide	4–8	>16	3–4 hr
N-acetylprocainamide	1–10	?	6 hr

The amide analogue of procaine is known as procainamide, an antiarrhythmic agent given orally or by intramuscular injection in doses of 200–1000 mg. The major metabolite, N-acetylprocainamide, has efficacy similar to that of its parent and has a longer plasma half-life. The following colorimetric procedure measures only procainamide, whereas the fluorometric, gas chromatographic and liquid chromatographic methods are designed to quantitate results within a reasonable period of time. Procainamide and N-acetylprocainamide may also be assayed individually using EMIT reagents.

Plasma Procainamide by Colorimetry

Principle:
Procainamide is extracted from alkalinized plasma into an organic solvent. After evaporation of the solvent, the residue is subjected to a diazotization reaction and the resulting chromogen is analyzed by visible spectrophotometry.

Reagents:
Stock solution – 1 mg/mL procainamide in methanol
Plasma standards – 2, 5, 10 and 20 mg/L
Sodium chloride – solid NaCl
5 mol/L Hydrochloric acid
0.1% Sodium nitrite
0.5% Ammonium sulfamate
Marshall's reagent – 0.1% N-(1-naphthyl)ethylenediamine dihydrochloride (Fisher reagent N-30)

Instrumental Conditions:
Visible spectrophotometer set to 550 nm

Procedure:
1. Transfer 1 mL plasma to a 15 ml screw-cap tube. Add approximately 0.25 g NaCl, 0.2 mL 5 mol/L NaOH and 0.5 mL water and vortex.
2. Add 10 mL dichloromethane and shake to extract. Centrifuge and transfer 8 mL of the organic layer to a 15 mL centrifuge tube.

3. Evaporate the dichloromethane to dryness at 40°C. under a stream of nitrogen. Place the tube in an ice bath and add 2 mL 1 mol/L HCl and 1 mL 0.1% NaNO$_2$.
4. Vortex briefly and place in the ice bath for 10 min. Add 1 mL 0.5% ammonium sulfamate and vortex.
5. Add 1 mL Marshall's reagent, vortex and allow to stand at room temperature for 15 min. Measure the absorbance of the solution at 550 nm against a plasma blank.

Calculation:

Calculation is based on a response factor derived from a standard curve. A quality control specimen containing 5 mg/L procainamide is analyzed daily.

Evaluation:

Sensitivity: 0.5 mg/L
Linearity: 0.5–25 mg/L
C.V.: 4.5%
Relative recovery: not established

Interferences:

Other primary aromatic amines will interfere with this procedure, although the major metabolite of procainamide (a secondary amine) does not. Hemolysis or lipemia do not result in interference.

References:

1. D.S. Sitar, D.N. Graham, R.E. Rangno et al. Modified colorimetric method for procainamide in plasma. Clin. Chem. 22: 379–380, 1976.
2. L.C. Mark, H.J. Kayden, J.M. Steele et al. The physiological disposition and cardiac effects of procaine amide. J. Pharm. Exp. Ther. 102: 5–15, 1951.

Plasma Procainamide and N-Acetylprocainamide by Fluorescence Spectrophotometry

Principle:

Procainamide and its metabolite are extracted from alkalinized plasma into toluene. After back extraction into aqueous acid, the two substances are measured individually in the fluorometer at different pH values.

Reagents:

Stock solutions – 1 mg/mL procainamide in methanol
                   1 mg/mL N-acetylprocainamide in methanol
Plasma standards – 2, 5 and 10 mg/L for each drug
Sodium chloride – solid NaCl
5 mol/1 Sodium hydroxide
Extraction solvent – toluene/isoamyl alcohol, 98.7:1.3 by volume
0.1 mol/L Hydrochloric acid

Instrumental Conditions:

Fluorescence spectrophotometer set to the following conditions:

	Excite	Analyze
Nacetylprocainamide	282 nm	340 nm
procainamide	298 nm	358 nm

Procedure:

1. Transfer 2 mL plasma to a 15 mL screw-cap tube. Add about 250 mg NaCl and 250 µL 5 mol/L NaOH and vortex.
2. Add 10 mL extraction solvent and shake for 30 seconds. Centrifuge and transfer 8 mL of the solvent layer to a clean tube.
3. Add 3 mL 0.1 mol/L HCl and shake to extract. Centrifuge and transfer 2.5 mL of the aqueous layer to a quartz cuvette.
4. Analyze for N-acetylprocainamide by reading in the fluorometer against a plasma blank under the specified conditions.
5. Add 100 µL 5 mol/L NaOH to each cuvette and mix. Analyze for procainamide by reading in the fluorometer against a plasma blank under the specified conditions.

Calculation:

Calculation is based on a response factor derived from a standard curve. A quality control specimen containing 5 mg/L of each drug is analyzed daily.

Evaluation:

Sensitivity: 0.1 mg/L for both drugs
Linearity: 0.1–10 mg/L for both drugs
C.V.: 10% for both drugs
Relative recovery: 94–103% for both drugs

Interferences:

Neither drug interferes significantly with the determination of the other. Ten other drugs commonly administered to cardiac patients did not interfere with the assay.

References:

1. E. Matusik and T.P. Gibson. Fluorometric assay for N-acetylprocainamide. Clin. Chem. 21: 1899–1902, 1975.
2. R. Baselt and S. Voll. Unpublished results, 1977.

Plasma Procainamide and N-Acetylprocainamide by Gas Chromatography

Principle:

Procainamide, N-acetylprocainamide and an internal standard are extracted from alkalinized plasma with dichloromethane. The concentrated residue is analyzed by flame-ionization gas chromatography.

Reagents:

Stock solution – 1 mg/mL procainamide in methanol
$\qquad$ 1 mg/mL N-acetylprocainamide in methanol
Plasma standards – 2, 5 and 10 mg/L for each drug
Internal standard – 5 mg/L p-amino-N-(2-dipropylaminoethyl)benzamide (Squibb and Sons) in water
5 mol/L Sodium hydroxide
Dichloromethane
Ethyl acetate

Instrumental Conditions:

Gas chromatograph with flame-ionization detector
1.6 m × 1 mm i.d. glass column containing 3% OV-17 on 80/100 mesh Chromosorb W-HP
Injector, 255°C.; detector, 255°C.
Column temperature program: initial, 210°C.
$\qquad$ increase, 2°C./min
$\qquad$ final, 250°C.
Nitrogen flow rate, 40 mL/min

Procedure:

1. Transfer 1 mL plasma to a 15 mL screw-cap tube. Add 1 mL internal standard and 0.2 mL 5 mol/L NaOH and vortex.
2. Add 5 mL dichloromethane and shake for 15 seconds. Centrifuge and transfer the organic layer to a 15 mL conical centrifuge tube.
3. Evaporate to dryness under a stream of nitrogen at 40°C. Dissolve the residue in 50 µL ethyl acetate and inject 5 µL into the gas chromatograph.

	Retention time (min)
procainamide	2
internal standard	4
N-acetylprocainamide	5.5

Calculation:

Calculation is based on a response factor derived from a standard curve. A quality control specimen containing 5 mg/L of each drug is analyzed daily.

Evaluation:

Sensitivity: <1 mg/L
Linearity: 1–20 mg/L
C.V.: 4–5%
Relative recovery: not established

Interferences:

Normal plasma components do not interfere with the assay. Other drugs were not studied for potential interferences.

References:

1. J. Elson, J.M. Strong, W.K. Lee and A.J. Atkinson, Jr. Antiarrhythmic potency of N-acetylprocainamide. Clin. Pharm. Ther. 17: 134–140, 1975.
2. T.P. Gibson, J. Matusik, E. Matusik et al. Acetylation of procainamide in man and its relationship to isonicotinic acid hydrazide acetylation phenotype. Clin. Plarm. Ther. 17: 395–399, 1975.

Plasma Procainamide and N-Acetylprocainamide by Liquid Chromatography

Principle:

Procainamide, its metabolite and an internal standard are extracted from alkalinized plasma with dichloromethane. The concentrated extract is analyzed by liquid chromatography with detection at 254 nm.

Reagents:

Stock solutions –
  1 mg/mL procainamide in methanol
  1 mg/mL N-acetylprocainamide in methanol
Plasma standards – 2, 5 and 10 mg/L for each drug
Internal standard – 9 mg/L pheniramine in water
0.1 mol/L Ammonium hydroxide
Dichloromethane
Mobile phase – 0.1% acetic acid and 20% 0.1 mol/L ammonium acetate in acetonitrile

Instrumental Conditions:

Liquid chromatograph with 254 nm ultraviolet detector
25 cm × 2 mm i.d. stainless-steel column containing 5 μm silica gel
Column temperature, ambient
Solvent flow rate, 1 mL/min

Procedure:

1. Transfer 2 mL plasma to a 15 mL polypropylene screw-cap tube. Add 1 mL internal standard and 0.5 mL 0.1 mol/L NH$_4$OH and vortex.
2. Extract with 10 mL dichloromethane and centrifuge. Discard the aqueous phase and transfer the lower solvent layer to a 15 mL conical polypropylene centrifuge tube.
3. Evaporate the solvent to a volume of 0.3–0.5 mL under a stream of nitrogen at 55°C. Vortex briefly and inject 100 μL into the chromatograph.

	Retention time (min)
internal standard	4
procainamide	5
N-acetylprocainamide	6

Calculation:

Calculation is based on a response factor derived from a standard curve. A quality control specimen containing 5 mg/L of each drug is analyzed daily.

Evaluation:

Sensitivity: 0.1 mg/L
Linearity: 0.1–8.0 mg/L
C.V.: 2–3%
Relative recovery: 97–106%

Interferences:

Normal plasma components do not interfere with the assay. Other drugs were not studied for potential interferences.

Reference:

A.G. Butterfield. J.K. Cooper and K.K. Midha. Simultaneous determination of procainamide and N-acetylprocainamide in plasma by high-performance liquid chromatography. J. Pharm. Sci. 67: 839–842, 1978.

PROPOXYPHENE

	Plasma Concentrations (mg/L)			
	Therapeutic	Toxic	Fatalities	T½
propoxyphene	0.1–0.4	0.5–2	1–17	3 hr
norpropoxyphene	0.1–1.5	2–10	2–30	17 hr

Propoxyphene is a narcotic analgesic that is structurally related to methadone. It is easily prescribed and widely used, aften in combination with aspirin or acetaminophen. The major metabolite, norpropoxyphene, has less than one-half the analgesic activity of propoxyphene but accumulates in plasma and may be nearly as toxic.

Propoxyphene and norpropxyphene may be detected at toxic levels using the Urine Drug Screen by Thin-Layer Chromatography (p. 41) or the Serum Drug Screen by Gas Chromatography (p. 43). The following gas chromatographic procedure is specifically designed for measurement of therapeutic concentrations, however, and offers better accuracy, sensitivity and specificity. Reagents are available commercially for determination of propoxyphene in urine by EMIT.

Plasma Propoxyphene and Norpropoxyphene by Gas Chromatography

Principle:

Propoxyphene, norpropoxyphene and an internal standard are extracted from alkalinized plasma with an organic solvent. The drugs are back-extracted into dilute acid and the aqueous layer is adjusted to a strongly alkaline pH to convert norpropoxphene to an amide. A final extraction into toluene is performed and the concentrated extract is analyzed by flame-ionization gas chromatography.

Reagents:

Stock solutions –
   1 mg/mL propoxyphene in methanol
   1 mg/mL norpropoxyphene in methanol
Plasma standards – 0.2, 0.5, 1 and 2 mg/L for each drug
Internal standard – 20 mg/L SKF-525A (Smith, Kline and French) in water
Ammonium hydroxide – concentrated NH_4OH
Extraction solvent – heptane/isoamyl alcohol, 98.5:1.5 by volume
0.1 mol/L Hydrochloric acid
10 mol/L Sodium hydroxide
Toluene – chromatographic grade

Instrumental Conditions:

Gas chromatograph with flame-ionization detector
2 m × 2 mm i.d. glass column containing 2% OV-1 on 100/120 mesh Chromosorb G-HP
Injector, 250°C.; detector, 300°C.
Column temperature program: initial, 200°C.
                             8°C./min increase
                             final, 250°C.
Nitrogen flow rate, 30 mL/min

Procedure:

1. Transfer 2 mL plasma to a 15 mL screw-cap tube. Add 0.2 mL internal standard and 2 drops conc. NH_4OH and vortex.
2. Add 9 mL extraction solvent and shake for 30 seconds. Centrifuge and transfer the upper organic layer to a clean tube.
3. Extract the solvent with 1 mL 0.1 mol/L HCl. Centrifuge and discard the upper organic layer.
4. Add 1 drop 10 mol/L NaOH to the aqueous layer and vortex for 10 seconds. Extract with 1 mL toluene.
5. Centrifuge and transfer the toluene layer to a 15 mL conical centrifuge tube. Evaporate to a volume of about 100 μL at 40°C. under a stream of nitrogen.
6. Inject 2–4 μL into the gas chromatograph.

	Retention time (min)
propoxyphene	4
internal standard	5
norpropoxyphene	7

Calculation:

Calculation is based on a response factor derived from a standard curve. A quality control specimen containing 0.5 mg/L of each drug is analyzed daily.

Evaluation:

Sensitivity: 0.05 mg/L
Linearity: 0.2–2.0 mg/L
C.V.: 4–6% within-run
Relative recovery: not established

Interferences:

Normal plasma components do not interfere with the assay. Other commonly used or abused drugs have not been found to interfere.

References:

1. K. Verebely and C.E. Inturrisi. The simultaneous determination of propoxyphene and norpropoxyphene in human biofluids using gas-liquid chromatography.
2. R. Baselt and C. Stewart. Unpublished results, 1976.

PROPRANOLOL

	Therapeutic Plasma Concentrations (mg/L)	T½
propranolol	0.06–0.40	2–3 hr
4-hydroxypropanolol	0.02–0.16	<2 hr

Propranolol is a β-adrenergic blocking agent that is used frequently as an antihypertensive and antiarrhythmic agent. It is administered orally or by intravenous injection in doses of 30–320 mg or 1–3 mg, respectively. Propranolol undergoes extensive metabolism and at least one of the metabolites, 4-hydroxypropranolol, has pharmacological activity. This metabolite is present in plasma, especially after oral administration of the drug, but has a shorter half-life than its parent. The spectrofluorometric method that follows is convenient and capable of individually measuring the parent drug and the metabolite. The gas chromatographic and liquid chromatographic techniques provide more specificity, but are limited to measuring only propranolol and require detectors that are not routinely available in many laboratories.

Plasma Propranolol and 4-Hydroxypropranolol by Fluorescence Spectrophotometry

Principle:
Propranolol and its metabolite are extracted from alkalinized plasma into toluene and re-extracted into aqueous acid. The final extract is analyzed sequentially for the two drugs by fluorescence spectrophotometry.

Reagents:
Stock solutions –
   1 mg/mL propranolol in methanol
   1 mg/mL 4-hydroxypropranolol in methanol
Plasma standards –
   0.05, 0.10, 0.20 and 0.40 mg/L for propranolol
   0.02, 0.04, 0.08 and 0.16 mg/L for 4 hydroxypropranolol
10% Potassium carbonate
Toluene
Acid solution – 0.005 mol/L acetic acid and 50 g/L ethylene glycol in water (pH 3.7)

Instrumental Conditions:
Fluorescence spectrophotometer set to the following conditions:

	Excite	Analyze
propranolol	290 nm	358 nm
4-hydroxypropranolol	320 nm	510 nm

Procedure:

1. Transfer 1 mL plasma to a 15 mL screw-cap tube. Add 1 mL 10% K_2CO_3 and 6 mL toluene and shake to extract.
2. Centrifuge and transfer 5 mL of the upper organic layer to a clean tube. Add 1.5 mL of the acid solution and shake to extract.
3. Centrifuge and transfer the aqueous layer to a quartz cuvette. Read against a plasma blank in the fluorometer using the specified conditions.

Calculation:

Calculation is based on a response factor derived from a standard curve. A quality control specimen containing each drug at a mid-range concentration is analyzed daily.

Evaluation:

Sensitivity: 0.015 mg/L
Linearity: 0.015–0.400 mg/L
C.V.: 3–4%
Relative recovery: 96–100%

Interferences:

Quinidine and procainamide are known to cause positive interference with this procedure, whereas normal plasma components and other common cardiovascular drugs do not.

Reference:

P.S. Rao, L.C. Quesada and H.S. Mueller. A simple micromethod for simultaneous determination of plasma propranolol and 4-hydroxypropranolol. Clin. Chim. Acta 88: 355–361, 1978.

Plasma Propranolol by Electron-Capture Gas Chromatography

Principle:

Propranolol and an internal standard are extracted from alkalinized plasma with an organic solvent. The concentrated extract is subject to a derivatization step, and the trifluoro-acetylated drugs are analyzed by electron-capture gas chromatography.

Reagents:

Stock solution – 1 mg/mL propranolol in methanol
Plasma standards – 0.05, 0.10, 0.20 and 0.40 mg/L
Internal standard – 2 mg/L oxprenolol (W.S. Merrell Co.) in water
5 mol/L Sodium hydroxide
Benzene
1 mol/L Trimethylamine in benzene
Trifluoroacetic anhydride
0.5 mol/L Phosphate buffer (pH 6.0)

Instrumental Conditions:

Gas chromatograph with electron-capture detector

1.5 m × 2 mm i.d. glass column containing 2% OV-17 on 80/100 mesh Chromosorb W Injector, 230°C.; column, 170°C.; detector, 270°C.
Nitrogen flow rate, 30 mL/min

Procedure:

1. Transfer 1 mL plasma to a 15 mL screw-cap tube. Add 100 μL internal standard and 100 μL 5 mol/L NaOH and vortex.
2. Add 3 mL benzene and shake to extract. Centrifuge and transfer the upper organic layer to a 5 mL glass-stoppered conical centrifuge tube.
3. Evaporate benzene to a volume of about 50 μL at 40°C. under a stream of nitrogen. Add 25 μL 1 mol/L trimethylamine in benzene and 50 μL trifluoroacetic anhydride and vortex.
4. Stopper the tube and heart at 50°C. for 5 min. Cool and add 1 mL 0.5 mol/L phosphate buffer.
5. Vortex for 30 seconds and centrifuge. Inject 1–5 μL of the upper benzene layer into the gas chromatograph.

	Retention time (min)
internal standard	3
propranolol	9

Calculation:

Calculation is based on a response factor derived from a standard curve. A quality control specimen containing 0.20 mg/L propranolol is analyzed daily.

Evaluation:

Sensitivity: 0.001 mg/L
Linearity: 0.005–0.500 mg/L
C.V.: 3–10%
Relative recovery: not established

Interferences:

Normal plasma constituents do not interfere with the assay, nor do other commonly prescribed cardiovascular drugs.

Reference:

T. Walle. GLC determination of propranolol, other β-blocking drugs, and metabolites in biological fluids and tissues. J. Pharm. Sci. 63: 1885–1891, 1974.

Plasma Propranolol by Liquid Chromatography

Principle:

Propranolol is extracted from plasma at physiologic pH with dichloromethane containing an internal standard. The concentrated extract is analyzed by liquid chromatography with fluorescent emission detection.

Reagents:

Stock solution – 1 mg/mL propranolol in methanol
Plasma standards – 0.05, 0.10, 0.20 and 0.40 mg/L
0.1 mol/L Phosphate buffer (pH 7.4)
Extraction solvent – 0.16 mg/L cyclomethycaine (Eli Lilly and Co.) in dichloromethane
Methanol
Mobile phase – 0.02 mol/L pH 7.0 acetate buffer-acetonitrile, 30:70

Instrumental Conditions:

Liquid chromatograph with a fluorescence detector set to excite at 276 nm and equipped
    with a 340 nm emission cutoff filter
30 cm × 4 mm i.d. stainless-steel column containing, μBondapak CN (Waters Associates)
Column temperature, ambient
Solvent flow rate, 2 mL/min

Procedure:

1. Transfer 0.5 mL plasma to a 15 mL screw-cap tube. Add 0.5 mL 0.1 mol/L phosphate
    buffer and 5 mL extraction solvent and vortex for 10 seconds.
2. Centrifuge and transfer 4 mL of the organic layer to a 12 mL conical centrifuge tube.
3. Dissolve the residue in 100 μL methanol and inject 50 μL into the chromatograph.

	Retention time (min)
propranolol	10.0
internal standard	13.5

Calculation:

Calculation is based on a response factor derived from a standard curve. A quality control
specimen containing 0.20 mg/L propranolol is analyzed daily.

Evaluation:

Sensitivity: 0.01 mg/L
Linearity: 0.01–0.15 mg/L
C.V.: 1–6%
Relative recovery: 97–108%

Interferences:

No interference was noted from plasma components or commonly prescribed cardiovascular drugs. 4-Hydroxypropranolol elutes at 7.7 minutes and thus does not interfere with
the assay.

Reference:

G. Nygard, W.H. Shelver and S.K. Wahba Khalil. Sensitive high-pressure liquid chromatographic determination
of propranolol in plasma. J. Pharm. Sci. 68: 379–381, 1979.

QUINIDINE

| | Plasma Concentrations (mg/L) | | |
	Therapeutic	Toxic	T½
quinidine	1–5	>8	4–9 hr
3-hydroxyquinidine	0.2–1.0	?	?

Quinidine is a stereoisomer of quinine that has been used for many years as an antiarrhythmic agent. Due to its natural fluorescence, it has commonly been determined in plasma by fluorometry, either directly on a deproteinized specimen or after solvent extraction. Both techniques yield clinically useful values, although the solvent extraction method is somewhat more reproducible and is less subject to interference by plasma constituents and quinidine metabolites. The plasma of patients on chronic quinidine therapy contains several substances that fluoresce like quinidine and that contribute to the value obtained with fluorometric techniques; dihydroquinidine is present in commercial quinidine preparations in amounts of 3–11% and the quinidine metabolites, 3-hydroxy-quinidine and 2'-quinidinone, are present in plasma to the extent to 20–50% and 2–3%, respectively, of the quinidine concentration. Since 3-hydroxyquinidine is pharmacologically active and is found in appreciable amounts in plasma, it is reasonable to measure its concentration when using a more specific method such as the liquid chromatographic procedure that is presented. This procedure is better suited to pharmacokinetic studies than the fluorometric methods. Quinidine may also be determined in plasma using commercially available EMIT or fluorescence immunoassay reagents.

Plasma Quinidine by Direct Fluorescence Spectrophotometry

Principle:
Plasma is deproteinized with metaphosphoric acid and the supernatant is subjected to analysis by fluorescence spectrophotometry.

Reagents:
Stock solution – 1 mg/mL quinidine in methanol
Plasma standards – 2, 4 and 8 mg/L
20% Metaphosphoric acid

Instrumental Conditions:
Fluorescence spectrophotometer set to excite at 360 nm
Measure fluorescence at 445 nm

Procedure:

1. Transfer 100 µL plasma to a 12 mL graduated centrifuge tube. Dilute to 4 mL with water and vortex.
2. Add 1 mL 20% metaphosphoric acid and vortex. Allow to stand for 15 min.
3. Centrifuge and transfer the supernatant to a cuvette. Determine the fluorescence against a plasma blank under the specified conditions.

Calculation:

Calculation is based on a response factor derived from a standard curve. A quality control specimen containing 3 mg/L quindine is analyzed daily.

Evaluation:

Sensitivity: 0.1 mg/L
Linearity: 1–10 mg/L
C.V.: not established
Relative recovery: 92–104%

Interferences:

Normal patient plasma yields a background fluorescence that is variable but low. Quinidine metabolites contribute significantly to the apparent concentration determined by this method. Quinine and other drugs which fluoresce may interfere in this assay.

Reference:

B.B. Brodie and S. Udenfriend. The estimation of quinine in human plasma with a note on the estimation of quinidine. J. Pharm. Exp. Ther. 78: 154–158, 1943.

Plasma Quinidine by Double-Extraction Fluorescence Spectrophotometry

Principle:

Quinidine is extracted from alkalinized plasma with an organic solvent. The drug is returned to aqueous acid and is analyzed by fluorescence spectrophotometry.

Reagents:

Stock solution – 1 mg/mL quinidine in methanol
Plasma standards – 2, 4 and 8 mg/L
0.1 mol/L Sodium hydroxide
Toluene
0.1 mol/L Sulfuric acid

Instrumental Conditions:

Fluorescence spectrophotometer set to excite at 360 nm
Measure fluorescence at 445 nm

Procedure:

1. Transfer 0.5 mL plasma to a 15 mL screw-cap tube. Add 1 mL 0.1 mol/L NaOH and 7.5 mL toluene and shake to extract.
2. Centrifuge and transfer 5 mL of the toluene layer to a clean tube. Extract with 5 mL 0.1 mol/L H_2SO_4.
3. Centrifuge and transfer 3 mL of the lower aqueous layer to a cuvette. Read in the fluorometer against a plasma blank under the specified conditions.

Calculation:

Calculation is based on a response factor derived from a standard curve. A quality control specimen containing 3 mg/L quinidine is analyzed daily.

Evaluation:

Sensitivity: 0.1 mg/L
Linearity: 1–10 mg/L
C.V.: not established
Relative recovery: 95–110%

Interferences:

Normal patient plasma yields a consistently low background fluorescence. Quinidine metabolites contribute significantly to the apparent concentration determined by this method. Quinine and other drugs that fluoresce may interfere in this assay.

Reference:

G. Cramer and B. Isaksson. Quantitative determination of quinidine in plasma. Scand. J. Clin. Lab. Invest. 15: 553–556, 1963.

Plasma Quinidine and 3-Hydroxyquinidine by Liquid Chromatography

Principle:

Quinidine and its major metabolite are extracted from alkalinized plasma with toluene containing quinine as an internal standard. The concentrated extract is analyzed by liquid chromatography with ultraviolet absorbance detection at 254 nm.

Reagents:

Stock solutions –
   1 mg/mL quinidine in methanol
   1 mg/mL 3-hydroxyquinidine (Research Triangle Institute) in methanol
Plasma standards –
   2, 4 and 8 mg/L for quinidine
   0.2, 0.5 and 1.0 mg/L for 3-hydroxyquinidine
Internal standard solution – 0.25 mg/L quinine in toluene
6 mol/L Sodium hydroxide
Mobile phase – 10% methanol, 0.85% concentrated H_3PO_4 and 10 mol/L KH_2PO_4 in water

Instrumental Conditions:

Liquid chromatograph with 254 nm ultraviolet detector

25 cm × 2 mm i.d. stainless-steel column containing C_{18} Micropak MCH-10 (Varian Instruments)

Column temperature, ambient

Solvent flow rate, 1 mL/min

Procedure:

1. Transfer 100 μL plasma to a 13 × 100 mm test tube. Add 50 μL 6 mol/L NaOH and vortex.
2. Add 2 mL internal standard solution and vortex for 15 seconds. Centrifuge and transfer the upper organic layer to a 12 × 75 mm tube.
3. Evaporate to dryness under a stream of nitrogen at room temperature. Dissolve the residue in 100 μL mobile phase and inject 20 μL into the chromatograph.

	Retention time (min)
3-hydroxyquinidine	1.0
quinidine	4.2
internal standard	6.4

Calculation:

Calculation is based on a response factor derived from a standard curve. A quality control specimen containing 3 mg/L quinidine and 0.6 mg/L 3-hydroxyquinidine is analyzed daily.

Evaluation:

Sensitivity: 0.1 mg/L

Linearity: 1–15 mg/L for quinidine; 0.2–9 mg/L for 3-hydroxyquinidine

C.V.: 3–6% between run

Relative recovery: 91–105%

Interferences:

No interference was observed due to normal plasma components or by 21 commonly prescribed drugs. Dihydroquinidine, present in commercial quinidine preparations, co-elutes with the internal standard but results in only a 0.1 mg/L concentration difference in routine practice.

Reference:

N. Weidner, J.H. Ladenson, L. Larson et al. A high-pressure liquid chromatography method for serum quinidine and (3S)-3-hydroxyquinidine. Clin. Chim. Acta 91: 7–13, 1979.

SALICYLATE

Plasma Salicylate Concentrations after Aspirin Ingestion (mg/L)		
Single Dose	High Dose Therapy	Toxicity
25–100	50–350	>500

Acetylsalicylic acid (aspirin) is the drug substance most frequently utilized by humans and one of the leading causes of accidental poisoning in children. The salicylate ion is the primary active form of aspirin in vivo and most analytical procedures are designed to measure this metabolite. The familiar colorimetric and ultraviolet spectrophotometric procedures for plasma salicylate determination are described. Additionally, several alternative techniques are presented that offer advantages in terms of sensitivity or specificity. These include a very sensitive fluorometric assay, a gas chromatographic method designed for simultaneous salicylate, aspirin and salicylamide measurement, and a liquid chromatographic technique capable of simultaneous determination of salicylate and acetaminophen.

Plasma Salicylate by Colorimetry

Principle:
Plasma is diluted with water and then reacted with Trinder's reagent, which both precipitates protein and produces a visible color with any salicylate ion that is present. The color change is measured at 540 nm.

Reagents:
Stock solution – 1 mg/mL salicylate ion in water
Plasma standards – 50, 100, 200 and 400 mg/L
Trinder's reagent – dissolve 4 g ferric nitrate nonahydrate and 4 g mercuric chloride in 12 mL 1 mol/L HCl and q.s. to 100 mL with water; filter and store at room temperature

Instrumental Conditions:
Visible spectrophotometer set to 540 nm

Procedure:
1. Transfer 0.5 mL plasma to a 15 mL conical centrifuge tube and add 5 mL water. Add 5 mL Trinder's reagent and vortex.
2. Allow the mixture to stand for 5 min and then centrifuge to precipitate protein. Transfer 3 mL of the supernatant to a cuvette and determine the absorbance at 540 nm against a plasma blank treated in the same manner.

Calculation:

Calculation is based on a response factor derived from a standard curve. A quality control specimen containing 200 mg/L salicylate is analyzed daily.

Evaluation:

Sensitivity: 30 mg/L
Linearity: 50–400 mg/L
C.V.: not established
Relative recovery: 95–105%

Interferences:

Lipemic, icteric or hemolyzed specimens may yield false positive results. The procedure responds to inactive metabolites that may be present in plasma and tends to yield higher values than more specific methods. It has been used on urine as a rapid screening technique for possible salicylate intoxication.

Reference:

P. Trinder. Rapid determination of salicylate in biological materials. Biochem. J. 57: 301–303, 1954.

Plasma Salicylate by Ultraviolet Spectrophotometry

Principle:

The drug is extracted from acidified plasma with chloroform which is filtered and then back-extracted with dilute alkali. The aqueous layer is acidified and extracted with ether. After evaporation of the ether, the residue is dissolved in dilute acid and the absorbance of this solution measured at 301 nm in an ultraviolet spectrophotometer.

Reagents:

Stock solution – 1 mg/mL salicylate ion in water
Plasma standards – 50, 100, 200 and 400 mg/L
1 mol/L Hydrochloric acid
Chloroform
4% Sodium bicarbonate – prepare fresh
25% Hydrochloric acid
Ether
0.05 mol/L Sulfuric acid

Instrumental Conditions:

Ultraviolet spectrophotometer set to 301 nm

Procedure:

1. Transfer 1 mL plasma to a 60 mL separatory funnel and add 0.5 mL 1 mol/L HCl. Extract with 25 mL CHCl$_3$ and allow layers to separate.
2. Filter the CHCl$_3$ layer through Whatman #1 filter paper into a 25 mL graduated

cylinder, collecting 20 mL. Extract this with 2 mL fresh 4% $NaHCO_3$ and allow layers to separate.

3. Transfer the upper aqueous layer to a 35 mL screw-cap tube and add 0.5 mL 25% HCl. Extract with 20 mL ether and centrifuge to separate layers.

4. Transfer 18 mL of the ether layer to a 50 mL beaker and evaporate to dryness at low heat under a stream of nitrogen. Do not continue heating once evaporation is complete.

5. Dissolve the residue in 3 mL 0.05 mol/L H_2SO_4 and measure in the spectrophotometer at 301 nm against a plasma blank treated in the same manner.

Calculation:

Calculation is based on a response factor derived from a standard curve. A quality control specimen containing 200 mg/L salicylate is analyzed daily.

Evaluation:

Sensitivity: 25 mg/L
Linearity: 25–400 mg/L
C.V.: not established
Relative recovery: not established

Interferences:

Other weak acid drugs that show significant ultraviolet absorbance in the area of 300 nm may cause positive interference with this method.

Reference:

K. Atermann, M. Holzbecher and H.A. Ellenberger. Salicylate levels in a stillborn infant born to a drug-addicted mother, with comments on pathology and analytical methodology. Clin. Tox. 16: 263–268, 1980.

Plasma Salicylate by Fluorescence Spectrophotometry

Principle:

Salicylate is extracted from acidified plasma into ether and re-extracted into a pH 10 buffer. The buffer solution is then analyzed by fluorometry. The assay is suitable for the measurement of low therapeutic concentrations of salicylate in small plasma specimens.

Reagents:

Stock solution – 1 mg/mL salicylate ion in water
Plasma standards – 10, 20, 50 and 100 mg/L
3 mol/L Hydrochloric acid
Ether
0.5 mol/L Borate buffer – 31.4 g boric acid and 35 mL 10 mol/L NaOH diluted to 1 L with water (pH 10.0)

Instrumental Conditions:

Fluorescence spectrophotometer set to excite at 310 nm
Measure fluorescence at 400 nm

Procedure:

1. Transfer 100 μL plasma to a 15 mL screw-cap tube. Add 2 mL 3 mol/L HCl and 10 mL ether and shake to extract.
2. Centrifuge and transfer 8 mL of the ether layer to a clean tube. Extract with 3 mL pH 10 borate buffer.
3. Centrifuge and discard the ether layer. Evaporate the residual ether from the aqueous layer under a stream of air.
4. Transfer the aqueous layer to a cuvette and determine the fluorescence against a plasma blank.

Calculation:

Calculation is based on a response factor derived from a standard curve. A quality control specimen containing 50 mg/L salicylate is analyzed daily.

Evaluation:

Sensitivity: 1 mg/L
Linearity: 10–400 mg/L
C.V.: not established
Relative recovery: 93–103%

Interferences:

Normal plasma components do not interfere with the assay, nor do the conjugated metabolites of acetylsalicylic acid. Gentisic acid, a salicylate metabolite, exhibits negligible fluorescence under the conditions described. Other drugs have not been studied for potential interference.

Reference:

M.A. Chirigos and S. Udenfriend. A simple fluorometric procedure for determining salicylic acid in biologic tissues. J. Lab. Clin. Med. 54: 769–772, 1959.

Plasma Salicylate, Aspirin and Salicylamide by Gas Chromatography

Principle:

The drugs and an internal standard, m-toluic acid, are extracted into ether from acidified plasma. The evaporated residue is subjected to trimethylsilyl derivatization and the solution is analyzed by flame-ionization gas chromatography.

Reagents:

Stock solutions – 1 mg/mL methanol solutions of salicylic acid, aspirin and salicylamide
Plasma standards – 20, 50 and 100 mg/L for salicylic acid; 2, 5 and 10 mg/L for aspirin; 4, 10 and 20 mg/L for salicylamide

Internal standard – 100 mg/L m-toluic acid in 0.2 mol/L pH 7.4 phosphate buffer
5% Potassium bisulfate
Ether
Anhydrous sodium sulfate
BSTFA – bis(trimethylsilyl)trifluoroacetamide (Pierce Chemical Co.)

Instrumental Conditions:

Gas chromatograph with flame-ionization detector
1.8 m × 4 mm i.d. glass column containing 5% OV-17 on 80/100 mesh Gas Chrom Q
Injector, 200°C.; detector, 250°C.
Column temperature program: initial, 160°C; 2°C./min increase; final, 200°C.
Nitrogen flow rate, 50 mL/min

Procedure:

1. Transfer 1 mL plasma to a 15 mL screwcap tube. Add 100 μL internal standard and 1 mL 5% potassium bisulfate and vortex.
2. Extract with 7 mL ether. Centrifuge and transfer the ether layer to a clean tube.
3. Add a small amount of solid Na_2SO_4 to the ether and vortex. Transfer the ether to a 12 mL centrifuge tube and evaporate to dryness at 30°C. under a stream of nitrogen.
4. Add 40 μL BSTFA to the tube and heat at 50°C. for 1 hour. Inject 1 μL of this solution into the gas chromatograph.

	Retention time (min)
internal standard derivative	5
salicylic acid derivative	8
aspirin derivative	12
salicylamide derivative	17

Calculation:

Calculation is based on a response factor derived from a standard curve. A quality control specimen containing each drug at a mid-range concentration is analyzed daily.

Evaluation:

Sensitivity: 0.5 mg/L
Linearity: 1–20 mg/L
C.V.: not established
Relative recovery: 92–104%

Interferences:

Normal plasma components do not interfere with the assay. Other drugs were not studied for potential interference.

Reference:

M.J. Rance, B.J. Jordan and J.D. Nichols. A simultaneous determination of acetylsalicylic acid, salicylic acid and salicylamide in plasma by gas liquid chromatography. J. Pharm. Pharmacol. 27: 425–429, 1975.

Plasma Salicylate and Acetaminophen by Liquid Chromatography

Principle:

Salicylic acid and acetaminophen are extracted into an organic solvent containing an internal standard. The concentrated extract is analyzed by liquid chromatography with ultraviolet absorbance detection at 248 nm.

Reagents:

Stock solution – 1 mg/mL methanol solutions of salicylic acid and acetaminophen

Plasma standards – 50, 100 and 200 mg/L for salicylate and acetaminophen

Extraction solvent – 20 mg/L 8-chlorotheophylline (K & K Chemicals) in chloroform/ isopropanol, 1:1

Sodium chloride – solid NaCl

Methanol

Mobile phase – 30 mL 2-propanol in 970 mL 0.02 mol/L pH 2.9 phosphoric acid

Instrumental Conditions:

Liquid chromatograph with 248 nm ultraviolet detector

25 cm × 4 mm i.d. stainless-steel column containing ODS-Sil-X-1 (Perkin Elmer)

Column temperature, 40°C.

Solvent flow rate, 1.5 mL/min

Procedure:

1. Transfer 50 µL plasma to a 1.5 mL plastic centrifuge tube. Add 0.5 mL extraction solvent and 0.1–0.2 g solid NaCl and vortex for 2 min.
2. Centrifuge and transfer the supernatant to a glass tube. Evaporate to dryness at 40°C. under a stream of nitrogen.
3. Dissolve the residue in 50 µL methanol and inject 2–5 µL into the chromatograph.

	Retention time (min)
acetaminophen	2.2
salicylate	2.9
internal standard	4.2

Calculation:

Calculation is based on a response factor derived from a standard curve. A quality control specimen containing salicylate and acetaminophen at mid-range concentrations is analyzed daily.

Evaluation:

Sensitivity: 10 mg/L for each drug

Linearity: 50–1000 mg/L for salicylate; 10–300 mg/L for acetaminophen

C.V.: 3–6% day-to-day

Relative recovery: 96–108% for each drug

Interferences:

Normal plasma constituents do not interfere with the assay. Eight other commonly used drugs did not interfere, although theophylline was found to co-elute with salicylate. Phenacetin has a retention time of 6 min and may be measured by this technique.

Reference:

J.N. Micelli, M.K. Aravind, S.N. Cohen and A.K. Done. Simultaneous measurements of acetaminophen and salicylate in plasma by liquid chromatography. Clin. Chem. 25: 1002–1004, 1979.

SOLVENTS

	Blood or Plasma Concentrations (mg/L)	
	Controlled Industrial Exposure	Fatalities
benzene	<0.2	1–38
carbon tetrachloride	<1	20–260
chloroform	<5	10–48
dichloromethane	<12	200–500
toluene	<2	10–20
trichloroethylene	<7	3–110

Human exposure to the common organic solvents often is a result of an accident involving careless handling of industrial or domestic chemical products. However, intentional abuse of the materials for the purpose of experiencing their euphoric effects occurs among children and young adults. It is useful to have available a convenient screening technique to determine the presence or absence of these substances in suspected instances of solvent exposure. The following gas chromatographic procedure involves equilibration of a specimen in a closed container and headspace analysis of the vapor sample with flame-ionization detection.

Blood Solvents by Gas Chromatography

Principle:

Whole blood is diluted with water and the specimen is allowed to equilibrate in a sealed container at a constant temperature. A sample of the headspace vapor is analyzed by flame-ionization gas chromatography.

Reagents:

Stock solutions – 1 mg/mL water solutions of benzene, carbon tetrachloride, chloroform, dichloromethane, toluene and trichloroethylene

Blood standards – 2, 5 and 10 mg/L for each of the above (prepare fresh from stock solution)

Instrumental Conditions:

Gas chromatograph with flame-ionization detector
2 m × 2 mm i.d. glass column containing 2% OV-17 on 100/120 mesh Chromosorb G-HP
Injector, 150°C.; column, 60°C.; detector, 150°C.
Nitrogen flow rate, 20 mL/min

Procedure:

1. Transfer 2 mL blood to a 10 mL serum bottle and add 2 mL water.
2. Seal the bottle by placing aluminum foil over a rubber septum and inserting the septum. Allow the bottle to equilibrate at 37°C. for 10 min. (room temperature may be used although sensitivity is diminished).
3. Withdraw 1 mL of the headspace vapor into a 2 mL glass syringe equipped with a 23 gauge metal needle and inject into the gas chromatograph.

	Retention time (min)
dichloromethane	1.3
chloroform	2.0
carbon tetrachloride	2.2
benzene	2.5
trichloroethylene	2.8
toluene	4.9

Calculation:

Calculation is based on a standard curve prepared each time an assay is performed. Control specimens are not applicable due to the volatility of the analytes. The results of this procedure should be considered semi-quantitative.

Evaluation:

Sensitivity: 1 mg/L
Linearity: 2–30 mg/L
C.V.: not established
Relative recovery: not established

Interferences:

Normal plasma components do not interfere with the assay. Many other volatile organic compounds are detected with this technique and may interfere.

Reference:

R. Baselt and C. Barrett, unpublished results, 1975.

SULFIDE

Blood Sulfide Concentrations (mg/L)	
Normal Subjects	Fatalities
<0.05	0.9–3.8

The most common source of sulfide ion in episodes of human poisoning is gaseous hydrogen sulfide, a product of organic decomposition and a byproduct of certain industrial processes. Determination of sulfide in whole blood or plasma is the only known chemical confirmation of sulfide poisoning. This is best performed by initial isolation of the sulfide ion using microdiffusion, followed by either colorimetry or ion-specific proteintiometry. Sulfide is rapidly lost from biologic specimens and therefore analysis should take place soon after specimen collection.

Blood Sulfide by Colorimetry

Principle:
Inorganic sulfide is isolated from whole blood by Conway microdiffusion. The isolated ion is reacted with a chromogenic reagent and the resulting colored solution is analyzed at 670 nm in a spectrophotometer.

Reagents:
Stock solution – 1 mg/mL sulfide ion in water
Blood standards – 0.5, 1.0 and 2.0 mg/L (prepare fresh)
0.1 mol/L Sodium hydroxide
0.5 mol/L Sulfuric acid
Ferric chloride solution – 200 mg $FeCl_3$ in 100 mL 10% HCl
N,N-dimethyl-p-phenylenediamine solution – 100 mg in 100 mL 50% HCl
Color reagent – 1 volume of $FeCl_3$ solution to 1 volume of N,N-dimethyl-p-phenylene-diamine solution (prepare fresh)

Instrumental Conditions:
Visible spectrophotometer set to 670 nm

Procedure:
1. Lubricate edges of Conway diffusion cells with stopcock grease. Add 3 mL 0.1 mol/L NaOH to the center well
2. Add 4 mL blood to the outer compartment of the cell. Add 4 mL 0.5 mol/L H_2SO_4 to the outer compartment and rapidly close the cell.

265

3. Tilt gently to mix and leave for 3–4 hours at room temperature (or for 1–2 hr in a 37°C. oven).
4. Transfer 2 mL of the reagent from the center well to a 12 mL centrifuge tube. Add 2 mL of the color reagent and vortex.
5. Allow to stand for 10 minutes and measure the absorbance at 670 nm against a blood blank.

Calculation:

Calculation is based on a standard curve prepared each time an assay is performed. This procedure cannot be controlled by the usual methods due to the instability of sulfide in biologic fluids.

Evaluation:

Sensitivity: 0.5 mg/L
Linearity: 0.5–2.0 mg/L
C.V.: not established
Relative recovery: 92–104%

Interferences:

Normal blood components do not interfere with the assay. The method is relatively specific for sulfide ion in freshly drawn specimens.

References:

1. J.M. Debevere and J.P. Voets. A rapid microdiffusion method for the determination of sulfides in biological fluids. Lab. Prac. 21: 713–714, 1972.
2. E.J. Conway. Microdiffusion Analysis and Volumetric Error, Crosby Lockwood, London, 1962.

Blood Sulfide by Ion-Specific Potentiometry

Principle:

Sulfide is isolated from blood by microdiffusion according to the previous procedure. The concentration of the ion is determined by direct potentiometric measurement with a cyanide-specific electrode.

Reagents:

Stock solution – 1 mg/mL sulfide ion in water
Blood standards – 0.1, 0.5 and 1.0 mg/L (prepare fresh)
0.5 mol/L Sulfuric acid
0.1 mol/L Sodium hydroxide
10% Lead acetate solution – 1 g $Pb(C_2H_3O_2)_2$ in 10 mL 0.1 mol/L NaOH

Instrumental Conditions:

pH Meter equipped with cyanide-specific electrode (Orion Research)

Procedure:

1. Process the blood specimen by Conway microdiffusion according to the previous procedure.
2. Stabilize the cyanide electrode by placing in 0.1 mol/L NaOH for 30 minutes or until a constant voltage reading is attained.
3. Determine the electrode response to the NaOH solution from the center well of the Conway cell and compare it to blood standards and a negative control blood processed in the same manner.
4. Add 1 drop 10% lead acetate solution to each NaOH solution after recording the initial reading. A significant change in electrode potential is confirmation of the presence of sulfide in the solution. An initial positive reading that is unaffected by lead acetate addition is indicative of the presence of cyanide.

Calculation:

Calculation is based on a standard curve prepared each time an assay is performed. This procedure cannot be controlled by the usual methods due to the instability of sulfide in biological fluids.

Evaluation:

Sensitivity: 0.01 mg/L
Linearity: 0.1–1.0 mg/L
C.V.: not established
Relative recovery: not established

Interferences:

Although cyanide is known to interfere in this procedure, the addition of lead acetate to the final solution will determine its presence or absence. Although fresh whole blood contains less than 0.05 mg/L inorganic sulfide, decomposed specimens may contain up to 0.4 mg/L of the ion.

Reference:

B.H. McAnalley, W.T. Lowry, R. Oliver and J.C. Garriott. Determination of inorganic sulfide and cyanide in blood using specific ion electrodes. J. Analyt. Tox. 3: 119–124, 1979.

TETRACYCLIC ANTIDEPRESSANTS

	Plasma Concentrations (mg/L)		
	Therapeutic	Toxic	T½
amoxapine	0.01–0.09	0.5–2.0	8 hr
8-hydroxyamoxapine	0.16–0.51	0.5–2.0	33 hr
loxapine	0.002–0.030	0.2–2.0	3–4 hr
8-hydroxyloxapine	0.010–0.090	?	?
8-hydroxyamoxapine	0.004–0.090	?	?
maprotiline	0.17–0.72	0.5–2.0	36–105 hr
mianserin	0.01–0.16	0.1–0.5	6–39 hr
trazodone	0.07–1.68	2.0–5.0	7–8 hr

The tetracyclic antidepressants are a diverse group of drugs used in the treatment of depression. In general, they have fewer anticholinergic side effects and exhibit lower cardiac toxicity than the tricyclic antidepressents. Loxapine produces the lowest therapeutic plasma concentrations of this group, and a method employing electron-capture gas chromatography is presented for its determination. The other drugs may be measured using liquid chromatography with ultraviolet detection.

Plasma Loxapine and Metabolites by Electron-Capture Gas Chromatography

Principle:

The drugs and an internal standard, 8-methoxyloxapine, are extracted from alkalinized plasma with ethyl acetate. The organic layer is back-extracted with dilute acid, the acid layer made alkaline, and extracted with ethyl acetate. The organic solvent is evaporated to dryness and the residue reacted first with trifluoroacetic anhydride to derivatize secondary amines and then with a silylating reagent to derivatize phenolic groups. The reaction mixture is analyzed by electron-capture gas chromatography.

Reagents:

Stock solutions – 1 mg/mL solutions of loxapine, 8-hydroxyloxapine and 8-hydroxyamoxapine in methanol

Plasma standards – 5, 10, 25 and 50 µg/L for each of the above drugs

Internal standard – 500 mg/mL 8-methoxyloxapine (Lederle) in water

1 mol/L pH 9.7 carbonate buffer – 9 parts 1 mol/L Na_2CO_3 plus 1 part 1 mol/L $NaHCO_3$

Ethyl acetate

0.1 mol/L Hydrochloric acid

TFAA solution – ethyl acetate/trifluoroacetic anhydride, 5:2 by volume (prepare fresh)

N-trimethylsilyldiethylamine (Pierce Chemical)

Instrumental Conditions:

Gas chromatograph with electron-capture detector

1.8 m × 2 mm i.d. glass column containing 3% SP-2100 on 100/200 mesh Supelcoport (Supelco)

Injector, 280°C.; column, 255°C.; detector, 300°C.

Argon/methane (95:5) flow rate, 30 mL/min

Procedure:

1. Transfer 2 mL plasma to a 15 mL screw-cap tube. Add 0.2 mL internal standard, 1 mL 1 mol/L carbonate buffer and 5 mL ethyl acetate. Shake to extract and centrifuge to separate layers.
2. Transfer the upper organic layer to a clean tube and add 1 mL 0.1 mol/L HCl. Shake to extract and centrifuge. Discard the upper organic layer and add 4 mL ethyl acetate. Shake, centrifuge and discard the upper organic layer.
3. Add 1 mL 1 mol/L carbonate buffer and 4 mL ethyl acetate. Shake to extract and centrifuge. Transfer the upper organic layer to a 5 mL Reacti-vial (Pierce Chemical) and evaporate to dryness in a 40°C. heating block under a stream of nitrogen.
4. Add 100 μL TFAA solution and allow to stand for 10 min at room temperature. Evaporate to dryness under a stream of nitrogen. Add 20 μL N-trimethylsilyldie-thylamine, cap the vial, and heat at 60°C. for 3 hr. Cool and inject 1–2 μL into the chromatograph.

	Retention time (min)
loxapine	4.0
internal standard	7.8
8-hydroxyloxapine	8.3
8-hydroxyamoxapine	13.0

Calculation:

Calculation is based on a response factor derived from a standard curve. A quality control specimen containing each drug or metabolite at a concentration of 15 μg/L is analyzed daily.

Evaluation:

Sensitivity: 1 μg/L

Linearity: 5–25 μg/L

C.V.: 8–11%

Relative recovery: not established

Interferences:

Normal plasma components do not interfere with the assay. This method may also be used for amoxapine and its metabolites, amoxapine eluting at 6.0 minutes. Other therapeutic agents have not been studied for possible interference.

Reference:

T.B. Cooper and R.G. Kelly. GLC analysis of loxapine, amoxapine, and their metabolites in serum and urine. J. Pharm. Sci. 68: 216–219, 1979.

Plasma Tetracyclic Antidepressants by Liquid Chromatography

Principle:

The drugs and an internal standard, a trazodone analogue, are extracted from alkalinized plasma with an organic solvent mixture. The solvent is evaporated to dryness and the residue is dissolved in dilute phosphoric acid. Analysis is by liquid chromatography with ultraviolet detection at 214 nm.

Reagents:

Stock solutions – 1 mg/mL methanol solutions of amoxapine, 8-hydroxyamoxapine, maprotiline, mianserin and trazodone

Plasma standards – 25, 50, 100, 250 and 500 μg/L for each of the above

Internal standard – 20 mg/L 2-[3-(4-m-chlorophenyl-1-piperazinyl)-propyl]-5-methyl-4-phenyltriazol-3-(2H)-one (Roussel Laboratories, Wiltshire, England) in methanol

2 mol/L Sodium hydroxide

Extraction solvent – hexane/isoamyl alcohol, 99:1 by volume

0.5 g/L Phosphoric acid

Mobile phase – pH 4.7 50 mmol/L potassium dihydrogen phosphate buffer/acetonitrile, 72:28 by volume

Instrumental Conditions:

Liquid chromatograph with 214 nm ultraviolet detector 30 cm × 4.6 mm i.d. stainless-steel column containing μBondapak C_{18} (Waters Associates)

Column temperature, 60°C.

Solvent flow rate, 2.5 mL/min

Procedure:

1. Transfer 1 mL plasma to a siliconized 15 mL screw-cap tube and add 100 μL internal standard and 0.5 mL 2 mol/L NaOH. Vortex.
2. Add 5 mL extraction solvent and place on a rotator for 15 min. Centrifuge and transfer the upper organic layer to a siliconized 12 mL conical centrifuge tube. Evaporate to dryness under a stream of dry air at 40°C.
3. Dissolve the residue in 400 μL 0.5 g/L H_3PO_4 and inject 100 μL into the chromatograph.

	Retention time (min)
8-hydroxyamoxapine	2.3
trazodone	5.3
maprotiline	7.0
amoxapine	9.0
mianserin	9.0
internal standard	12.6

Calculation:

Calculation is based on a response factor derived from a standard curve. A quality control specimen containing the appropriate drugs at mid-level concentrations is analyzed daily.

Evaluation:

Sensitivity: 5 µg/L
Linearity: 25–200 µg/L
C.V.: 4.7–7.6% day-to-day
Relative recovery: not established

Interferences:

Normal plasma components do not interfere with the assay. Over 20 commonly prescribed therapeutic agents were tested and were found not to interfere, with the exception of lorazepam, which co-elutes with amoxapine and mianserin.

References:

1. S.H.Y. Wong and S.W. Waugh. Determination of the antidepressants maprotiline and amoxapine, and their metabolites, in plasma by liquid chromatography. Clin. Chem. 29: 314–318, 1983.
2. S.H.Y. Wong, S.W. Waugh, M. Draz and N. Jain. Liquid-chromatographic determination of two antidepressants, trazodone and mianserin, in plasma. Clin. Chem. 30: 230–233, 1984.

THALLIUM

	Thallium Concentrations (mg/L)	
	Normal Subjects	Clinical Intoxication
blood	<0.005	0.1–8
urine	<0.002	1–20

Thallium salts are commercially available for use in insecticides, rodenticides and dipilatories. Most of the poisonings seen clinically are the result of accidental ingestion of these substances. Elevated thallium concentrations in either blood or urine are indicative of excessive exposure to this toxic metal, since normal concentrations are extremely low. The following colorimetric procedure is useful for the semi-quantitative screening of urine in suspected cases of acute poisoning. A more specific flame atomic absorption spectrometric procedure is also presented that is applicable to thallium determination in both blood and urine.

Urine Thallium by Colorimetry

Principle:
Urine is treated with bromine water to convert thallium ion to the trivalent thallic form. Excess bromine is removed with sulfosalicylic acid and brilliant green is added to complex the thallium. The complex is extracted into toluene and measured colorimetrically at 460 nm.

Reagents:
Stock solution – 1 mg/mL thallium ion
Urine standards – 1, 2, 5 and 10 mg/L (prepare fresh)
6 mol/L Hydrochloric acid
Bromine water – prepare fresh by saturating deionized water with bromine
200 g/L Sulfosalicylic acid
2 g/L brilliant green – extract the solution 3 times with one-half the volume of toluene, discarding the toluene each time
Toluene

Instrumental Conditions:
Visible spectrophotometer set to 460 nm

Procedure:
1. Transfer 5 mL urine to a 15 mL screw-cap tube. Add 1.5 mL 6 mol/L HCl and 1 mL bromine water. Vortex and allow to stand for 5 min.

2. Add 1 mL 200 g/L sulfosalicylic acid and vortex. Further add 0.25 mL 2 g/L brilliant green and vortex.
3. Add 5 mL toluene and place on a rotator for 5 min. Centrifuge to separate layers and measure the absorbance of the upper toluene layer at 460 nm against a reagent block.

Calculation:

Calculation is based on a standard curve prepared with each set of specimens.

Evaluation:

Sensitivity: 1 mg/L
Linearity: 1–10 mg/L
C.V.: not established
Relative recovery: 96–100%

Interferences:

Normal urine can contain interfering substances, resulting in apparent thallium concentrations as high as 5 mg/L. Therefore, this should be considered a semi-quantitative, presumptive technique and all positive results should be confirmed by a more specific method.

References:

1. J.N.M. de Wolf and J.B. Lenstra. The determination of thallium in urine. Pharm. Weekblad. 99: 377–382, 1964.
2. N.W. Wakid and N.K. Cortas. Chemical and atomic absorption methods for thallium in urine compound. Clin. Chem. 30: 587–588, 1984.

Blood and urine Thallium by Atomic Absorption Spectrometry

Principle:

Blood and urine are treated with diethldithiocarbamate to chelate ionic thallium. The chelate is extracted into methylisobutylketone and the extract is analyzed by flame atomic absorption spectrometry.

Reagents:

Stock solution – 1 mg/mL thallium ion
Aqueous standards – 0.2, 0.5, 1.0, 2.0 and 4.0 mg/L (prepare fresh)
2.5 mol/L Sodium hydroxide
DDC solution – 1% sodium diethyldithiocarbamate in water
5% Triton X-100
MIBK – methylisobutylketone

Instrumental Conditions:

Atomic absorption spectrometer with air-acetylene oxidizing flame
Thallium hollow cathode lamp
Measure absorption at 276.7 nm

Procedure:

Blood:

1. Transfer 5 mL citrated or heparinized whole blood to a 15 mL screw-cap tube. Add 1 mL DDC solution and 1 mL 5% Triton X-100 and vortex.
2. Let stand for 10 min. Add 3 mL MIBK and shake to extract.
3. Centrifuge and aspirate the MIBK layer into the flame of the spectrometer. Compare to aqueous standards processed in the same manner.

Urine:

4. Transfer 5 mL urine to a 15 mL screw-cap tube. Adjust to pH 6.0–7.5 by adding 2.5 mol/L NaOH.
5. Add 1 mL DDC solution and vortex. Add 3 mL MIBK and shake to extract.
6. Centrifuge and aspirate the MIBK layer into the flame of the spectrometer. Compare to aqueous standards processed in the same manner.

Calculation:

Calculation is based on a standard curve prepared with each set of specimens.

Evaluation:

Sensitivity: 0.1 mg/L
Linearity: 0.2–4.0 mg/L
C.V.: 3–5% within-run
Relative recovery: not established

Interferences:

Normal biological fluids contain only trace amounts of thallium. Other metals do not interfere, but to prevent thallium contamination all glassware should be soaked overnight in 25% nitric acid and reagent blanks should be analyzed frequently. The use of EDTA as a blood anticoagulant causes a slight reduction in the recovery of thallium.

References:

1. E. Berman. Determination of cadmium, thallium and mercury in biological materials by atomic absorption. At. Abs. Newsl. 6: 57–60, 1967.
2. F. Amore. Determination of cadmium, lead, thallium, and nickel in blood by atomic absorption spectrometry. Anal. Chem. 46: 1597–1599, 1974.

THEOPHYLLINE

Plasma Concentrations (mg/L)		
Therapeutic	Toxic	T½
10–20	>25	3–10 hr

Theophylline has been used for many years as a bronchodilator in the control of asthma. It is commonly administered by intravenous infusion in acute therapy, and by oral dosing for chronic care. Monitoring of plasma theophylline concentrations is very frequently requested, both to prevent toxicity from the drug and to ascertain that an adequate dosage has been prescribed. The drug may be conveniently assayed by a variety of procedures, each offering certain advantages in terms of simplicity of performance, specificity or small sample volume. Techniques based on ultraviolet spectrophotometry, gas chromatography and liquid chromatography are presented. The latter procedure may also be used for the measurement of plasma caffeine concentrations. Reagents are also available commercially for determination of theophylline in plasma by radiommunoassay, fluorescence immuno-assay and EMIT.

Plasma Theophylline by Ultraviolet Spectrophotometry

Principle:
Theophylline is extracted from 50 µL of plasma into an organic solvent. A back-extraction into dilute alkali is performed and the absorbance of the solution is determined in an ultraviolet spectrophotometer.

Reagents:
Stock solution – 1 mg/mL theophylline in methanol
Plasma standards – 5, 10 and 20 mg/L
Extraction solvent – chloroform/isopropanol, 20:1 by volume
0.03 mol/L Sodium hydroxide
2 mol/L Ammonium chloride

Instrumental Conditions:
Ultraviolet recording spectrophotometer with 1.4 mL quartz cuvettes
Record spectrum from 340 to 220 nm

Procedure:
1. Transfer 50 µL plasma to a 16 × 125 mm glass tube and add 150 µL water. Add 4 mL extraction solvent and vortex for 30 seconds.
2. Centrifuge and discard upper aqueous phase. Transfer 3 mL of the organic layer to a clean tube.

3. Add 0.5 mL 0.3 mol/L NaOH and vortex for 30 seconds. Centrifuge and transfer 0.4 mL of the aqueous phase to a 1.4 mL quartz cuvette.
4. Add 20 µL 2 mol/L NH$_4$Cl to the cuvette and mix. Record the absorbance spectrum of the solution against a plasma blank from 340 to 220 nm.
5. Record the absorbance at the 275 nm maximum and subtract the background absorbance at 300 nm.

Calculation:

Calculation is based on a response factor derived from a standard curve. A quality control specimen containing 15 mg/L theophylline is analyzed daily.

Evaluation:

Sensitivity: 2 mg/L
Linearity: 5–100 mg/L
C.V.: 6–8% between-run
Relative recovery: 87–104%

Interferences:

Normal plasma specimens yield a nonspecific absorbance peak at approximately 270 nm and therefore patient specimens must be analyzed against a drug-free specimen. Caffeine, salicylate and phenobarbital were found not to interfere even at toxic concentrations. Acetaminophen, sulfamethoxazole, theobromine and certain other drugs may interfere with the procedure. The complete ultraviolet spectrum should be recorded for each analysis in order to detect an atypical absorbance curve, and the analysis repeated using a more specific technique if interference is suspected.

Reference:

D.C. Hohnadel, T.H. Grove and P. Alonzo. A micro method for the ultraviolet spectrophotometric determination of theophylline. J. Analyt. Tox. 2: 141–145 1978.

Plasma Theophylline by Gas Chromatography

Principle:

Theophylline is extracted from acidified plasma using an organic solvent that contains the internal standard, a xanthine derivative. The concentrated extract is analyzed by gas chromatography on a special liquid phase.

Reagents:

Stock solution – 1 mg/mL theophylline in methanol
Plasma standards – 5, 10 and 20 mg/L
Extraction solvent – dichloromethane/hexane/acetic acid, 80:20:0.1 by volume, containing 1.5 mg/L 3-isobutyl-1-methylxanthine (Aldrich)
Ammonium sulfate
Chloroform

Instrumental Conditions:

Gas chromatograph with flame-ionization detector
2 m × 4 mm i.d. glass column containing 2% SP2510-DA on 100/120 mesh Supelcoport
    (Supelco, Inc.)
Injector, 300°C.; column, 245°C.; detector, 300°C.
Nitrogen flow rate, 50 mL/min

Procedure:

1. Transfer 1 mL plasma to a 15 mL screw-cap tube. Add about 0.8 g solid $(NH_4)_2SO_4$ and vortex.
2. Add 10 mL extraction solvent and shake to extract. Centrifuge and decant the organic layer into a 12 mL conical centrifuge tube.
3. Evaporate to dryness under a stream of nitrogen at 50°C. Dissolve the residue in 50 µL chloroform and inject 10 µL into the chromatograph.

	Retention time (min)
caffeine	0.6
theobromine	1.6
theophylline	3.7
internal standard	4.2

Calculation:

Calculation is based on a response factor derived from a standard curve. A quality control specimen containing 15 mg/L theophylline is analyzed daily.

Evaluation:

Sensitivity: 2.5 mg/L
Linearity: 2.5–30 mg/L
C.V.: 6% day-to-day
Relative recovery: not established

Interferences:

Normal plasma constituents do not interfere with the assay. Several commonly prescribed anticonvulsant drugs were found not to interfere, although carbamazepine elutes between theophylline and the internal standard and could lead to inaccuracies.

Reference:

H.A. Schwertner. Analysis for underivatized theophylline by gas-chromatography on a silicone stationary phase, SP-2510-DA. Clin. Chem. 25: 212–214, 1979.

Plasma Theophylline by Liquid Chromatography

Principle:

Plasma is deproteinized by addition of the internal standard solution. The supernatant is analyzed by reversed-phase liquid chromatography with detection at 254 nm. Only 30 µL of plasma is required for this assay and the procedure is applicable to the simultaneous determination of caffeine.

Reagents:

Stock solution – 1 mg/mL theophylline in methanol

Plasma standards – 5, 10 and 20 mg/L

Internal standard solution – 40 mg/L β-hydroxyethyltheophylline (ICN Pharmaceuticals) in acetonitrile

Acetate buffer – 10 mmol/L sodium acetate adjusted to pH 4.0 with glacial acetic acid (prepare fresh)

Mobile phase – acetonitrile/acetate buffer, 7:93 by volume

Instrumental Conditions:

Liquid chromatograph with 254 nm ultraviolet detector (273 nm is preferred if a variable wavelength is available)

30 cm × 4 nm i.d. stainless-steel column containing μBondapak C_{18} (Waters Associates)

Column temperature, ambient

Solvent flow rate, 2 mL/min

Procedure:

1. Transfer 30 μL plasma to a plastic micro-centrifuge tube. Add 30 μL internal standard solution and vortex.
2. Centrifuge and inject 5 μL of the supernatant into the chromatograph.

	Retention time (min)
theobromine	4.5
theophylline	6.0
internal standard	7.5
caffeine	10.5

Calculation:

Calculation is based on a response factor derived from a standard curve. A quality control specimen containing 15 mg/L theophylline is analyzed daily.

Evaluation:

Sensitivity: 0.2 mg/L

Linearity: 5–40 mg/L

C.V.: 2.2% within-run

Relative recovery: not established

Interferences:

Normal plasma components do not interfere with the assay. Specimens containing high caffeine concentrations may yield an apparent theophylline concentration of up to 3.5 mg/L. Other drugs were not observed to interfere. Other xanthines and their metabolites may be assayed using this procedure.

Reference:

J.J. Orcutt, P.O. Kozak, Jr., S.A. Gillman and L.H. Cummins. Micro-scale method for theophylline in body fluids by reversed-phase, high-pressure liquid chromatography. Clin. Chem. 23: 599–601, 1977.

THIOCYANATE

Thiocyanate Concentrations in Plasma (mg/L) and Urine (mg/24 hr)			
	Nonsmokers	Smokers	Nitroprusside Infusion
plasma	1–4	3–12	6–29
urine	1–4	7–17	?

Thiocyanate is the major metabolite of cyanide, being produced via the liver enzyme rhodanase in the presence of a sufficient supply of sulfur. Thiocyanate is present in the body fluids of healthy subjects as a result of normal metabolic processes. Since cyanide is a component of cigarette smoke, thiocyanate concentrations tend to be elevated in smokers; however, subjects who suffer from tobacco amblyopia actually have lower than normal thiocyanate levels and are thought to have an impaired ability to detoxify cyanide. Other sources of cyanide are the antihypertensive drug nitroprusside, cyanogenetic glycosides in laetrile, fires, industrial processes and of course intentional poisonings with cyanide compounds. The following colorimetric procedure for determination of thiocyanate in plasma and urine is convenient and specific.

Plasma and Urine Thiocyanate by Colorimetry

Principle:

Thiocyanate is removed from the specimen by absorption on an ion-exchange column. The eluate is treated with a halogenating reagent and allowed to react with a pyridine-barbituric acid chromogenic solution. The absorbance of the final solution is measured at 580 nm in the spectrophotometer.

Reagents:

Stock solution – 1 mg/mL thiocyanate ion in water

Aqueous standards – 1, 3, 6 and 12 mg/L

0.1 mol/L Sodium hydroxide – 4 g NaOH per L

1 mol/L Sodium perchlorate – 140 g $NaClO_4.H_2O$ per L

0.5 mol/L Acetic acid – 28.5 mL conc. acetic acid per L

50 mmol/L Sodium hypochlorite – 5 mL 0.5 mol/L NaClO in 0.1 mol/L NaOH diluted to 50 mL with water (stable for 1 month if refrigerated)

Chromogenic reagent – dissolve 6 g barbituric acid in 30 mL pyridine and 64 mL water; add 6 mL conc. HCl (stable for 1 week if refrigerated)

Ion-exchange column – 4 cm × 0.7 cm i.d. column containing 100/120 mesh Lewatit MP7080 (EM Laboratories, Elsmford, NY 10523)

Instrumental Conditions:

Visible spectrophotometer set to 580 nm

Procedure:

Resin preparation:

1. Wash resin in water and suspend in 1 mol/L HCl. Filter and wash with water until pH of washings exceeds 4.5.
2. Spread resin on a glass plate and dry at 100°C. for 12 hr. Suspend in water and let stand 15 min.
3. Decant off water and resuspend resin in 1 mol/L NaOH. Let stand 15 min and wash with water until washings are a neutral pH. Fill resin column to a height of 2.5 cm.

Sample analysis:

1. Dilute 0.5 mL plasma or urine with 5 mL 0.1 mol/L NaOH and apply to the ion-exchange column. Wash column 3 times with 5 mL portions of water.
2. Elute the column with 8 mL 1 mol/L $NaClO_4$. Transfer 4 mL of the eluate to a 12 mL centrifuge tube.
3. Add 0.2 mL 0.5 mol/L acetic acid and vortex. Add 0.1 mL 50 mmol/L NaClO and vortex.
4. Within 1 min add 0.5 mL chromogenic reagent and vortex. After 5–15 min measure the absorbance in the spectrophotometer against a water blank that has been processed in the same manner.

Calculation:

Calculation is based on a response factor derived from a standard curve. A quality control specimen consisting of an aqueous solution containing 3 mg/L thiocyanate is analyzed daily.

Evaluation:

Sensitivity: 0.5 mg/L
Linarity: 1–12 mg/L
C.V.: 2.3% between-day
Relative recovery: 98–105%

Interferences:

Normal plasma components do not interfere with the assay. Cyanide will be measured as thiocyanate if present; normal plasma and urine cyanide concentrations are very low, but this interference may be avoided by washing the column two times with 5 mL of 0.1 mol/L HCl prior to elution with $NaClO_4$. Certain antibiotics, including benzylpenicillin, cloxacillin and cephalothin, interferred when present at very high concentrations (2 g/L); this problem may be avoided by washing the column 3 times with 5 mL of 4 mol/L NH_4Cl prior to elution with $NaClO_4$.

Reference:

P. Lundquist, J. Martensson, B. Sorbo and S. Ohman. Method for determining thiocyanate in serum and urine. Clin. Chem. 25: 678–681, 1979.

THIOPENTAL

Plasma Concentrations (mg/L)

Anesthetic Levels	Fatal Intoxication
7–130	6–392

Thiopental is an intravenous anesthetic inducing agent that has seen widespread usage since its introduction in 1935. The wide range of concentrations observed in therapeutic usage result from the large amounts of the drug that are sometimes used and the fact that it is occasionally used as the sole anesthetic agent in short surgical procedures. Plasma concentrations exceeding 7 mg/L are generally associated with unconsciousness and respiratory depression. Since the drug is converted to a small extent to pentobarbital, it is desirable that a method for thiopental be capable of measuring the metabolite. The following gas chromatographic procedure has the sensitivity and specificity required for monitoring anesthetic levels of thiopental or for pharmacokinetic studies.

Plasma Thiopental by Gas Chromatography

Principle:
Thiopental and an internal standard are extracted from plasma with an organic solvent. After several clean-up steps, the concentrated extract is analyzed by flame-ionization gas chromatography. The procedure is applicable to the determination of the pentobarbital metabolite of thiopental.

Reagents:
Stock solution – 1 mg/mL thiopental in methanol
Plasma standards – 5, 10, 20 and 40 mg/L
Internal standard – 10 mg/L butethal (butobarbitone) in isopropanol
1.5 mol/L Sodium dihydrogen phosphate
Hexane
2.5 mol/L Sodium hydroxide
6 mol/L Hydrochloric acid
Dichloromethane
Carbon tetrachloride

Instrumental Conditions:
Gas chromatograph with flame-ionization detector
1.8 m × 4 mm i.d. glass column containing 5% OV-1 on 100/120 mesh
  Chromosorb W

Injector, 230°C.; column, 205°C.; detector, 230°C.
Nitrogen flow rate, 45 mL/min

Procedure:

1. Transfer 1 mL plasma to a 15 mL screw-cap tube. Add 1 mL internal standard and 1 mL 1.5 mol/L NaH_2PO_4 and vortex.
2. Extract with 10 mL hexane by shaking for 30 seconds. Centrifuge and transfer the hexane layer to a clean tube.
3. Extract the hexane with 4 mL 2.5 mol/L NaOH. Centrifuge and discard the upper hexane layer.
4. Wash the aqueous layer with 3 mL hexane. Centrifuge and discard the hexane.
5. Add 2 mL 6 mol/L HCl to the aqueous layer and vortex. Extract with 3 mL dichloromethane.
6. Centrifuge and discard the upper aqueous layer. Transfer the organic phase to a 5 mL conical centrifuge tube and evaporate to dryness under a stream of nitrogen at 40°C.
7. Dissolve the residue in 10 μL CCl_4 and inject 1 μL into the chromatograph.

	Retention time (min)
internal standard	1.8
pentobarbital	2.0
thiopental	3.2

Calculation:

Calculation is based on a response factor derived from a standard curve. A quality control specimen containing 10 mg/L thiopental is analyzed daily.

Evaluation:

Sensitivity: 0.1 mg/L
Linearity: 5–30 mg/L (also linear over the range 0.1–5 mg/L when 2 mL plasma and 0.25 mL internal standard are used)
C.V.: 3–5%
Relative recovery: not established

Interferences:

Normal plasma components do not interfere with the assay. Less than 2% of the thiopental present in a specimen is converted to pentobarbital during the performance of this procedure, and so there is minimal effect on apparent pentobarbital concentrations. Other drugs were not studied for potential interference.

Reference:

M.J. Van Hamme and M.M. Ghoneim. A sensitive gas chromatograph assay for thiopentone in plasma. Brit. J. Anesth. 50: 143–145, 1978.

THIORIDAZINE

	Plasma Concentrations (mg/L)	
	Therapeutic	Fatal Intoxication
thioridazine	0.2–2.6	1–13
mesoridazine	0.1–1.4	?
sulforidazine	0.0–0.5	?
ring sulfoxide	0.0–3.8	?

Thioridazine is a popular antipsychotic phenothiazine derivative that is administered orally in doses of 100–800 mg daily. The drug is metabolized primarily by oxidation of either or both sulfur atoms to a series of sulfoxide and sulfone derivatives; these metabolites are pharmacologically active and accumulate to a certain degree in plasma. When using the fluorometric assay for phenothiazines (p. 233), the value that is obtained represents the sum of the parent drug and the metabolites. Occasionally, it may be necessary to employ a more specific procedure to investigate the disposition of the drug in a particular patient or to distinguish between acute and chronic usage. The following gas and liquid chromatographic procedures allow the detection of the major thioridazine metabolites in plasma specimens from patients undergoing therapy with the drug.

Plasma Thioridazine and Metabolites by Gas Chromatography

Principle:
Thioridazine and its pharmacologically active metabolites are extracted from alkalinized plasma into an organic solvent mixture. After several clean-up steps, the final extract is analyzed by flame-ionization gas chromatography, using chlorpromazine as internal standard.

Reagents:
Stock solutions – 1 mg/mL methanol solutions of chlorpromazine, thioridazine, mesoridazine, sulforidazine and thioridazine ring sulfoxide
Plasma standards – 1, 5 and 10 mg/L for each drug (prepare fresh)
pH 7.8 0.1 mol/L Phosphate buffer
Extraction solvent – heptane/toluene, 4:1 by volume
0.1 mol/L Hydrochloric acid
Internal standard solution – extraction solvent freshly prepared to contain 100 µL of the chlorpromazine stock solution in 1.5 mL

Instrumental Conditions:

Gas chromatograph with flame-ionization detector
1.8 m × 2 mm i.d. glass column containing 3% OV-17 on 100/120 mesh Chromosorb Q
Injector, 325°C.; column, 275°C.; detector, 325°C.
Helium flow rate, 100 mL/min

Procedure:

1. Transfer 4 mL plasma to a 15 mL screw-cap tube. Add 1 mL pH 7.8 phosphate buffer.
2. Extract with 10 mL of the extraction solvent. Centrifuge and transfer the solvent layer to a clean tube.
3. Extract with 2 mL 0.1 mol/L HCl. Centrifuge and discard the upper organic layer.
4. Transfer 1.5 mL of the aqueous layer to a 3 mL conical glass-stoppered centrifuge tube. Add 0.8 mL 2 mol/L NaOH and vortex.
5. Extract with 100 µL of the internal standard solution. Centrifuge and remove most of the lower aqueous layer with a disposable pipet.
6. Recentrifuge and inject 2–3 µL of the organic phase into the chromatograph. The electrometer attenuation will need to be adjusted following elution of the internal standard to provide higher sensitivity for detection of thioridazine and its metabolites.

	Retention time (min)
internal standard	0.8
thioridazine	3.6
mesoridazine	8.3
sulforidazine	9.7
thioridazine ring sulfoxide	12.8

Calculation:

Calculation is based on a response factor derived from a standard curve. This procedure cannot be controlled by the usual procedures due to the instability of phenothiazine drugs in biological specimens.

Evaluation:

Sensitivity: 0.3 mg/L
Linearity: 0.5–10 mg/L
C.V.: 5–8%
Relative recovery: not established

Interferences:

Normal plasma constituents do not interfere with the assay. Four other phenothiazines were distinguishable from thioridazine and its metabolites. The use of chlorpromazine as internal standard necessitates that this drug be absent from patient specimens analyzed by this technique.

Reference:

E.C. Dinovo, L.A. Gottschalk, B.R. Nandi and P.G. Geddes. GLC analysis of thioridazine, mesoridazine and their metabolites. Anal. Chem. 65: 667–669, 1976.

Plasma Thioridazine and Mesoridazine by Liquid Chromatography

Principle:

Thioridazine, mesoridazine and an internal standard, trifluoperazine, are extracted from plasma into chlorobutane. The drugs are partitioned into aqueous acid and analyzed by reversed-phase liquid chromatography, with detection at 263 nm.

Reagents:

Stock solutions – 1 mg/mL methanol solutions of thioridazine and mesoridazine
Plasma standards – 0.25, 0.5, 1 and 2 mg/L for each drug (prepare fresh)
Internal standard – 100 mg/L trifluoperazine in water
pH 7.4 Phosphate buffer – 82 mL 0.067 mol/L NaH_2PO_4 and 18 mL 0.067 mol/L KH_2PO_4
1-Chlorobutane
0.2 mol/L Sulfuric acid
Mobile phase – 66 parts methanol and 34 parts 1% acetic acid containing 0.005 mol/L heptanesulfonic acid sodium salt, by volume

Instrumental Conditions:

Liquid chromatograph with 263 nm ultraviolet detector
25 cm × 4 mm i.d. stainless-steel column containing µBondapak C_{18} (Waters Associates)
Column temperature, ambient
Solvent flow rate, 2 mL/min

Procedure:

1. Transfer 2 mL plasma to a 13 × 100 mm glass tube. Add 100 µL internal standard and 0.5 mL pH 7.4 phosphate buffer and vortex.
2. Add 3 mL chlorobutane and vortex for 1 min. Centrifuge and transfer the organic layer to a clean tube.
3. Add 100 µL 0.2 mol/L H_2SO_4 and vortex for 1 min. Centrifuge and inject 25 µL of the lower aqueous layer into the chromatograph.

	Retention time (min)
mesoridazine	3.9
thioridazine	8.5
internal standard	11.7

Calculation:

Calculation is based on a response factor derived from a standard curve. This procedure cannot be controlled by the usual methods due to the instability of phenothiazine derivatives in biological fluids.

Evaluation:

Sensitivity: 0.25 mg/L
Linearity: 0.25–10 mg/L
C.V.: not established
Relative recovery: not established

Interferences:

Normal plasma constituents do not interfere with the assay. This is a preliminary procedure that has not been applied to the determination of patient specimens; other drugs or thioridazine metabolites have not been studied for potential interference.

Reference:

J.R. McCutcheon. Reverse-phase HPLC determination of thioridazine and mesoridazine in whole blood. J. Analyt. Tox. 3: 105–107, 1979.

THIOXANTHENES

	Therapeutic Plasma Concentrations (mg/L)
chlorprothixene	0.04–0.10
thiothixene	0.01–0.10

The thioxanthene derivatives, which include chlorprothixene and thiothixene, are analogues of the phenothiazines and are used in a similar manner as antipsychotic agents. The fluorometric technique presented has the necessary sensitivity to measure the very low therapeutic plasma concentrations of these drugs, but is somewhat nonspecific. Metabolites of the drugs contribute to the fluorescence and the final result may be nearly twice the actual parent drug concentration. The result is clinically useful, however, since the plasma metabolites are believed to have pharmacological activity.

Plasma Thioxanthenes by Fluorescence Spectrophotometry

Principle:
The thioxanthene derivatives are extracted from alkalinized plasma into an organic solvent. After back-extraction into dilute acid, the drugs are oxidized to fluorescent products and analyzed by spectrophotofluorometry.

Reagents:
Stock solutions – 1 mg/mL methanol solutions of chlorprothixene and thiothixene
Plasma standards – 0.02, 0.05, 0.10 and 0.20 mg/L of the appropriate drug
1 mol/L Sodium hydroxide
Extraction solvent – heptane/isoamyl alcohol, 98.7:1.3 by volume
0.05 mol/L Sulfuric acid
pH 5 Phosphate buffer – 50% saturated KH_2PO_4
0.1% Potassium permanganate
0.1% Hydrogen peroxide

Instrumental Conditions:
Fluorescence spectrophotometer set to excite at 280 nm
Record the emission spectrum from 370–470 nm

	Emission peak
chlorprothixene	450 nm
thiothixene	435 nm

Procedure:

1. Transfer 2 mL plasma to a 15 mL screw-cap tube. Add 1 mL 1 mol/L NaOH and vortex.
2. Add 10 mL extraction solvent and shake for 30 seconds. Centrifuge and transfer 9 mL of the upper organic layer to a clean tube.
3. Add 3 mL 0.05 mol/L H_2SO_4 and shake to extract. Centrifuge and transfer 2 mL of the lower aqueous layer to a clean tube.
4. Add 1 mL pH 5 phosphate buffer and 0.2 mL 0.1% $KMnO_4$ and vortex. Let stand 5 min.
5. Add 0.2 mL 0.1% H_2O_2 and vortex. Transfer to a cuvette and determine the fluorescent emission under the described conditions. Subtract the emission of the plasma blank from all results.

Calculation:

Calculation is based on a response factor derived from a standard curve. A quality control specimen containing 0.05 mg/L of the appropriate drug is analyzed daily.

Evaluation:

Sensitivity: 0.005 mg/L
Linearity: 0.02–0.50 mg/L
C.V.: not established
Relative recovery: not established

Interferences:

This procedure is applicable to the determination of most thioxanthene derivatives as well as thioridazine. Several drugs, including desipramine, haloperidol and levomepromazine, did not cause significant interference.

References:

1. T. Mjorndal and L. Oreland. Determination of thioxanthenes in plasma at therapeutic concentrations. Acta Pharm. Tox. 29: 295–302, 1971.
2. R. Baselt and C. Stewart. Unpublished results, 1977.

TOBRAMYCIN

Serum Concentrations (mg/L)		
Therapeutic	Toxic	T½
4–10	>12 (peak)	2–4 hr
	>2 (trough)	

Tobramycin is a frequently prescribed aminoglycoside antibiotic. Reagents are commercially available for determination of the drug in serum by radioimmunoassay, EMIT and fluorescence immunoassay, but occasionally it may be necessary to use a technique with more specificity. The following liquid chromatographic method is well suited for the routine analysis of tobramycin.

Serum Tobramycin by Liquid Chromatography

Principle:

An internal standard, sisomycin, dissolved in acetonitrile is added to serum, causing protein precipitation. The supernatant is treated with a derivatizing reagent to form a trinitrophenyl derivative of tobramycin and the internal standard. The drugs are isolated using a Bond-Elut extraction column and analyzed by liquid chromatography with detection at 340 nm.

Reagents:

Stock solution – 1 mg/mL tobramycin in water
Serum standards – 2, 5, 10 and 25 mg/L
Internal standard – 10 mg sisomycin per L of acetonitrile
Tris buffer – 2 mol/L Trizma base (Sigma), pH 10.3 (dissolve 24.2 g in 100 mL water)
Derivatizing reagent – 2,4,6-trinitrobenzene-1-sulfonic acid, 250 g/L (dissolve 2.5 g in 10 mL acetonitrile)
Wash buffer – methanol/100 mmol/L K_2HPO_4, 1:1 (adjust to pH 8.5 with H_3PO_4
Acetonitrile – Burdick-Jackson
Methanol – Burdick-Jackson
Mobile phase – 700 mL acetonitrile plus 300 mL 50 mmol/L pH 3.5 phosphate buffer (dissolve 6.8 g KH_2PO_4 in 1 L water and adjust to pH 3.5 with H_3PO_4)

Instrumental Conditions:

Liquid chromatograph with 340 nm wavelength detector
Ultrasphere Octyl 5 micron column, 25 cm × 4.6 mm i.d. (Altex Scientific)
Column temperature, 50°C.
Solvent flow rate, 3.0 mL/min

Vac-Elut vacuum chamber with Bond-Elut C_{18} extraction columns (Analytichem International)

Procedure:

1. Transfer 50 µL serum to a disposable plastic microtube and add 25 µL Tris buffer and 100 µL internal standard. Vortex and centrifuge at 15,000 X g for 1 min.
2. Decant the supernatant into a clean microtube and add 30 µL derivatizing reagent. Cap and vortex and heat at 70°C. for 30 min.
3. Pretreat the Bond-Elut column with 2 column volumes of methanol and 2 of water. Disconnect the vacuum and fill column with 700 µL of wash buffer followed by 200 µL of derivatized sample.
4. Turn on the vacuum and add 3 volumes of wash buffer to the column. Disconnect the vacuum and place a 10 × 75 mm glass tube under the column.
5. Elute the drugs from the column with 300 µL acetonitrile and inject 50 µL of the eluate into the chromatograph.

Calculation:

Calculation is based on a response factor derived from a standard curve. A quality control specimen containing 20 mg/L tobramycin is analyzed daily.

Evaluation:

Sensitivity: 0.2 mg/L
Linearity: 1–25 mg/L
C.V.: 4.6–5.1% day-to-day
Relative recovery: 94–99%

Interferences:

None of the more than 30 drugs studied, including gentamicin, amikacin and kanamycin, was found to interfere. The method correlated well with a commercial radioimmunoassay (Gamma Coat).

Reference:

P.M. Kabra, P.K. Bhatnager, M.A. Nelson et al. Liquid-chromatographic determination of tobramycin in serum with spectrophotometric detection. Clin. Chem. 29: 672–674, 1983.

TRANYLCYPROMINE

Therapeutic Plasma Concentrations (mg/L)	T½
0.01–0.04	2 hr

Tranylcypromine, a structural analogue of amphetamine, is marketed as the racemate for use as an antidepressant drug. One of the mechanisms of its pharmacological effects is believed to be the inhibition of monoamine oxidase in the central nervous system, resulting in increased levels of biologic amines. The very low therapeutic plasma concentrations of this drug require a sensitive method for its detection. The following electron-capture gas chromatographic procedure involves the preparation of a halogenated derivative of tranylcypromine, but is easy to perform.

Plasma Tranylcypromine by Electron-Capture Gas Chromatography

Principle:
Tranylcypromine and an internal standard, N-propylamphetamine, are extracted into toluene from alkalinized plasma. Both drugs are derivatized with trichloroacetyl chloride and the concentrated extract is anlyzed by electron-capture gas chromatography.

Reagents:
Stock solution – 1 mg/mL tranylcypromine in methanol
Working solution – 0.1 mg/mL tranylcypromine in methanol
Plasma standards – 0.005, 0.010, 0.020 and 0.040 mg/L
Internal standard – 1 mg/L N-propylamphetamine in water (see p. 20 for preparation)
10 mol/L Sodium hydroxide
Toluene
Derivatizing reagent – add 10 µL trichloroacetyl chloride to 1 mL toluene (prepare fresh)

Instrumental Conditions:
Gas chromatograph with electron-capture detector
2 m × 2 mm i.d. glass column containing 2% OV-1 on 100/120 mesh Chromosorb G-HP
Injector, 250°C.; column 185°C.; detector, 300°C.
5% Methane in argon flow rate, 33 mL/min

Procedure:
1. Transfer 2 mL plasma to a 15 mL screw-cap tube. Add 50 µL internal standard and vortex.

2. Add 1 drop 10 mol/L NaOH and 2.5 mL toluene and shake for 30 seconds. Centrifuge and transfer the upper solvent layer to a 15 mL graduated centrifuge tube.
3. Add 10 μL derivatizing reagent and vortex. Evaporate the solvent to a volume of approximately 100 μL under a stream of nitrogen at 50°C.
4. Inject 2 μL into the chromatograph.

	Retention time (min)
tranylcypromine derivative	3.1
internal standard derivative	4.1

Calculation:

Calculation is based on a response factor derived from a standard curve. A quality control specimen containing 0.010 mg/L tranylcypromine is analyzed daily.

Evaluation:

Sensitivity: 0.001 mg/L
Linearity: 0.001–0.100 mg/L
C.V.: 14.5% day-to-day
Relative recovery: 88–107%

Interferences:

Drug-free specimens should be analyzed frequently to establish freedom from interference by plasma components and reagent impurities. Of five other phenylethylamine derivatives studied for interference, only methamphetamine (retention time, 3.0 min) was found to present a problem.

Reference:

R.C. Baselt, C.B. Stewart and E. Shaskan. Determination of serum and urine concentrations of tranylcypromine by electron-capture gas-liquid chromatography. J. Analyt. Tox. 1: 215–217, 1977.

TRICYCLIC ANTIDEPRESSANTS

	Plasma Concentrations (mg/L)		
	Therapeutic	Toxic	T½
amitriptyline	0.04–0.16	0.5–2.0	15 hr
desipramine	0.01–0.28	0.5–2.0	17 hr
doxepin	0.01–0.15	0.5–2.0	7 hr
imipramine	0.01–0.11	0.3–1.8	14 hr
nortriptyline	0.01–0.38	0.5–2.0	27 hr
protriptyline	0.07–0.17	0.5–2.0	74 hr

The tricyclic antidepressants are a group of chemically and pharmacologically related substances that are extensively used in psychotherapy to counteract depression. The N-desmethyl metabolites of the drugs (desipramine and nortriptyline are metabolites of imipramine and amitriptyline, respectively) are active and tend to accumulate in plasma. Most of these agents may be detected qualitatively in plasma or urine at toxic levels using the procedures described under the Basic Drug Screen section (p. 40). A flame-ionization gas chromatographic method that is optimized for the tricyclic antidepressants is presented here for the quantitative determination of toxic concentrations of these drugs. For therapeutic monitoring purposes, the nitrogen-selective gas chromatographic and the liquid chromatographic procedures are equally suitable, although the latter technique offers the advantage of simultaneous analysis of all of the drugs in common usage.

Plasma Tricyclic Antidepressants by Gas Chromatography

Principle:

The tricyclic antidepressants and an internal standard are extracted from alkalinized plasma with an organic solvent. The drugs are back-extracted into dilute acid and then returned to toluene. The secondary amine drugs are derivatized to render them less polar and all compounds are analyzed by flame-ionization gas chromatography. The procedure is suitable for the detection of toxic concentrations of these drugs.

Reagents:

Stock solutions – 1 mg/mL solutions of amitriptyline, desipramine, doxepin, imipramine, nordoxepin, nortriptyline and protriptyline
Plasma standards – 0.2, 0.5, 1 and 2 mg/L
Internal standards – 80 mg/L promazine HCl (Wyeth Labs) in water
0.5 mol/L Sodium hydroxide
Extraction solvent – heptane/isoamyl alcohol, 98.3:1.7 by volume
0.1 mol/L Hydrochloric acid

pH 9.8 Buffer – 24.8 g Na_2CO_3 and 25.2 g $NaHCO_3$ in 500 mL water
Toluene
Trifluoroacetic anhydride

Instrumental Conditions:

Gas chromatograph with flame-ionization detector
2 m × 2 mm i.d. glass column containing 2% OV-17 on 100/120 mesh Chromosorb G-HP
Injector, 250°C.; column, 240°C.; detector, 300°C.
Nitrogen flow rate, 33 mL/min

Procedure:

1. Transfer 2 mL plasma to a 15 mL screw-cap tube. Add 100 µL internal standard and 0.5 mL 0.5 mol/L NaOH and vortex.
2. Add 10 mL extraction solvent and shake for 30 seconds. Centrifuge and transfer the organic layer to a clean tube.
3. Extract the solvent with 1 mL 0.1 mol/L HCl. Centrifuge and discard the upper organic layer.
4. Transfer the aqueous layer to a 15 mL glass-stoppered centrifuge tube and evaporate any traces of organic solvent under a stream of nitrogen.
5. Add 0.5 mL pH 9.8 buffer and 1 mL toluene and shake to extract. Centrifuge and transfer the upper organic layer to a 12 mL conical centrifuge tube.
6. Add 10 µL trifluoroacetic anhydride to the toluene and evaporate the solvent to approximately 100 µL under a stream of nitrogen at 40°C.
7. Inject 2 µL of the concentrated solvent into the chromatograph.

	Retention time (min)
amitriptyline	3.2
imipramine	3.4
doxepin	3.9
internal standard	5.9
nortriptyline derivative	6.2
desipramine derivative	7.3
nordoxepin derivative	7.3
protriptyline	7.3

Calculation:

Calculation is based on a response factor derived from a standard curve. A quality control specimen containing the appropriate drugs at concentrations of 1 mg/L is analyzed daily.

Evaluation:

Sensitivity: 0.1 mg/L
Linearity: 0.2–5 mg/L
C.V.: not established
Relative recovery: not established

Interferences:

Normal plasma components do not interfere with the assay. Desipramine, nordoxepin and protriptyline all elute at the same time and would need to be distinguished using another technique. Other basic drugs would be extracted with this method and could interfere, although the common drugs are separated from the tricyclics.

References:

1. D.N. Bailey and P.I. Jatlow. Gas-chromatographic analysis for therapeutic concentrations of imipramine and desipramine in plasma, with use of a nitrogen detector. Clin. Chem. 22: 1697–1701, 1976.
2. R. Baselt and C. Stewart. Unpublished results, 1977.

Plasma Tricyclic Antidepressants by Nitrogen-Specific Gas Chromatography

Principle:

The tricyclics are extracted together with an internal standard from alkalinized plasma into an organic solvent. The drugs are partitioned into dilute acid and then re-extracted into a small volume of organic solvent. The final extract is analyzed by isothermal gas chromatography using a nitrogen-phosphorus detector.

Reagents:

Stock solution – 1 mg/mL methanol solutions of amitriptyline, desipramine, imipramine and nortriptyline
Plasma standards – 0.025, 0.050, 0.100, 0.200 and 0.400 mg/L of the appropriate drugs
Internal standard – 3 mg/L amitriptyline HCl or protriptyline HCl in water
0.25 mol/L Sodium hydroxide
Extraction solvent – heptane/isoamyl alcohol, 98.5:1.5 by volume
0.1 mol/L Hydrochloric acid
pH 9 Buffer – 24.8 g Na_2CO_3 and 25.2 g $NaHCO_3$ in 500 mL water
Toluene/isoamyl alcohol, 85:15 by volume

Instrumental Conditions:

Gas chromatograph with nitrogen-phosphorus detector
1.8 m × 2 mm i.d. glass column containing 3% OV-17 on 100/120 mesh Supelcoport
Injector, 260°C.; column, 240°C.; detector, 260°C.
Helium flow rate, 22 mL/min
Hydrogen flow rate, 5 mL/min; air flow rate, 85 mL/min

Procedure:

1. Transfer 2 mL plasma to a screw-cap tube. Add 100 μL internal standard (use amitriptyline for imipramine-desipramine analysis and protriptyline for amitriptyline-nortriptyline analysis) and 1 mL 0.25 mol/L NaOH and vortex.
2. Add 10 mL extraction solvent and place on a tilted rotator at slow speed for 15 min. Centrifuge and transfer the organic layer to a clean tube.
3. Extract with 1.2 mL 0.1 mol/L HCl. Centrifuge and discard upper organic layer.
4. Transfer the aqueous layer to a 3 mL conical glass-stoppered centrifuge tube, taking care to avoid contamination by the organic layer. Add 0.5 mL pH 9 buffer and vortex.

5. Add 50 µL toluene/isoamyl alcohol (85:15) and stopper the tube, wetting the ground glass interface with a drop of solvent. Place on the rotator for 15 minutes.
6. Centrifuge and discard the lower aqueous layer. Recentrifuge and inject 2–5 µL of the upper solvent layer into the chromatograph.

	Retention time (min)
amitriptyline	3.9
imipramine	4.4
nortriptyline	4.6
desipramine	5.2
protriptyline	5.4

Calculation:

Calculation is based on a response factor derived from a standard curve. A quality control specimen containing 0.050 mg/L of the appropriate drugs is analyzed daily.

Evaluation:

Sensitivity: 0.001 mg/L
Linearity: 0.005–0.400 mg/L
C.V.: 4–6%
Relative recovery: not established

Interferences:

Normal plasma components do not interfere with the assay. Other basic drugs do not interfere, with the exception of trihexyphenidyl, which co-elutes with imipramine. Not all of the tricyclic derivatives may be simultaneously analyzed; the identity of the drug to be analyzed must be known and the internal standard chosen accordingly. With the proper internal standard, doxepin and protriptyline may also be determined using this procedure.

References:

1. T.B. Cooper, D. Allen and G.M. Simpson. A sensitive glc method for the determination of imipramine and desmethylimipramine using a nitrogen detector. Psychopharm. Comm. 1: 445–454, 1975.
2. T.B. Cooper, D. Allen and G.M. Simpson. A sensitive method for the determination of amitriptyline and nortriptyline in human plasma. Psychopharm. Comm. 2: 105–116, 1976.

Plasma Tricyclic Antidepressants by Liquid Chromatography

Principle:

The tricyclics and an internal standard are extracted from alkalinized plasma into an organic solvent. The drugs are returned to dilute acid and an aliquot is analyzed by ion-pair reversed-phase liquid chromatography, with detection at 254 nm. Each of the drugs may be analyzed in the presence of others.

Reagents:

Stock solutions – 1 mg/mL methanol solutions of amitriptyline, desipramine, doxepin, imipramine and nortriptyline

Plasma standards – 0.025, 0.050, 0.100, 0.200 and 0.400 mg/L of the appropriate drugs

Internal standard – 1 mg/L β-naphthylamine in 0.1 mol/L HCl

1.5 mol/L Sodium hydroxide

Extraction solvent – hexane/isoamyl alcohol, 99:1 by volume

0.1 mol/L Hydrochloric acid

Mobile phase – 41% methanol, 15% acetonitrile and 44% 0.1 mol/L pH 6.5 phosphate buffer containing 5 mmol/L pentanesulfonic acid.

All glassware should be cleaned before use by sonication in a 99:1 hexane/n-propylamine mixture followed by rinsing with the extraction solvent.

Instrumental Conditions:

Liquid chromatograph with 254 nm ultraviolet detector

30 cm × 3.9 mm i.d. stainless-steel column containing μBondapak C_{18} (Waters Associates)

Column temperature, ambient

Solvent flow rate, 1.5 mL/min

Procedure:

1. Transfer 2 mL plasma to a 30 mL polypropylene tube. Add 100 μL internal standard and 200 μL 1.5 mol/%L NaOH.
2. Add 10 mL extraction solvent and place on a tilted rotator at slow speed for 5 min. Centrifuge and transfer the organic layer to a 15 mL glass-stoppered conical centrifuge tube.
3. Add 200 μL 0.1 mol/L HCl and shake to extract. Centrifuge and discard the upper organic layer.
4. Inject 85 μL of the aqueous layer into the chromatograph.

	Retention time (min)
internal standard	4.5
doxepin	7.5
desipramine	8.8
nortriptyline	9.0
imipramine	11.0
amitriptyline	13.0

Calculation:

Calculation is based on a response factor derived from a standard curve. A quality control specimen containing 0.050 mg/L of the appropriate drugs is analyzed daily.

Evaluation:

Sensitivity: 0.005 mg/L

Linearity: 0.025–1.5 mg/L

C.V.: 3–7% day-to-day

Relative recovery: not established

Interferences:

Normal plasma components do not interfere with the assay. Of 48 basic drugs tested for interference, chlordiazepoxide, thioridazine and mesoridazine were found to interfere with doxepin determination, promazine with desipramine determination, and several anti-histamines (including promethazine) with nortriptyline determination.

Reference:

H.G. Proelss, H.J. Lohmann and D.G. Miles. High-performance liquid-chromatographic simultaneous determination of commonly used tricyclic antidepressants. Clin. Chem. 24: 1948–1953, 1978.

TUBOCURARINE

Plasma Concentrations (mg/L)

99% Paralysis	50% Paralysis	0% Paralysis
0.7	0.5	0.2

Tubocurarine is an alkaloid derived from the South American plant *Chondrodendron tomentosum*. It is a quaternary ammonium compound that is utilized clinically as a neuromuscular blocking agent during surgery. When administered intravenously, initial serum concentrations are as high as 6 mg/L and the muscle relaxant effects last for up to 1.5 hours. The spectrophotometric method presented is capable of measuring tubocurarine in plasma at the higher therapeutic levels. A specific radioimmunoassay has been used for determination of a much wider range of tubocurarine plasma concentrations, but the reagents for this assay are not commercially available at this time.

Plasma Tubocurarine by Ultraviolet Spectrophotometry

Principle:
Tubocurarine is isolated from plasma using a paired-ion extraction technique. The drug is returned from the organic solvent into dilute acid and the solution is analyzed by ultraviolet spectrophotometry.

Reagents:
Stock solution – 1 mg/mL tubocurarine in water
0.1 mol/L Glycine buffer – 7.5 g glycine and 5.9 g NaCl dissolved in 1 L water
KI-glycine buffer – 6 mL 0.1 mol/L glycine buffer, 4 mL 0.1 mol/L NaOH and 12.8 g KI
Ethylene dichloride
0.01 mol/L Hydrochloric acid

Instrumental Conditions:
Ultraviolet spectrophotometer set to 280.5 nm

Procedure:
1. Transfer 5 mL plasma to a 15 mL screw-cap tube. Add 1 mL KI-glycine buffer and 7 mL ethylene dichloride and shake for 2 min.
2. Centrifuge and discard the upper aqueous layer. Transfer 5 mL of the organic layer to a clean tube.
3. Add 0.5 mL 0.01 mol/L HCl and shake for 30 seconds. Centrifuge and transfer the upper aqueous layer to a small test tube.

4. Evaporate any traces of the organic solvent under a stream of air. Transfer the aqueous layer to a microcuvette and read in the spectrophotometer at 280.5 nm against a plasma blank.

Calculation:

Calculation is based on a response factor derived from a standard curve. A quality control specimen containing 0.7 mg/L tubocurarine is analyzed daily.

Evaluation:

Sensitivity; 0.1 mg/L
Linearity: 0.2–4.0 mg/L
C.V.: not established
Relative recovery: not established

Interferences:

Drug-free plasma specimens yield a small, reproducible background absorbance at 280.5 nm, that must be subtracted from the readings for patient specimens. Normal plasma concentrations of histamine, creatinine, acetylcholine, epinephrine and thiopental did not interfere with the assay. Other basic drugs that are utilized during surgery should be studied for potential interference.

References:

1. B.T. Elert and E.N. Cohen. A micro spectrophotometric method for the analysis of minute concentrations of d-tubocurarine chloride in plasma. Amer. J. Med. Tech. 28: 125–134, 1962.
2. E.N. Cohen. Quantitative determination of d-tubocurarine in body tissues and fluids. J. Lab. Clin. Med 62: 979–984, 1963.

VALPROIC ACID

Therapeutic Plasma Concentrations (mg/L)	T1/2
50–100	7–15 hr

Valproic acid is a relatively new anticonvulsant drug, having been first introduced into therapy in 1963. The compound is administered in large oral doses, usually as the sodium salt. The pure acid is a volatile, clear liquid and so it is desirable to use an analytical procedure that does not involve evaporation steps. The technique presented is very convenient and rapid, but requires a dedicated column in the gas chromatograph. An advantage is that the method is easily adapted to analysis of ethosuximide in plasma.

Plasma Valproic Acid by Gas Chromatography

Principle:

Valproic acid and an internal standard are extracted into chloroform from acidified plasma. The organic layer is analyzed directly by flame-ionization gas chromatography on SP-1000. This micro-scale procedure requires only 100 µL of plasma.

Reagents:

Stock solution – 1 mg/mL valproic acid in water
Plasma standards – 10, 20, 50, 100 and 200 mg/L
Internal standard – 60 mg/L caproic acid in 3 mol/L HCl
Chloroform

Instrumental Conditions:

Gas chromatograph with flame-ionization detector
1.5 m × 2 mm i.d. glass column containing 10% SP-1000 on 100/120 mesh Chromosorb W
Injector, 240°C.; column, 160°C.; detector, 240°C.
Nitroten flow rate, 50 mL/min

Procedure:

1. Transfer 100 µL plasma to a plastic micro-centrifuge tube. Add 100 µL internal standard and 100 µL chloroform and vortex for 30 seconds.
2. Centrifuge and inject 5 µL of the lower chloroform layer into the chromatograph.

	Retention time (min)
internal standard	2.5
valproic acid	3.5

Calculation:

Calculation is based on a response factor derived from a standard curve. A quality control specimen containing 80 mg/L valproic acid is analyzed daily.

Evaluation:

Sensitivity: 5 mg/L
Linearity: 10–200 mg/L
C.V.: 2–5%
Relative recovery: not established

Interferences:

Normal plasma components do not interfere with the assay. No other drugs, including other anticonvulsants, have been observed to interfere in this procedure. Ethosuximide elutes at 8–10 minutes and may be determined by this method using α,α-dimethyl-β-methylsuccinimide (Aldrich) as internal standard.

References:

1. D.J. Berry and L.A. Clarke. Determination of valproic acid (dipropylacetic acid) in plasma by gas-liquid chromatography. J. Chrom. 156: 301–307, 1978.
2. G.A. Peyton S.C. Harris and J.E. Wallace. Determination of valproic acid by flame-ionization gas-liquid chromatography. J. Analyt. Tox. 3: 108–110, 1979.
3. J. Wall. Personal communication, 1978.

VERAPAMIL

Plasma Concentrations (mg/L)

	Therapeutic	Toxic	T½
verapamil	0.1–0.8	>2	3–7 hr
norverapamil	0.0–0.6	?	?

Verapamil (Isoptin) is a synthetic papaverine derivative, first introduced in 1962 as an antianginal agent. It has since been found to have antiarrhythmic and antihypertensive properties, attributable to its ability to inhibit transmembrane calcium flux in excitable tissues. Single intravenous doses of 5–10 mg are used for hypertensive crises, while daily oral maintenance doses range from 240–480 mg.

Two analytical procedures are presented for the analysis of verapamil and its demethylated active metabolite, norverapamil, in plasma. The first involves nitrogen-specific gas chromatography while the second employs high-pressure liquid chromatography with fluorescence detection.

Verapamil and Norverapamil by Nitrogen-Specific Gas Chromatography

Principle:

The drugs and two internal standards are extracted from alkalinized plasma with an organic solvent mixture. The solvent is filtered and back-extracted with dilute acid. The acid layer is then alkalinized and extracted with ether. After drying with sodium sulfate, the ether is evaporated to dryness and the residue reconstituted in ethanol. Analysis is by packed column gas chromatography with nitrogen-specific detection.

Reagents:

Stock solutions – 1 mg/mL verapamil in methanol
                1 mg/mL norverapamil in methanol
Plasma standards – 0.05, 0.1, 0.2, 0.5 and 1.0 mg/L for each drug
Internal standard mixture – dissolve 25 mg prazepam (Warner-Lambert) and 10.8 mg D-517 HCl (Knoll Pharmaceutical) in 100 mL ethanol; dilute 1 mL of this to 100 mL with water
0.5 mol/L Sodium hydroxide
Extraction solvent – heptane/2-butanol, 96:4 by volume
1 mol/L Sulfuric acid
4.4 mol/L Sodium hydroxide
Ether

Sodium sulfate, anhydrous
Ethanol

Instrumental Conditions:

Gas chromatograph with nitrogen-phosphorus detector
1.2 m × 2 mm i.d. glass column containing 3% SP-2250 on 100/120 mesh Chromosorb W-HP
Injector, 290°C.; column, 290°C.; detector, 300°C.
Helium flow rate, 40 mL/min

Procedure:

1. Transfer 2 mL plasma to a 35 mL screw-cap glass tube. Add 0.2 mL internal standard solution and 4 mL 0.5 mol/L NaOH and vortex. Add 15 mL extraction solvent and place on a rotator for 15 min.
2. Centrifuge to separate layers and filter 12 mL of the upper solvent layer through Whatman #1 filter paper into a clean tube. Add 4 mL 1 mol/L H_2SO_4, shake for 2 min to extract and centrifuge.
3. Discard the upper solvent layer and transfer 3 mL of the acid layer to a 15 mL screw-cap tube. Add 2.5 mL 4.4 mol/L NaOH, vortex and extract with 5 mL ether.
4. Centrifuge and transfer the ether layer to a clean tube. Add 1 g Na_2SO_4 and vortex. Filter the ether through Whatman #1 filter paper into a 12 mL conical centrifuge tube.
5. Evaporate the ether to dryness at 40°C. under a stream of dry air. Dissolve the residue in 50 μL ethanol and inject 3 μL into the gas chromatograph.

	Retention time (min)
prazepam (i.s.)	1.2
D-517 (i.s.)	3.1
verapamil	3.9
norverapamil	4.8

Calculation:

Calculation is based on a response factor derived from a standard curve. Drug concentrations under 1 mg/L should be calculated using D-517 as internal standard, while those over 1 mg/L should be based on prazepam. A quality control specimen containing verapamil and norverapamil at mid-level concentrations is analyzed daily.

Evaluation:

Sensitivity: 0.025 mg/L
Linearity: 0.05–5.0 mg/L
C.V.: 7–11% day-to-day
Relative recovery: 91–109%

Interferences:

None of the more than 30 commonly prescribed drugs checked was found to interfere except for midazolam, which co-elutes with prazepam. Other verapamil metabolites and endogenous plasma components were not found to interfere.

Reference:

J. Vasiliades, K. Wilkerson, D. Ellul et al. Gas-chromatographic determination of verapamil and norverapamil, with a nitrogen-selective detector. Clin. Chem. 28: 638–641, 1982.

Plasma Verapamil and Norverapamil by Liquid Chromatography

Principle:

Verapamil, its demethylated metabolite, and an internal standard are extracted from alkalinized plasma with methyl t-butyl ether. The extract is analyzed by liquid chromatography with fluorescent detection.

Reagents:

Stock solutions – 1 mg/mL verapamil in methanol
                               1 mg/mL norverapamil in methanol
Plasma standards – 0.05, 0.1, 0.2, 0.5 and 1.0 mg/L for each drug
Internal standard – 0.2 mg/L 5,6-benzoquinoline (Aldrich) in water (dilute from a 1 g/L
     solution in water/methanol, 80:20 by volume)
4 mol/L Sodium hydroxide
Methyl t-butyl ether
Mobile phase – 3 mmol/L potassium bromide and 0.004% perchloric acid in methanol

Instrumental Conditions:

Liquid chromatograph with fluorescence detector (excitation at 203 nm, no emission cutoff
     filter)
12.5 cm × 5 mm i.d. stainless steel Spherisorb 5 silica column
Column temperature, ambient
Solvent flow rate, 2 mL/min

Procedure:

1. Transfer 100 μL plasma to a small glass tube and add 50 μL internal standard and 50 μL 4 mol/L NaOH. Vortex briefly.
2. Add 200 μL methyl t-butyl ether and vortex for 30 seconds. Centrifuge for 2 min and inject 100 μL of the upper solvent layer into the chromatograph.

	Retention time (min)
norverapamil	2.5
verapamil	4.0
internal standard	5.5

Calculation:

Calculation is based on a response factor derived from a standard curve. A quality control specimen containing verapamil and norverapamil at mid-level concentrations is analyzed daily.

Evaluation:

Sensitivity: 0.002 mg/L
Linearity: 0.1–1.0 mg/L
C.V.: 1.2–4.8% day-to-day
Relative recovery: not established

Interferences:

Over 20 commonly prescribed drugs or their metabolites were studied for potential interference and were found not to interfere. Endogenous plasma components did not cause interference.

Reference:

S.C.J. Cole, R.J. Flanagan, A. Johnston and D.W. Holt. Rapid high-performance liquid chromatographic method for the measurement of verapamil and norverapamil in blood plasma or serum. J. Chrom. 218: 621–629, 1981.

VOLATILES

	Blood or Plasma Concentrations (mg/dL)	
	Social Intoxication	Clinical Intoxication
acetone	–	40–150
ethanol	–	180–780
isopropanol	40–250	40–440
methanol	–	20–400
	–	

The group of substances known as the volatiles includes the chemicals listed above. Acetaldehyde and some common laboratory solvents are sometimes included in this group. Ethanol is very frequently involved in clinical poisonings, often in combination with therapeutic agents, while isopropanol and methanol are occasionally observed in accidental and intentional intoxication. Acetone is a major metabolite of isopropanol, but is also present in the plasma of subjects in diabetic coma, in concentrations up to 40 mg/dL. The procedure which follows describes a very convenient gas chromatographic means of assaying these substances in plasma or other body fluids. The column used allows the separation of acetone and methanol, which are difficult to distinguish with the customary Porapak Q column packing.

Plasma Volatiles by Gas Chromatography

Principle:
Plasma is diluted with an equal volume of the internal standard, an aqueous solution of methyl ethyl ketone. The mixture is injected directly into a gas chromatograph equipped with a flame-ionization detector.

Reagents:
Stock solutions – 100 mg/mL aqueous solutions of acetone, ethanol, isopropanol and methanol
Plasma standards – 20, 50, 100, 200 and 400 mg/dL for each chemical
Internal standard solution – 2 mL methyl ethyl ketone per L of water

Instrumental Conditions:
Gas chromatograph with replaceable glass injector sleeve and flame-ionization detector
6′ × ⅛″ stainless-steel column containing 0.2% Carbowax on 60/80 mesh Carbopack C (Supelco)
Injector 200°C.; column, 125°C.; detector, 200°C.
Nitrogen flow rate, 17 mL/min

Procedure:

1. Transfer 100 µL plasma or whole blood to a plastic micro-centrifuge tube. Add 100 µL internal standard and vortex.
2. Inject 0.5 µL of the solution into the gas chromatograph using a 5 µL direct-injection syringe (Hamilton #7105 N) that has been pre-loaded with 0.5 µL of water. Withdraw the needle and immediately rinse the syringe with water.

	Retention time (min)
methanol	0.6
ethanol	0.9
acetone	1.1
isopropanol	1.3
internal standard	2.3

Calculation:

Calculation is based on a response factor derived from a standard curve. A quality control specimen containing 100 mg/dL of each chemical is analyzed daily.

Evaluation:

Sensitivity: 5 mg/dL
Linearity: 10–400 mg/dL
C.V.: 2–4%
Relative recovery: not established

Interferences:

The injection technique must be standardized in order to obtain reproducible results. The glass insert for the injector should be replaced after every 10–20 injections, replacing the septum at the same time. Acetaldehyde co-elutes with methanol in this procedure; if this presents a problem, a column containing Porapak Q will resolve these two substances.

References:

1. C.H. Hine and K. Parker. In Alcohol and the Impaired Driver, American Medical Association, Chicago, 1968, pp. 84–87.
2. R. Baselt and C. Barrett. Unpublished results. 1975.

WARFARIN

Plasma Concentrations (mg/L)	T½
1–7	47 hr

Warfarin is a synthetic vitamin K antagonist that is administered as an anticoagulant drug in daily oral doses of 2–25 mg. The compound is also used as a rodent and predator poison and is found in commercial animal baits in a concentration of 0.025%. Although acute poisoning with warfarin is rare, since a single dose is usually insufficient to cause a significant anticoagulant effect, toxicity can occur during chronic therapeutic administration. The drug's effects may be easily monitored by measuring the patient's prothrombin time, but it may be more informative to determine the plasma warfarin level. This information is especially useful in patients with a genetic resistance to anticoagulant drugs. An ultraviolet spectrophotometric procedure is presented that is relatively specific for unchanged warfarin in the presence of its 7-hydroxy metabolite. A liquid chromatographic technique is also included that has better sensitivity for low therapeutic levels of warfarin, and that is free from interference by warfarin metabolites.

Plasma Warfarin by Ultraviolet Spectrophotometry

Principle:
Warfarin is extracted from acidified plasma into ethylene dichloride, and back-extracted into dilute alkali. The extract is analyzed by ultraviolet spectrophotometry.

Reagents:
Stock solution – 1 mg/mL warfarin in methanol
Plasma standards – 1, 2, 4 and 8 mg/L
3 mol/L Hydrochloric acid
Ethylene dichloride
pH 7.25 0.5 mol/L Phosphate buffer
2.5 mol/L Sodium hydroxide

Instrumental Conditions:
Ultraviolet spectrophotometer
Record spectrum from 360 to 290 nm
Measure absorbance at 360 nm and 308 nm

Procedure:

1. Transfer 2 mL plasma to a 15 mL screw-cap tube. Add 0.5 mL 3 mol/L HCl and 10 mL ethylene dichloride and shake for 30 seconds.
2. Centrifuge and discard the upper aqueous phase. Add 3 mL pH 7.25 phosphate buffer and shake.
3. Centrifuge and discard the upper aqueous phase. Transfer 9 mL of the organic layer to a clean tube.
4. Extract with 4 mL 2.5 mol/L NaOH. Centrifuge and transfer the aqueous layer to a quartz cuvette.
5. Determine the absorbance of the solution at 308 nm against a plasma blank. Subtract the background reading at 360 nm.

Calculation:

Calculation is based on a response factor derived from a standard curve. A quality control specimen containing 3 mg/L warfarin is analyzed daily.

Evaluation:

Sensitivity: 1 mg/L
Linearity: 1–20 mg/L
C.V.: not established
Relative recovery: not established

Interferences:

The procedure is relatively specific for unchanged warfarin in plasma, but is inaccurate at concentrations below 1 mg/L warfarin in plasma. Other acidic drugs that absorb in the same region of the ultraviolet spectrum as warfarin, such as dicumarol, thiopental and salicylate, may interfere.

Reference:

R.A. O'Reilly, P.M. Aggeler, M.S. Hoag and L. Leong. Studies on the coumarin anticoagulant drugs: the assay of warfarin and its biological application. Thromb. Diath. Haem. 8: 82–95, 1962.

Plasma Warfarin by Liquid Chromatography

Principle:

Warfarin and an internal standard, p-chlorowarfarin, are extracted from acidified plasma into ether. The concentrated extract is analyzed by reversed-phase liquid chromatography, with detection at 308 nm.

Reagents:

Stock solution – 1 mg/mL warfarin in methanol
Plasma standards – 0.5, 1, 2 and 4 mg/L
Internal standard – 12 mg/L p-chlorowarfarin (Aldrich) in water
0.25 mol/L Sulfuric acid
Ether

Methanol
Mobile phase – methanol/0.5% acetic acid, 1:1 by volume

Instrumental Conditions:

Liquid chromatograph with 308 nm ultraviolet detector
25 cm × 2.2 mm i.d. stainless-steel column containing Micro Pak CH-10 (Varian)
Column temperature, ambient
Solvent flow rate, 1 mL/min

Procedure:

1. Transfer 1 mL plasma into a 15 mL screw-cap tube. Add 100 µL internal standard and 0.5 mL 0.25 mol/L H_2SO_4 and vortex.
2. Extract with 5 mL ether by gentle agitation for 10 min. Centrifuge and transfer ether layer to a 5 mL conical centrifuge tube.
3. Evaporate ether to dryness under a stream of nitrogen at 40°C. Dissolve the residue in 25 µL methanol and inject 15 µL into the chromatograph.

	Retention time (min)
warfarin	3.3
internal standard	6.0

Calculation:

Calculation is based on a response factor derived from a standard curve. A quality control specimen containing 2 mg/L warfarin is analyzed daily.

Evaluation:

Sensitivity: 0.1 mg/L
Linearity: 0.1–4.0 mg/L
C.V.: 2–4%
Relative recovery: not established

Interferences:

Normal plasma components do not interfere with the assay. Fifty other drugs were studied for potential interference and were found not to co-elute with warfarin or the internal standard. The known metabolites of warfarin all eluted in 2 minutes or less and did not interfere with the determination of warfarin.

Reference:

T.D. Bjornsson, T.F. Blaschke and P.J. Meffin. High-pressure liquid chromatographic analysis of drugs in biological fluids. I: warfarin. J. Pharm. Sci. 66: 142–144, 1977.

ZINC

Normal Serum Concentrations (mg/L)
0.5–1.5

Zinc is an essential trace element, necessary for the proper functioning of several enzymes and in insulin and prophyrin metabolism. Subnormal zinc levels have been reported in patients with dietary deficiencies, atherosclerosis, malignant tumors, myocardial infarctions and acute and chronic infections. Elevated levels have been associated with excessive dietary exposure, systemic lupus erythematosis and polymyositis. Serum zinc levels are estimated to be 16% higher than plasma levels due to platelet destruction; from 75–88% of total zinc in whole blood is contained in the red cells and hemolysis will therefore cause elevation of serum values. The following atomic absorption procedure is rapid and specific for serum zinc.

Serum Zinc by Atomic Absorption Spectrometry

Principle:
Serum is deproteinized with trichloroacetic acid and the supernatant is analyzed by atomic absorption spectrometry.

Reagents:
Stock solution – 1 mg/mL zinc ion (Fisher reference standard)
Aqueous standards – 0.5, 1.0 and 2.0 mg/L
25% Trichloroacetic acid

Instrumental Conditions:
Atomic absorption spectrometer with air-acetylene oxidizing flame
Zinc hollow cathode lamp
Measure absorption at 213.8 nm

Procedure:
1. Obtain patient specimen in a disposable plastic syringe and transfer to a 12 × 75 mm plastic tube. Allow to clot and transfer serum to a clean plastic tube.
2. Transfer 1 mL serum to a 16 × 125 mm plastic tube. Add 9 mL 25% trichloroacetic acid and vortex for 10 seconds.
3. Heat at 37°C. for 10 minutes. Centrifuge and decant supernatant to a clean plastic tube.
4. Aspirate into the flame of the atomic absorption spectrometer. Subtract the value of a reagent blank. Compare to aqueous standards analyzed in the same manner as the specimen.

Calculation:

Calculation is based on a response factor derived from a standard curve. A quality control specimen consisting of normal pooled serum is analyzed daily.

Evaluation:

Sensitivity: 0.1 mg/L
Linearity: 0.1–4.0 mg/L
C.V.: 6%
Relative recovery: 94–103%

Interferences:

The method is highly specific for zinc. Caution must be taken during sampling and handling of the specimen to avoid contact with zinc-containing materials. Vacuum collection tubes with rubber stoppers and glass vessels should be especially avoided.

References:

1. N. Weissman and W.J. Pileggi. Inorganic ions. In Clinical Chemistry, Principles and Techniques (R.J. Henry, D.C. Cannon and J.W. Winkelman, eds.), Harper and Row, New York, 2nd ed., 1978, pp. 704–705.
2. R. Perkins and R. Baselt. Unpublished results, 1979.

INDEX TO SUPPLIERS

A. *Immunoassay Kits*

The following are some of the major suppliers of reagents for immunoassay drug determinations:

1. Radioimmunoassay

Clinical Assays (Cambridge, MA 02139)
    digitoxin
    digoxin
    gentamicin
    phenobarbital
    phenytoin
    theophylline

Diagnostic Products (Los Angeles, CA 90064)
    amikacin
    digitoxin
    digoxin
    gentamicin
    kanamycin
    sisomicin
    tobramycin

Roche Diagnostics (Nutley, NJ 07110 or Basel, Switzerland)
    amphetamines
    barbiturates
    cocaine metabolite
    marijuana
    methadone
    methaqualone
    morphine
    phencyclidine

2. Enzyme Immunoassay

Syva (Palo Alto, CA 94304 or Maidenhead, Berkshire, England SL6 1RD)
    Urine assays:
    amphetamine
    barbiturates
    benzodiazepine metabolite
    cocaine metabolite
    marijuana
    methadone
    opiates

phencyclidine
propoxyphene

Serum Assays:
amikacin
barbiturate
benzodiazepine
carbamazepine
digoxin
ethosuximide
gentamicin
lidocaine
methotrexate
phenobarbital
phenytoin
primidone
procainamide
N-acetylprocainamide
quinidine
theophylline
tobramycin

3. Fluorescene Immunoassay

Abbott Laboratories (Abbott Park, IL 60064)
Urine Assays:
amphetamines
barbiturates
benzodiazepines
cannabinoids
cocaine
opiates
phencyclidine

Serum Assays:
acetaminophen
amikacin
carbamazepine
dibekacin
digitoxin
digoxin
disopyramide
ethanol
ethosuximide
gentamicin
kanamycin
lidocaine
methotrexate

netilmicin
phenobarbital
phenytoin
primidone
procainamide
NAPA
quinidine
salicylate
streptomycin
theophylline
tobramycin
tricyclic antidepressants
valproate
vancomycin

Ames Division (Elkhart, IN 46515)
amikacin
carbamazepine
disopyramide
ethosuximide
gentamicin
kanamycin
netilmicin
phenobarbital
phenytoin
primidone
procainamide
NAPA
quinidine
sisomicin
theophylline
tobramycin
valproate

B. Internal Standards

Many of the internal standards used in chromatographic assays are available from Aldrich Chemical Company (Milwaukee, WI 53233 or Gillingham, Dorset, England SP8 4JL) or other major chemical supply houses. Some internal standards are rarely-used or European pharmaceuticals; these are often obtained from U.S. pharmaceutical houses (see Physicians' Desk Reference).

C. Primary Standards

Most pharmaceuticals may be obtained (often gratis) in pure form by writing directly to the commercial suppliers listed in the most current edition of Physicians' Desk

Reference (Medical Economics Co., Oradell, NJ 07649). Other major suppliers of less common substances are listed below:

Drugs and metabolites – Applied Science Laboratories, Inc.
(especially drugs of   P.O. Box 440
abuse)   State College, PA 16801 or
                        9 New Street
                        Carnforth, Lancashire
                        England LA5 9BX

                        Research Triangle Institute
                        Box 12194
                        Research Triangle Park, NC 27709
drugs   – USP Reference Standards
                        12601 Twinbrook Parkway
                        Rockville, MD 20852
pesticides   – U.S. Environmental Protection Agency
                        Chemical Reference
                            Standards and Quality Control
                        Chemistry Lab, Rm. 101
                        Bldg. 306, ARC-East
                        Beltsville, MD 20705
trace metal   – Fisher Scientific Company
reference solutions   711 Forbes Avenue
                        Pittsburgh, PA 15219

D. *Proficiency Testing Programs*

1. **College of American Pathologists**

7400 N. Skokie Blvd.
Skokie, IL 60077
quarterly, approx. $500 per year
Therapeutic Drug Monitoring (Series 2)
  Each of the four annual shipments includes six serum specimens, each of which may contain up to nine of the following drugs:
  amikacin
  carbamazepine
  chloramphenicol
  digoxin
  disopyramide
  ethosuximide
  gentamicin
  lidocaine
  lithium
  methotrexate
  nortriptyline
  phenobarbital

phenytoin
primidone
procainamide
N-acetylprocainamide
propranolol
quinidine
salicylate
theophylline
tobramycin
valproate

Toxicology Survey (Series 2)

Each of the four annual shipments includes four serum specimens and one urine specimen, each of which may contain up to six of the following drugs:

acetaminophen
acetone
amitriptyline
ambarbital
amoxapine
amphetamine
benzoylecgonine
butalbital
cannabinoids
chlordiazepoxide
chlorpheniramine
cimetidine
cocaine
codeine
desalkylflurazepam
desipramine
diazepam
doxepin
ethanol
ethchlorvynol
glutethimide
imipramine
isopropanol
lidocaine
loxapine
meperidine
meprobamate
methadone and metabolite
methamphetamine
methanol
methaqualone and metabolite
morphine
norcodeine
nordiazepam

nordoxepin
normeperidine
norpropoxyphene
nortriptyline
oxazepam
oxycodone
pentobarbital
phencyclidine
phenobarbital
phenytoin
primidone
propoxyphene
quinidine
salicylamide
salicylate
secobarbital
theophylline
thioridazine
trichloroethanol
valproate

2. U.S. Dept. of HEW

Public Health Service
Center for Disease Control
Atlanta, GA 30333
quarterly, no charge

Drug Monitoring
   Each of the four annual shipments includes four serum specimens (two for emergency toxicology and two for therapeutic monitoring), each of which may contain up to three of the following drugs:
   Toxicology
   acetaminophen
   amitriptyline
   diazepam
   ethanol
   glutethimide
   imipramine
   phenobarbital
   propoxyphene
   salicylate
   secobarbital

   Therapeutic Monitoring
   carbamazepine
   ethosuximide
   phenobarbital

phenytoin
primidone
theophylline
valproate

Endocrinology – includes digoxin
Chemistry Profile – includes iron, lithium, magnesium

3. Americal Association for Clinical Chemistry

725 K Street, N.W.
Washington, D.C. 20006
monthly, $600 per year

Therapeutic Drug Monitoring
    Each of the twelve annual shipments includes one to three serum specimens containing the following drugs:

Vial A
carbamazepine
ethosuximide
lithium
phenobarbital
phenytoin
primidone
valproate

Vial B
caffeine
digoxin
disopyramide
gentamicin
lidocaine
methotrexate
procainamide
NAPA
quinidine
theophylline

Vial C
acetaminophen
amikacin
amitriptyline
chloramphenicol
desipramine
gentamicin
imipramine
nortriptyline

salicylate
tobramycin

Toxicology

Each of the twelve annual shipments includes a urine specimen containing four or five of the following drugs:

acetaminophen
acetone
amitriptyline
amphetamine
benzoylecgonine
butalbital
cannabinoids
cocaine
codeine
desipramine
diazepam
diphenhydramine
ethanol
imipramine
isopropanol
methadone
methaqualone
methanol
morphine and metabolite
nordiazepam
norpropoxyphene
nortriptyline
oxazepam
phenacetin
phencyclidine
phenobarbital
phenylpropanolamine
propoxyphene
salicylate
secobarbital

4. National Highway Traffic Safety Administration

Transportation Systems Center
Kendall Square
Cambridge, MA 02142
quarterly, no charge

Blood Alcohol

Each of the quarterly shipments includes four blood specimens containing ethanol at various concentrations.

E. Quality Control Materials

Quality control specimens for most assays may be prepared in the analyst's own laboratory at very low cost, but in many cases it may be more convenient or cost-effective to purchase these materials from commercial suppliers who have investigated the stability of their products. Some of the major suppliers are listed below:

Dade Divison
American Hospital Supply Corporation
Miami, FL 33152
   Radioimmunoassay Control (digoxin)
   Cation-Cal (includes copper, iron, lithium, magnesium, zinc)

General Diagnostics
Division of Warner-Lambert
Morris Plains, NJ 07950
   Validate (iron, lithium, magnesium)

Lederle
Pearl River, NY 10965
   (Available also from Fisher Scientific Co.)

   RIA Control (digoxin or digitoxin)
   Serum Toxicology (amobarbital, glutethimide, meprobamate, methaqualone, methyprylon, phenobarbital, phenytoin)
   Urine Toxicology (amobarbital, amphetamine, codeine, meperidine, methadone, methamphetamine, morphine, phenobarbital, secobarbital)
   Leder Eth (ethanol)
   Urine Chemistry II (arsenic, copper, lead, magnesium, mercury, salicylate, zinc)

Ortho Diagnostics
Raritan, NY 08869
   RIA Control (digoxin or digitoxin)
   Urine Control (arsenic, copper, lead, magnesium, mercury, salicylate, zinc)
   Toxicology Control Urine (amobarbital, amphetamine, codeine, meperidine, methadone and metabolite, methamphetamine, morphine, morphine glucuronide, phenobarbital, secobarbital)
   Toxicology Control Serum (amobarbital, glutethimide, meprobamate, methaqualone, methyprylon, phenobarbital, phenytoin)
   Anticonvulsant Control Serum (carbamazepine, ethosuximide, phenobarbital, phenytoin, primidone, theophylline)

Utak Laboratories
21704 W. Golden Triangle Road
Saugus, CA 91350
   Over 40 individual drugs and chemicals in lyophilized human serum:

acetaminophen
amobarbital – secobarbital
anticonvulsants (phenytoin, primidone and phenobarbital)
anticonvulsants (phenytoin, primidone, phenobarbital, carbamazepine and
  ethosuximide)
bromide
carbamazepine
chlordiazepoxide
diazepam
digoxin
disopyramide
ethanol
ethchlorvynol
ethosuximide
fluoride
glutethimide
hypnotics (secobarbital, methaqualone, meprobamate and methyprylon)
hypnotics (phenobarbital, glutethimide, chlordiazepoxide and salicylate)
hypnotics (pentobarbital, ethchlorvynol, carisoprodol and diazepam)
lidocaine
lithium
mephenytoin
meprobamate
methapyrilene and salicylamide
methaqualone
phenobarbital
phenytoin
primidone
procainamide
procainamide and N-acetylprocainamide
propranolol
quinidine
salicylate
sulfanilamide
theophylline
valproic acid

College of American Pathologists
7400 N. Skokie Blvd.
Skokie, IL 60076

The CAP Quality Assurance Service for therapeutic drug monitoring consists of control serum (prepared by Hyland Diagnostics) that is to be used as the routine quality control material for the appropriate assays. Each laboratory's data is charted by computer on a monthly or quarterly basis, and, in addition, is compared to other laboratories throughout the country. The control material contains the following analytes at two different concentrations:

carbamazepine
digoxin
ethosuximide
gentamicin
lidocaine
phenobarbital
phenytoin
primidone
procainamide
NAPA
propranolol
quinidine
theophylline
valproate

INDEX